Basic Pharmacokinetics

Basic Pharmacokinetics

Sunil S Jambhekar

MS, PhD, Professor
Department of Pharmaceutical Sciences
LECOM-Bradenton, School of Pharmacy
Bradenton, Florida, USA

and

Philip J Breen

PhD, Associate Professor
College of Pharmacy
University of Arkansas for Medical Sciences
Little Rock, Arkansas, USA

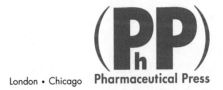

London • Chicago **Pharmaceutical Press**

Published by the Pharmaceutical Press
An imprint of RPS Publishing

1 Lambeth High Street, London SE1 7JN, UK
100 South Atkinson Road, Suite 200, Grayslake, IL 60030-7820, USA

©Pharmaceutical Press 2009

(**P̯P**) is a trade mark of RPS Publishing

RPS Publishing is the publishing organisation of the Royal
Pharmaceutical Society of Great Britain

First published 2009
Reprinted 2009

Typeset by Thomson Digital, Noida, India

Printed in Great Britain by J International, Padstow, Cornwall

ISBN 978 0 85369 772 5

A catalogue record for this book is available from the British Library.

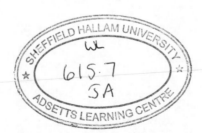

Contents

Preface

PHARMACOKINETICS AND BIOPHARMACEUTICS courses have been included in pharmacy curricula across the USA and in many other countries for the past several years. At present, there are a number of textbooks available for use by students and other readers. Most of these textbooks, although valuable and well written, concentrate on presenting the material in substantial mathematical depth, with much less emphasis needed on explanations that will facilitate understanding and the ability to use the pharmacokinetic equations which are introduced. Furthermore, also evident in currently available textbooks is a paucity of adequate explanation regarding factors influencing pharmacokinetic parameters present in these equations.

The intent of this textbook is to provide the reader with a basic intuitive understanding of the principles of pharmacokinetics and biopharmaceutics and how these principles, along with the equations presented in each chapter, can be applied to achieve successful drug therapy. It has been our intent to illustrate the application of pharmacokinetic principles and equations by providing the reader with data available in the literature. Additionally, when relevant, problem sets and problem-solving exercises, complete with keys, have been provided at the conclusion of each chapter. This approach will enable the reader to become adept at solving pharmacokinetic problems arising in drug therapy and to understand the applications and utility of equations in clinical practice.

Since pharmacokinetics is basically mathematical in nature, a chapter has been included to provide the reader with a basic review of the mathematical principles and graphing techniques necessary to understand pharmacokinetics. At the outset of each chapter, important objectives have been listed that will accentuate and identify the salient and indelible points of the chapter. When an important and clinically applicable equation appears in the text, a paragraph follows, explaining the significance and therapeutic applications of the equation. Additionally, this paragraph includes and explains the relevant factors that influence the parameters appearing in an equation. After the introduction of an important equation, a general profile illustrating the relationship between the two variables of an equation has been presented. This approach, we believe, will demystify key concepts in pharmacokinetics.

Derivations of key equations have been included to show their origins and to satisfy the inquisitive reader. However, students are not expected to memorize any of these derivations or to perform them in any problem set or problem solving exercise.

We remain cognizant that this edition of the textbook includes some references that may be considered by some viewers not to be the most current. We, however, believe that the chosen references are classic ones best suited to illustrate a particular point. Additionally, we fully recognize that this edition omits topics such as the Wagner and Nelson method for the determination of the absorption rate constant, urinary data analysis following the administration of a drug by an extravascular route, two-compartment model pharmacokinetics for an extravascularly administered drug, and metabolite kinetics.

Ultimately, though important topics, we consciously decided that these topics may be less important for entry level pharmacy programs.

Organization

As listed in the table of contents, the book is organized into 19 chapters, the last one appearing as an Appendix. The first chapter consists of an introduction to the principles necessary to understand pharmacokinetics as well as an overview of the subject matter. The remaining chapters are organized in an order that should be easy for the reader to follow, while still demonstrating the salient features of each topic. Clearance and other essential fundamental pharmacokinetic parameters have been introduced early in the book, since the student will need to apply these concepts in subsequent chapters. This has necessitated cross referencing concepts introduced in the first few chapters throughout the remainder of the book.

We have adopted a uniform set of notation throughout the textbook. This notation has been defined within the body of the book and also summarized in two glossaries in the Appendix.

Since the text is primarily targeted for the entry level pharmacy (PharmD) students in the United States and Canada, the book fulfills the current course requirements of schools of pharmacy in these countries. In addition, we believe that the book will prove to be of considerable value and utility for pharmaceutical scientists with no formal pharmacy education, medical students, graduate students in the pharmaceutical sciences, as well as for undergraduate and graduate students in the United States, the United Kingdom, and countries where the medium of instruction in colleges of pharmacy is English.

In conclusion, we wish to acknowledge our mentors, colleagues, and a number of former and current diligent and serious undergraduate and graduate students for their constructive comments, encouragement, suggestions, and support. We view them as partners in our quest to facilitate understanding of pharmacokinetics.

Dr Sunil S Jambhekar and Dr Philip J Breen,
February 2009

About the authors

Sunil S Jambhekar received his BPharm degree from Gujarat University, India and MS and PhD degrees in Pharmaceutics from the University of Nebraska. Prior to pursuing graduate education, Dr Jambhekar worked for four years as a research scientist at two major pharmaceutical companies in India.

Prior to assuming his current position, Dr Jambhekar served as an Assistant and Associate Professor of Pharmaceutics at the Massachusetts College of Pharmacy in Boston, where he was a recipient of the Trustee's Teacher of the Year award and the Scholarly Publication award. Subsequently he was appointed Professor of Pharmaceutics at South University School of Pharmacy in Savannah, Georgia.

Dr Jambhekar has taught undergraduate and graduate courses in pharmaceutics and pharmacokinetics. Additionally, he has directed the research and served on the thesis advisory committees of a number of graduate students. He has authored many peer-reviewed articles and book chapters as well as scientific presentations at national and international conferences. Dr Jambhekar has reviewed scientific books and research articles for many journals. He has been an invited external examiner for a number of doctoral candidates at colleges of pharmacy here and abroad.

Dr Jambhekar has been a Fulbright Scholar in the lecture/research category for India and currently is a Fulbright Senior Specialist and Fulbright Foundation grantee in the global/public health category. Dr Jambhekar is an active member of several professional organizations.

Dr Philip J Breen received his BS in Pharmacy and PhD degrees at the Massachusetts College of Pharmacy and Allied Health Sciences in Boston. For several years between undergraduate and graduate school, he was staff pharmacist and manager of a community pharmacy. For the past 20 years, Dr Breen has been Assistant and then Associate Professor at the College of Pharmacy of the University of Arkansas for Medical Sciences in Little Rock, where he teaches courses in both undergraduate and graduate pharmacokinetics. He was named Teacher of the Year at this college in 1989.

Dr Breen has numerous national presentations and publications to his credit, as well as several patents.

Dedication

To my family
SSJ
To Ginny and Danny
PJB

1

Introduction and overview

Objectives

Upon completion of this chapter, you will have the ability to:

- compare and contrast the terms *pharmacokinetics* and *biopharmaceutics*
- describe absorption, distribution, metabolism and excretion (ADME) processes in pharmacokinetics
- delineate differences between intravascular and extravascular administration of drugs
- explain the *compartmental model* concept in pharmacokinetics
- explain what is meant by the *order* of a reaction and how the order defines the equation determining the rate of the reaction
- compare and contrast a first-order and a zero-order process.

1.1 Use of drugs in disease states

The use of drugs to treat or ameliorate disease goes back to the dawn of history. Since drugs are *xenobiotics*, that is compounds that are foreign to the body, they have the potential to cause harm rather than healing, especially when they are used inappropriately or in the wrong dose for the individual patient being treated. What, then, is the right dose? The medieval physician/alchemist Paracelsus stated: "Only the dose makes a thing not a poison." This implies: "The dose of a drug is enough but not too much." It is the objective of this text to present some tools to allow the determination of the proper dose – a dose that will be therapeutic but not toxic in an individual patient, possessing a particular set of physiological characteristics.

At the same time that the disciplines of medicine and pharmacy strive to use existing drugs in the most effective manner, scientific researchers are engaged in the process of discovering new drugs that are safe and effective and which are significant additions to our armamentarium for the treatment or prevention of disease. This process is increasingly time-consuming, expensive, and often frustrating.

Here are two statistics about new drug approval:

- the average time for a new drug to be approved is between 7 to 9 years
- the cost of introducing a new drug is approximately $700 million to $1 billion.

Steps involved in the drug development process include:

1. The pharmacologically active molecule or drug entity must be synthesized, isolated or extracted from various possible sources (relying on the disciplines of medicinal chemistry, pharmacology, and toxicology).
2. The formulation of a dosage form (i.e. tablet, capsules, suspension, etc.) of this drug must be

accomplished in a manner that will deliver a recommended dose to the "site of action" or a target tissue (employing the principles of physical pharmacy and pharmaceutics).

3. A *dosage regimen* (dose and dosing interval) must be established to provide an effective concentration of a drug in the body, as determined by physiological and therapeutic needs (utilizing pharmacokinetics and biopharmaceutics).

Only a successful integration of these facets will result in successful drug therapy. For example, an analgesic drug with a high therapeutic range can be of little use if it undergoes a rapid decomposition in the gastrointestinal tract and/or it fails to reach the general circulation and/or it is too irritating to be administered parenterally.

Therefore, the final goal in the drug development process is to develop an optimal dosage form to achieve the desired therapeutic goals. The optimal dosage form is defined as one that provides the maximum therapeutic effect with the least amount of drug and achieves the best results consistently.

In other words, a large number of factors play an important role in determining the activity of a drug administered through a dosage form. It is one of the objectives of this book to describe these factors and their influence on the effectiveness of these drugs.

A variety of disciplines are involved in understanding the events that take place during the process by which a chemical entity (substance) becomes an active drug or a therapeutic agent.

1. Principles of physics, physical chemistry, and mathematics are essential in the formulation of an optimum dosage form.
2. An understanding of physiology and pharmacology is essential in the process of screening for active drug and in selecting an appropriate route of administration.
3. Knowledge of the principles of kinetics (rate processes), analytical chemistry and therapeutics is essential in providing an effective concentration of a drug at the "site of action."

Pharmacokinetics and biopharmaceutics are the result of such a successful integration of the various disciplines mentioned above.

The first such approach was made by Teorell (1937), when he published his paper on distribution of drugs. However, the major breakthrough in developing and defining this discipline has come since the early 1970s.

1.2 Important definitions and descriptions

Pharmacokinetics

"Pharmacokinetics is the study of kinetics of absorption, distribution, metabolism and excretion (ADME) of drugs and their corresponding pharmacologic, therapeutic, or toxic responses in man and animals" (American Pharmaceutical Association, 1972). Applications of pharmacokinetics studies include:

- bioavailability measurements
- effects of physiological and pathological conditions on drug disposition and absorption
- dosage adjustment of drugs in disease states, if and when necessary
- correlation of pharmacological responses with administered doses
- evaluation of drug interactions
- clinical prediction: using pharmacokinetic parameters to individualize the drug dosing regimen and thus provide the most effective drug therapy.

Please note that in every case, the use must be preceded by observations.

Biopharmaceutics

"Biopharmaceutics is the study of the factors influencing the bioavailability of a drug in man and animals and the use of this information to optimize pharmacological and therapeutic activity of drug products" (American Pharmaceutical Association, 1972). Examples of some factors include:

- chemical nature of a drug (weak acid or weak base)
- inert excipients used in the formulation of a dosage form (e.g. diluents, binding agents, disintegrating agents, coloring agents, etc.)

- method of manufacture (dry granulation and/or wet granulation)
- physicochemical properties of drugs (pK_a, particle size and size distribution, partition coefficient, polymorphism, etc.).

Generally, the goal of biopharmaceutical studies is to develop a dosage form that will provide consistent bioavailability at a desirable rate. The importance of a consistent bioavailability can be very well appreciated if a drug has a narrow therapeutic range (e.g. digoxin) where small variations in blood concentrations may result in toxic or subtherapeutic concentrations.

Relationship between the administered dose and amount of drug in the body

Only that fraction of the administered dose which actually reaches the systemic circulation will be available to elicit a pharmacological effect.

For an *intravenous solution*, the amount of drug that reaches general circulation is the dose administered. Moreover

$$\text{Dose} = X_0 = (\text{AUC})_0^\infty KV \qquad (1.1)$$

where $(\text{AUC})_0^\infty$ is the area under curve of plasma drug concentration versus time (AUC) from time zero to time infinity; K is the first-order elimination rate constant and V (or V_d) is the drug's volume of distribution.

Volume of distribution may be thought of as the apparent volume into which a given mass of drug would need to be diluted in order to give the observed concentration.

For the *extravascular route*, the amount of drug that reaches general circulation is the product of the bioavailable fraction (F) and the dose administered. Moreover,

$$F \times \text{Dose} = FX_0 = (\text{AUC})_0^\infty KV \qquad (1.2)$$

Equations 1.1 and 1.2 suggest that we must know or determine all the parameters (i.e. $(\text{AUC})_0^\infty$, K, V, F) for a given drug; therefore, it is important to know the concentration of a drug in blood (plasma or serum) and/or the amount (mass) of drug removed in urine (excretion data). A typical plasma concentration versus time profile (rectilinear, R.L.) following the administration of a drug by an extravascular route is presented in Fig. 1.1.

Onset of action

The time at which the administered drug reaches the therapeutic range and begins to produce the effect.

Duration of action

The time span from the beginning of the onset of action up to the termination of action.

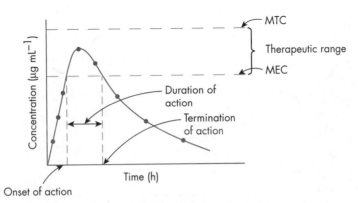

Figure 1.1 A typical plot (rectilinear paper) of plasma concentration versus time following the administration of a drug by an extravascular route. MTC, minimum toxic concentration; MEC, minimum effective concentration.

Table 1.1 The therapeutic range of selected drugs

Drug	Therapeutic use	Therapeutic range
Tobramycin (Nebcin, Tobrex)	Bactericidal–antibiotic	4–8 mg L^{-1}
Digoxin (Lanoxin)	Congestive heart failure (CHF)	1–2 µg L^{-1}
Carbamazepine (Tegretol)	Anticonvulsant	4–12 mg L^{-1}
Theophylline	Bronchial asthma	10–20 mg L^{-1}

Termination of action

The time at which the drug concentration in the plasma falls below the minimum effective concentration (MEC).

Therapeutic range

The plasma or serum concentration (e.g. µg mL^{-1}) range within which the drug is likely to produce the therapeutic activity or effect. Table 1.1 provides, as an example, the therapeutic range of selected drugs.

Amount of drug in the urine

One can monitor the drug in the urine in order to obtain selected *pharmacokinetic parameters* of a drug as well as other useful information such as the **bioavailability** of a drug.

Figure 1.2 represents a typical urinary plot, regardless of the route of drug administration.

1.3 Sites of drug administration

Sites of drug administration are classified into two categories:

- intravascular routes
- extravascular routes.

Intravascular routes

Intravascular administration can be:

- intravenous
- intra-arterial.

Important features of the intravascular route of drug administration

1. There is no absorption phase.
2. There is immediate onset of action.
3. The entire administered dose is available to produce pharmacological effects.

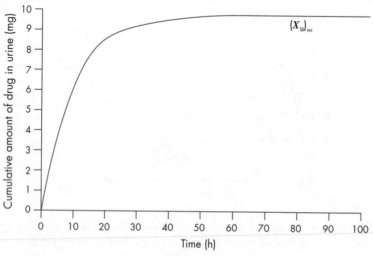

Figure 1.2 A typical plot (rectilinear paper) of the cumulative amount of drug in urine (X_u) against time.

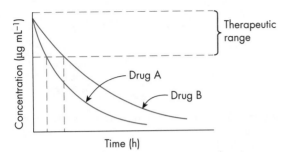

Figure 1.3   A typical plasma concentration versus time plot (rectilinear paper) following the administration of a dose of a drug by an intravascular route.

4. This route is used more often in life-threatening situations.
5. Adverse reactions are difficult to reverse or control; accuracy in calculations and administration of drug dose, therefore, are very critical.

A typical plot of plasma and/or serum concentration against time, following the administration of the dose of a drug by intravascular route, is illustrated in Fig. 1.3.

Extravascular routes of drug administration

Extravascular administration can be by a number of routes:

- oral administration (tablet, capsule, suspension, etc.)
- intramuscular administration (solution and suspension)
- subcutaneous administration (solution and suspension)
- sublingual or buccal administration (tablet)
- rectal administration (suppository and enema)
- transdermal drug delivery systems (patch)
- inhalation (metered dose inhaler).

Important features of extravascular routes of drug administration

1. An *absorption phase* is present.
2. The *onset of action* is determined by factors such as formulation and type of dosage form, route of administration, physicochemical properties of drugs and other physiological variables.
3. The *entire administered dose* of a drug *may not always reach the general circulation* (i.e. incomplete absorption).

Figure 1.4 illustrates the importance of the absorption characteristics when a drug is administered by an extravascular route.

In Fig. 1.4, please note the differences in the onset of action, termination of action and the duration of action as a consequence of the differences in the absorption characteristics of a drug owing to formulation differences. One may observe similar differences in the absorption characteristics of a drug when it is administered via different dosage forms or different extravascular routes.

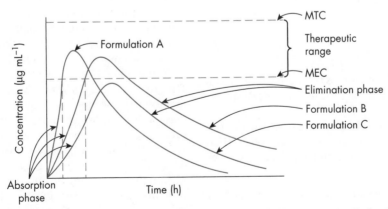

Figure 1.4   A typical plot (rectilinear paper) of plasma concentration versus time following the (oral) administration of an identical dose of a drug via identical dosage form but different formulations. MTC, minimum toxic concentration; MEC, minimum effective concentration.

1.4 Review of ADME processes

ADME is an acronym representing the pharmacokinetic processes of absorption, distribution, metabolism, and elimination.

Absorption

Absorption is defined as the process by which a drug proceeds from the site of administration to the site of measurement (usually blood, plasma or serum).

Distribution

Distribution is the process of reversible transfer of drug to and from the site of measurement (usually blood or plasma). Any drug that leaves the site of measurement and does not return has undergone elimination. The rate and extent of drug distribution is determined by:

1. how well the tissues and/or organs are perfused with blood
2. the binding of drug to plasma proteins and tissue components
3. the permeability of tissue membranes to the drug molecule.

All these factors, in turn, are determined and controlled by the physicochemical properties and chemical structures (i.e. presence of functional groups) of a drug molecule.

Metabolism

Metabolism is the process of a conversion of one chemical species to another chemical species (Fig. 1.5).

Usually, metabolites will possess little or none of the activity of the parent drug. However, there are exceptions. Some examples of drugs with therapeutically active metabolites are:

procainamide (Procan; Pronestyl) used as anti-dysrhythmic agent: active metabolite is *N*-acetyl procainamide

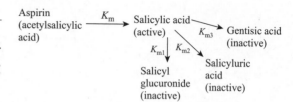

Figure 1.5   Metabolism of aspirin. K_m, metabolic rate constant.

propranolol HCl (Inderal) used as a non-selective β-antagonist: active metabolite is 4-hydroxypropranolol

diazepam (Valium) used for symptomatic relief of tension and anxiety: active metabolite is desmethyldiazepam.

Elimination

Elimination is the irreversible loss of drug from the site of measurement (blood, serum, plasma). Elimination of drugs occur by one or both of:

*   metabolism
*   excretion.

Excretion

Excretion is defined as the irreversible loss of a drug in a chemically unchanged or unaltered form. An example is shown in Fig. 1.6.

The two principal organs responsible for drug elimination are the *kidney* and the *liver*. The kidney is the primary site for removal of a drug in a chemically unaltered or unchanged form (i.e. excretion) as well as for metabolites. The liver is the primary organ where drug metabolism occurs. The lungs, occasionally, may be an important route of elimination for substances of high vapor pressure (i.e. gaseous anesthetics, alcohol, etc.). Another potential route of drug removal is a mother's milk. Although not a significant route for elimination of a drug for the mother, the drug may be consumed in sufficient quantity to affect the infant.

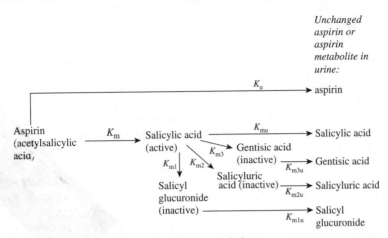

Figure 1.6   Renal excretion of aspirin and its metabolites. K_m, metabolic rate constant.

Disposition

Once a drug is in the systemic circulation (immediately for intravenous administration and after the absorption step in extravascular administration), it is distributed simultaneously to all tissues including the organ responsible for its elimination. The distinction between elimination and distribution is often difficult. When such a distinction is either not desired or is difficult to obtain, *disposition* is the term used. In other words, disposition is defined as all the processes that occur subsequent to the absorption of the drug. Hence, by definition, the components of the disposition phase are distribution and elimination.

1.5 Pharmacokinetic models

After administering a dose, the change in drug concentration in the body with time can be described mathematically by various equations, most of which incorporate exponential terms (i.e. e^x or e^{-x}). This suggests that ADME processes are "first order" in nature at therapeutic doses and, therefore, drug transfer in the body is possibly mediated by "passive diffusion." Therefore, there is a directly proportional relationship between the observed plasma concentration and/or the amount of drug eliminated in the urine and the administered dose

of the drug. This direct proportionality between the observed plasma concentration and the amount of drug eliminated and the dose administered yields the term "linear pharmacokinetics" (Fig. 1.7).

Because of the complexity of ADME processes, an adequate description of the observations is sometimes possible only by assuming a simplified model; the most useful model in pharmacokinetics is the compartment model. The body is conceived to be composed of mathematically interconnected compartments.

Compartment concept in pharmacokinetics

The compartment concept is utilized in pharmacokinetics when it is necessary to describe the plasma concentration versus time data adequately and accurately, which, in turn, permits

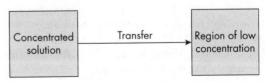

Rate of transfer varies with the concentration
in the left compartment

Figure 1.7   The principle of passive diffusion and the relationship between the rate of transfer and the administered dose of a drug.

us to obtain accurate estimates of selected fundamental pharmacokinetics parameters such as the apparent volume of drug distribution, the elimination half life and the elimination rate constant of a drug. The knowledge of these parameters and the selection of an appropriate equation constitute the basis for the calculation of the dosage regimen (dose and dosing interval) that will provide the desired plasma concentration and duration of action for an administered drug.

The selection of a compartment model solely depends upon the distribution characteristics of a drug following its administration. The equation required to characterize the plasma concentration versus time data, however, depends upon the compartment model chosen and the route of drug administration. The selected model should be such that it will permit accurate predictions in clinical situations. As mentioned above, the distribution characteristics of a drug play a critical role in the model selection process. Generally, the slower the drug distribution in the body, regardless of the route of administration, the greater the number of compartments required to characterize the plasma concentration versus time data, the more complex is the nature of the equation employed. On the basis of this observation, it is, therefore, accurate to state that if the drug is rapidly distributed following its administration, regardless of the route of administration, a one-compartment model will do an adequate job of accurately and adequately characterizing the plasma concentration versus time data.

The terms rapid and slow distribution refer to the time required to attain distribution equilibrium for the drug in the body. The attainment of distribution equilibrium indicates that the rate of transfer of drug from blood to various organs and tissues and the rate of transfer of drug from various tissues and organs back into the blood have become equal. Therefore, rapid distribution simply suggests that the rate of transfer of drug from blood to all organ and tissues and back into blood have become equal instantaneously, following the administration (intra- or extravascular) of the dose of a drug. Therefore, all organs and tissues are behaving in similar fashion toward the administered drug.

Slow distribution suggests that the distribution equilibrium is attained slowly and at a finite time (from several minutes to a few hours, depending upon the nature of the administered drug). Furthermore, it suggests that the vasculature, tissues and organs are not behaving in a similar fashion toward this drug and, therefore, we consider the body to comprise two compartments or, if necessary, more than two compartments.

Highly perfused systems, such as the liver, the kidney and the blood, may be pooled together in one compartment (i.e. the central compartment: compartment 1); and systems that are not highly perfused, such as bones, cartilage, fatty tissue and many others, can also be pooled together and placed in another compartment (i.e. the tissue or peripheral compartment: compartment 2). In this type of model, the rates of drug transfer from compartment 1 to compartment 2 and back to compartment 1 will become equal at a time greater than zero (from several minutes to a few hours).

It is important to recognize that the selection of the compartment model is contingent upon the availability of plasma concentration versus time data. Therefore, the model selection process is highly dependent upon the following factors.

1. The frequency at which plasma samples are collected. It is highly recommended that plasma samples are collected as early as possible, particularly for first couple of hours, following the administration of the dose of a drug.
2. The sensitivity of the procedure employed to analyze drug concentration in plasma samples. (Since inflections of the plasma concentration versus time curve in the low-concentration regions may not be detected when using assays with poor sensitivity, the use of a more sensitive analytical procedure will increase the probability of choosing the correct compartment model.)
3. The physicochemical properties (e.g. the lipophilicity) of a drug.

As mentioned above, only the distribution characteristics of a drug play a role in the selection of the compartment model. The chosen model, as well as the route of drug administration, by comparison, will contribute to the selection of an appropriate equation necessary to characterize the plasma concentration versus time data accurately. The following illustrations and examples, hopefully, will delineate some of the concepts discussed in this section.

Intravenous bolus administration, one-compartment model

Figure 1.8 is a semilogarithmic (S.L.) plot of plasma concentration versus time data for a drug administered as an intravenous bolus dose. A semilogarithmic plot derives its name from the fact that a single axis (the y-axis in this case) employs logarithmic co-ordinates, while the other axis (the x-axis) employs linear co-ordinates. The plotted curve is a straight line, which clearly indicates the presence of a single pharmacokinetic phase (namely, the elimination phase.) Since the drug is administered intravenously, there is no absorption phase. The straight line also suggests that distribution is instantaneous; thus the drug is rapidly distributed in the body. These data can be accurately and adequately described by employing the following mono-exponential equation

$$C_p = (C_p)_0 e^{-Kt} \qquad (1.3)$$

where C_p is the plasma drug concentration at any time t; and $(C_p)_0$ is the plasma drug concentration at time $t = 0$.

Please note that there is a single phase in the concentration versus time plot and one exponential term in the equation required to describe the data. This indicates that a one-compartment model is appropriate in this case.

Intravenous bolus administration, two-compartment model

Figure 1.9 clearly shows the existence of two phases in the concentration versus time data. The first phase (curvilinear portion) represents drug distribution in the body; and only after a finite time (indicated by a discontinuous perpendicular line) do we see a straight line. The time at which the concentration versus time plot begins to become a straight line represents the occurrence of distribution equilibrium. This suggests that drug is being distributed slowly and requires a two-compartment model for accurate characterization. The equation employed to characterize these plasma concentration versus time data will be biexponential (contain two exponential terms):

$$C_p = A e^{-\alpha t} + B e^{-\beta t} \qquad (1.4)$$

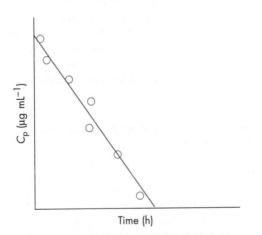

Figure 1.8   A typical plot (semilogarithmic) of plasma concentration (C_p) versus time following the administration of an intravenous bolus dose of a drug that is rapidly distributed in the body.

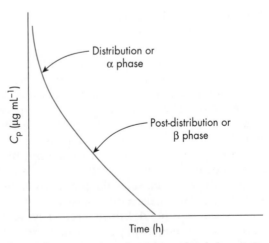

Figure 1.9   A typical semilogarithmic plot of plasma concentration (C_p) versus time following the administration of an intravenous bolus dose of a drug that is slowly distributed in the body.

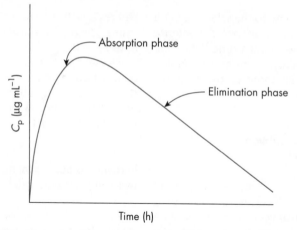

Figure 1.10   A typical semilogarithmic plot of plasma concentration (C_p) versus time following the extravascular administration of a dose of a drug that is rapidly distributed in the body.

where A and α are parameters associated with drug distribution and B and β are parameters associated with drug post-distribution phase.

Please note that there are two phases in the concentration versus time data in Fig. 1.9 and that an equation containing two exponential terms is required to describe the data. This indicates that a two-compartment model is appropriate in this case.

Extravascular administration: one-compartment model

The plasma concentration versus time profile presented in Fig. 1.10 represents a one-compartment model for a drug administered extravascularly. There are two phases in the profile: absorption and elimination. However, the profile clearly indicates the presence of only one phase in the post-absorption period. Since distribution is the sole property that determines the chosen compartment model and, since the profile contains only one phase in the post-absorption period, these data can be described accurately and adequately by employing a one-compartment model. However, a biexponential equation would be needed to characterize the concentration versus time data accurately. The following equation can be employed to characterize the data:

$$
\begin{aligned}
C_p &= \frac{K_a (X_a)_{t=0}}{V(K_a - K)} [e^{-Kt} - e^{-K_a t}] \\
&= \frac{K_a F X_0}{V(K_a - K)} [e^{-Kt} - e^{-K_a t}]
\end{aligned}
\tag{1.5}
$$

where K_a is the first-order absorption rate constant, K is the first-order elimination rate constant; $(X_a)_{t=0}$ is the amount of *absorbable* drug at the absorption site present at time zero; F is the absorbable fraction; and X_0 is the administered dose.

Please note that a one-compartment model will provide an accurate description since there is only one post-absorption phase; however, since there are two phases for the plasma concentration versus time data, a biexponential equation is required to describe the data accurately.

Extravascular route of drug administration, two-compartment model

Figure 1.11 clearly shows the presence of three phases in the plasma concentration versus time data for a drug administered by an extravascular route. Three phases include absorption, distribution and post-distribution. Please note that in the figure, there is a clear and recognizable distinction between the distribution and post-distribution phases. Furthermore, the plasma concentration

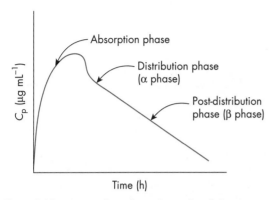

Figure 1.11 A typical semilogarithmic plot of plasma concentration (C_p) versus time following the extravascular administration of a dose of a drug that is slowly distributed in the body.

versus time profile, in the post-absorption period looks identical to that for an intravenous bolus two-compartment model (Fig. 1.9). These data, therefore, can be described accurately by employing a two-compartment model and the equation will contain three exponential terms (one for each phase: absorption, distribution, and post-distribution.)

It should be stressed that these compartments do not correspond to physiologically defined spaces (e.g. the liver is not a compartment).

If the chosen model does not adequately describe the observed data (plasma concentration), another model is proposed.

The model that is ultimately chosen should always be the simplest possible model which is still capable of providing an adequate description of the observed data. The kinetic properties of a model should always be understood if the model is used for clinical predictions.

Types of model in pharmacokinetics

There are several types of models used:

- one compartment
- two compartment
- three compartments or higher (not often used).

A basic model for absorption and disposition

A simple pharmacokinetic model is depicted in Figs 1.12 and 1.13. This model may apply to any extravascular route of administration.

The model is based on mass balance considerations:

1. The amount (e.g. mg) of unchanged drug and/or metabolite(s) can be measured in urine.
2. Drug and metabolite(s) in the body (blood, plasma or serum) are measured in concentration units (e.g. $\mu g\,mL^{-1}$).
3. Direct measurement of drug at the site of administration is impractical; however, it can be assessed indirectly.

Mass balance considerations, therefore, dictate that, at any time t, for the extravascular route:

$$F(\text{Dose}) = \text{absorbable amount at the absorption site}$$
$$+ \text{amount in the body}$$
$$+ \text{cumulative amount metabolized}$$
$$+ \text{cumulative amount excreted unchanged}$$

and for the intravascular route:

$$\text{Dose} = \text{amount in the body}$$
$$+ \text{amount metabolized}$$
$$+ \text{cumulative amount excreted unchanged.}$$

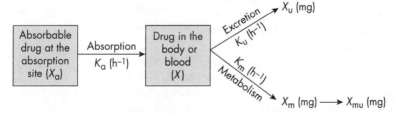

Figure 1.12 The principle of passive diffusion and the relationship between the rate of transfer and the administered dose of a drug following the administration of a drug by an extravascular route.

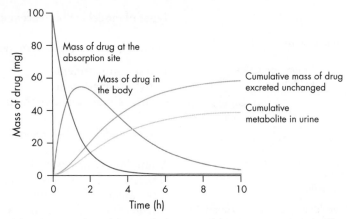

Figure 1.13 Amount of drug (expressed as a fraction of administered dose) over time in each of the compartments shown in Fig. 1.12.

Characteristics of a one-compartment model

1. Equilibrium between drug concentrations in different tissues or organs is obtained rapidly (virtually instantaneously), following drug input. Therefore, a distinction between distribution and elimination phases is not possible.
2. The amount (mass) of drug distributed in different tissues may be different.
3. Following equilibrium, changes in drug concentration in blood (which can be sampled) reflect changes in concentration of drug in other tissues (which cannot be sampled).

1.6 Rate processes

After a drug is administered, it is subjected to a number of processes (ADME) whose rates control the concentration of drug in the elusive region known as "site of action." These processes affect the onset of action, as well as the duration and intensity of pharmacological response. Some knowledge of these rate processes is, therefore, essential for a better understanding of the observed pharmacological activity of the administered drug.

Let us introduce the symbol Y as some function which changes with time (t). This means Y is a dependent variable and time (t) is an independent variable.

For the purpose of this textbook, the dependent variable (Y) is either mass of drug in the body (X), mass of drug in the urine (X_u) or the concentration of drug in plasma or serum (C_p or C_s, respectively). For a very small time interval, there will be a very small change in the value of Y as follows:

$$\frac{dY}{dt} = \frac{Y_2 - Y_1}{t_2 - t_1} \tag{1.6}$$

where dY/dt is the instantaneous rate of change in function Y with respect to an infinitesimal time interval (dt).

Order of a process

In the equation $dY/dt = KY^n$, the numerical value (n) of the exponent of the substance (Y) undergoing the change is the *order* of the process. Typical orders and types of process encountered in science include:

- zero order
- first order
- second order
- third order
- reversible
- parallel
- consecutive.

$$X \xrightarrow{K_0} \text{Product (b)}$$

where X is a substance undergoing a change

$$X \xrightarrow{K_0} X \text{ (in another location)}$$

where X is a substance undergoing transfer

Figure 1.14   Process of change (zero order).

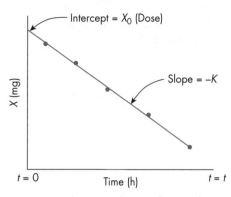

Figure 1.15   Rectilinear graph (R.L.) of zero-order process. X, concentration of drug; K, rate constant.

Zero- and first-order processes are most useful for pharmacokinetics.

Zero-order process

Figure 1.14 shows the process of change in a zero-order process.

The following is the derivation of the equation for a zero-order elimination process:

$$\frac{-dY}{dt} = K_0 Y^0 \tag{1.7}$$

where K_0 is the zero-order rate constant and the minus sign shows negative change over time (elimination).

Since $Y^0 = 1$,

$$\frac{-dY}{dt} = K_0 \tag{1.8}$$

This equation clearly indicates that Y changes at a constant rate, since K_0 is a constant (the zero-order rate constant). This means that the change in Y must be a function of factors *other than* the amount of Y present at a given time. Factors affecting the magnitude of this rate could include the amount of enzymes present, light or oxygen absorbed, and so on.

The integration of Eq. 1.8 yields the following:

$$Y = Y_0 - K_0 t \tag{1.9}$$

where Y is the amount present at time t and Y_0 is the amount present at time zero. (For example, Y_0 could stand for $(X)_{t=0}$, the mass of drug in the body at time zero. In the case of an intravenous injection, $(X)_{t=0}$ would be equal to X_0, the administered dose.)

Equation 1.9 is similar to other linear equations (i.e. $y = b - mx$, where b is the vertical axis intercept and $-m$ is the negative slope of the line) (Fig. 1.15).

Applications of zero-order processes

Applications of zero-order processes include administration of a drug as an intravenous infusion, formulation and administration of a drug through controlled release dosage forms and administration of drugs through transdermal drug delivery systems.

In order to apply these general zero-order equations to the case of zero-order drug elimination, we will make the appropriate substitutions for the general variable Y.

For example, substitution of X (mass of drug in the body at time t) for Y in Eq. 1.8 yields the zero-order elimination rate equation:

$$\frac{-dX}{dt} = K_0 \tag{1.10}$$

Whereas, the counterpart of the integrated Eq. 1.9 is $X = X_{t=0} - K_0 t$, or

$$X = X_0 - K_0 t \tag{1.11}$$

where $X_{t=0}$ is the amount of drug in the body at time zero. (For an intravenous injection, this equals the administered dose, X_0.)

the rate constant (K_0) for zero-elimination of drug

... e dX in Eq. 1.10 has units of mass and dt has units of time, K_0 must have units of *mass/time* (e.g. $\mathrm{mg\,h^{-1}}$). This can also be seen by the integrated Eq. 1.11: $K_0 t = X_0 - X$. Therefore,

$$K_0 = \frac{X_0 - X}{t - t_0} = \mathrm{mg\,h^{-1}}$$

First-order process

Figure 1.16 shows the process of change in a first-order process.

$$X \xrightarrow{\quad K \quad} \text{Product (b)}$$

where X is a substance undergoing a change

$$X \xrightarrow{\quad K \quad} X \text{ (in another location)}$$

where X is a substance undergoing transfer

Figure 1.16 Process of change (first order).

The following is the derivation of the equation for a first-order *elimination* process, since the negative sign indicates that the amount of Y is *decreasing* over time.

$$\frac{-dY}{dt} = KY^1 \tag{1.12}$$

where Y is again the mass of a substance undergoing a change or a transfer, and K is the first-order elimination rate constant. However, since by definition $Y^1 = Y$,

$$\frac{-dY}{dt} = KY \tag{1.13}$$

Equation 1.13 tells us that the rate at which Y changes (specifically, decreases) depends on the product of the rate constant (K) and the mass of the substance undergoing the change or transfer.

Upon integration of Eq. 1.13, we obtain:

$$Y = Y_0 e^{-Kt} \tag{1.14}$$

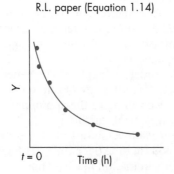

R.L. paper (Equation 1.14)

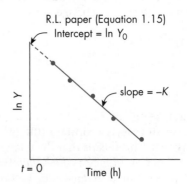

R.L. paper (Equation 1.15)
Intercept = $\ln Y_0$
slope = $-K$

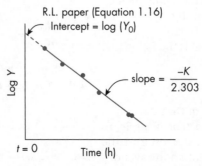

R.L. paper (Equation 1.16)
Intercept = $\log (Y_0)$
slope = $\dfrac{-K}{2.303}$

Figure 1.17 One-compartment intravenous bolus injection: three plots using rectilinear (R.L.) co-ordinates. K, rate constant; Y can stand for mass of drug in the body (X), concentration of drug in plasma, etc.

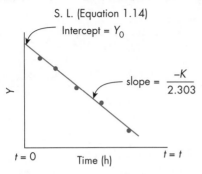

S. L. (Equation 1.14)

Intercept = Y_0

slope = $\dfrac{-K}{2.303}$

$t = 0$ \qquad Time (h) \qquad $t = t$

Figure 1.18 One-compartment intravenous bolus injection: plot using semilogarithmic (S.L.) co-ordinates. K, rate constant; Y can be X or C_p.

or

$$\ln Y = \ln Y_0 - Kt \tag{1.15}$$

or

$$\log Y = \log Y_0 - Kt/2.303 \tag{1.16}$$

The above three equations for a first-order process may be plotted on rectilinear co-ordinates (Fig. 1.17).

Use of semilogarithm paper (i.e. S.L. plot): Eq. 1.14 may be plotted (Y versus t) on semilogarithmic co-ordinates. It will yield a vertical axis intercept of Y_0 and a slope of $-K/2.303$ (Fig. 1.18).

Applications

First-order elimination is extremely important in pharmacokinetics since the majority of therapeutic drugs are eliminated by this process.

We apply the general first-or[der] above to the case of first-order dr[ug] by making the appropriate subst[itution] general variable Y.

For example, substitution of X (mass of drug in the body at time t) for Y in Eq. 1.12 yields the first-order elimination rate equation:

$$\frac{-dX}{dt} = KX^1 = KX \tag{1.17}$$

Upon integration of Eq. 1.17, we obtain:

$$X = X_0 e^{-Kt} \tag{1.18}$$

where X_0 is the dose of intravenously injected drug (i.v. bolus), or

$$\ln X = \ln X_0 - Kt \tag{1.19}$$

or

$$\log X = \log X_0 - Kt/2.303 \tag{1.20}$$

Unit for a first-order rate constant, K

Eq. 1.17

$$\frac{-dX}{dt} = KX$$

or $-dX/dt \times X^{-1} = K$, where units are $\mathrm{mg\,h^{-1}} \times \mathrm{mg^{-1}}$. So K has units of $\mathrm{h^{-1}}$.

Comparing zero- and first-order processes

Tables 1.2 and 1.3 compare zero-order and first-order processes.

Table 1.2 Comparison of zero-order and first-order reactions

Terms	Zero order	First order
$-dX/dt$	$=K_0$ (Eq. 1.10); rate remains constant	$=KX$ (Eq. 1.17); rate changes over time
rate constant	$=K_0$ (unit $= \mathrm{mg\,h^{-1}}$)	$=K$ (unit $= \mathrm{h^{-1}}$)
X	$X = X_0 - Kt$ (Eq. 1.11) (integrated equation)	$\ln X = \ln X_0 - Kt$ (Eq. 1.19) or $\log X = \log X_0 - Kt/2.303$ (Eq. 1.20) (integrated equation)
X_0	Assume is 100 mg or 100%	Assume is 100 mg or 100%
rate	$K_0 = 10\ \mathrm{mg\,h^{-1}}$	$K = 0.1\ \mathrm{h^{-1}}$ or 10% of the remaining X

Table 1.3   Values for parameters over time in zero- and first-order processes

Time (h)	Zero order		First order	
	X (mg)	dX/dt (mg h^{-1})	X (mg)	dX/dt (mg h^{-1})
0	100	–	100	–
1	90	10	90	10
2	80	10	81	9
3	70	10	72.9	8.10
4	60	10	65.61	7.29
5	50	10	59.05	6.56
6	40	10	53.14	5.91
7	30	10	47.82	5.32
8	20	10	43.04	4.78
9	10	10	38.74	4.30

2

Mathematical review

Objectives

Upon completion of this chapter, you will have the ability to:

- correctly manipulate arithmetic and algebraic expressions, expressing the result in the correct number of significant figures
- compare and contrast the terms *variable, constant* and *parameter*
- correctly manipulate the units in a calculation
- explain the interrelationship between *slope, rate,* and *derivative*
- construct sketches (profiles) illustrating pharmacokinetic equations.

2.1 Introduction

Pharmacokinetics is a mathematical subject. It deals in quantitative conclusions, such as a dose or a concentration of drug in the blood. There is a single correct numerical answer (along with many incorrect answers) for a pharmacokinetic problem. Therefore, pharmacokinetics meets Lord Kelvin's criterion (1889) for substantial scientific knowledge: "I often say that when you can measure what you are speaking about, and express it in numbers, you know something about it, but when you cannot express it in numbers your knowledge is of a meagre and unsatisfactory kind."

Pharmacokinetics concerns itself with a particular set of mathematical problems: the so-called "word problems." This type of problem presents additional challenges to the problem solver: translating the words and phrases into mathematical symbols and equations, performing the mathematical manipulations and finally translating the result into a clinically meaningful conclusion, such as the proper dosage regimen for the patient or the projected course of the blood concentration of drug over time.

The exact, and exacting, nature of the science of pharmacokinetics requires some degree of facility in mathematical manipulation. The objective of this section is to refamiliarize the reader with some fundamental mathematical concepts that were learned once but, perhaps, forgotten.

2.2 A brief history of pharmacokinetics

The mathematics of pharmacokinetics strongly resembles, and arises from, the mathematics of chemical kinetics, enzyme kinetics, and radioisotope (tracer) kinetics. Table 2.1 shows how, over the years, the mathematical theory of pharmacokinetics and that of its older siblings has been substantiated by experimental work. In fact, substantiation of a particular kinetic theory often

Table 2.1   Kinetics timeline

Date	Theoretical work	Experimental work
1670	Invention of calculus (independently by Newton and Leibnitz)	
1850		First experimentally determined chemical reaction rate (hydrolysis of sucrose in solution: rotation of polarized light changing over time)
1864–1877	Chemical reaction kinetics elucidated by van't Hoff	
mid 1800s		Existence of enzymes deduced from fermentation experiments
1896		Becquerel discovers "radio-activity" in uranium
1904	Radioisotope kinetics described in "Radioactivity" by Rutherford	
1913	Enzyme kinetics described by Michaelis and Menten	
1937	Birth of pharmacokinetics: two papers by Teorell	
1941		Invention of first spectrophotometer (Beckman DU)
1953	First pharmacokinetic book, *Der Blutspiegel* by Dost, expands pharmacokinetics	
1966	*Drugs and Tracer Kinetics* by Rescigno and Segré published	
1975	First pharmacokinetics textbook published: *Pharmacokinetics* by Gibaldi and Perrier	

had to wait on the development of an analytical instrument or technique. For pharmacokinetics, it was the development of the spectrophotometer that allowed the detection of concentrations of drug in the blood and comparison of these with values predicted by theory.

2.3 Hierarchy of algebraic operations

A basic requirement for the correct calculation of arithmetic and algebraic expressions is the adherence to the correct hierarchy, or order, of operations. Table 2.2 shows that parentheses have the

highest priority in directing which calculation is carried out first, followed by exponentiation, then multiplication or division (equal priority) and, finally, addition or subtraction (equal priority). The first row of this table show a calculation involving parentheses; while the last three rows of this table show a single calculation involving the other operations carried out in the proper order.

2.4 Exponents and logarithms

For many processes in nature, the rate of removal or modification of a species is proportional to,

Table 2.2   Hierarchy of arithmetic operations (in order from high to low)

Hierarchy number and operation	Examples	Comments
1. Parentheses	$(k_1 + k_2)(A) \neq k_1 + k_2 A$ $(2 + 3)(4) \neq 2 + 3 \cdot 4$ $20 \neq 14$	Without parentheses, you would multiply first and then add. Parentheses will override these lower hierarchy rules
	$((2)(5 + (3)(2)))(4 + 6) =$ $((2)(5 + 6))(4 + 6) =$ $((2)(11))(10) =$ $(22)(10) = 220$	Clear innermost parentheses first
2. Exponentiation	$2e^{-2 \cdot 3} + 5e^{-3 \cdot 0.5} =$ $2e^{-6} + 5e^{-1.5} =$ $2(0.00248) + 5(0.2231)$	Exponentiate before performing multiplication or addition (in order to exponentiate, you must first clear 2×3 and 3×0.5 inside the two exponential expressions)
3. Multiplication or division	$2(0.00248) + 5(0.2231)$ $= 0.00496 + 1.1155$	Next, do the multiplications
4. Addition or subtraction	$0.00496 + 1.1155 = 1.1205$	Finally, add terms

and driven by, the amount of that species present at a given time. This is true for the kinetics of diffusion, chemical reactions, radioactive decay and for the kinetics of the ADME processes of pharmaceuticals. Systems of this type are naturally described by exponential expressions. Consequently, in order to evaluate many pharmacokinetic expressions, it is necessary to have facility in the use of operations involving exponential expressions and their inverse expressions (logarithms). Table 2.3 displays the most common of these operations and illustrates their use with corresponding examples.

A logarithm is an exponent. A number raised to the power described by an exponent is called the base. Exponential processes in nature have the number e (equaling 2.7183...) for the base. For example, $e^1 = 2.7183....$. The inverse operation, "ln," will return the original exponent: ln $(e^1) = \ln(2.7183...) = 1$.

Since we humans have 10 digits and are used to counting in the decimal system, we often use the base 10, for which the inverse logarithmic operation is called "log." For example, $10^2 = 100$, and $\log(10^2) = \log(100) = 2$. In Table 2.3, we see the interconversion between expressions containing logs and expressions containing lns by use of the number 2.303, which is simply ln(10).

2.5 Variables, constants and parameters

Another fundamental mathematical concept important in pharmacokinetics is the difference between a variable and a constant. For the purposes of pharmacokinetics, a variable is something that changes *over time*. Conversely, a constant is time invariant. Box 2.1 presents some examples of variables and constants as well as rules showing whether an expression containing variables and/or constants will give rise to a variable or a constant.

There is, however, a special term used for a constant that may, in fact, be a variable under a particular set of circumstances. In particular for pharmacokinetics, a *parameter* is a value that is constant for a given individual receiving a particular drug. This value will most likely vary for the same subject receiving a different drug and may vary for different subjects receiving the same drug. This value may also vary for a given subject receiving a particular drug if it is measured over a long time period (e.g. months) or if a disease or drug interaction has occurred since the value was last calculated. For most pharmacokinetic calculations in this text, we will concern ourselves with a single subject or patient receiving a particular drug; therefore, the parameter will be a constant.

Table 2.3 Exponents and logarithms

Rule	Example
$n^a \cdot n^b = n^{a+b}$	$10^1 \cdot 10^2 = 10^3$
$\frac{n^a}{n^b} = n^{a-b}$	$\frac{10^4}{10^2} = 10^2$
$(n^a)^b = n^{ab}$	$(10^3)^2 = 10^6$
$\frac{1}{n^a} = n^{-a}$	$\frac{1}{10^2} = 10^{-2}$
$\sqrt[a]{n} = n^{1/a}$	$\sqrt{n} = n^{1/2}; \sqrt{100} = 100^{1/2} = 10$ $\sqrt[3]{n} = n^{1/3}; \sqrt[3]{1000} = 1000^{1/3} = 10$
$\log ab = \log a + \log b$	$\log 1000 = \log 10 + \log 100 = 3$
$\log\left(\frac{a}{b}\right) = \log a - \log b$	$\log 10 = \log 1000 - \log 100 = 1$
$\log(a^b) = b(\log a)$	$\log(10^2) = 2(\log 10) = 2$
$-\log\left(\frac{a}{b}\right) = +\log\left(\frac{b}{a}\right)$	$-\log\left(\frac{10}{1000}\right) = \log\left(\frac{1000}{10}\right) = 2$
$\log(10^a) = a$	$\log(10^3) = 3$
$\ln(e^a) = a$	$\ln(e^3) = 3$
$\log a = \frac{\ln a}{2.303}$	$\log 10 = \frac{\ln 10}{2.303} = 1$
$n^0 = 1$	$10^0 = e^0 = 1$
$\ln(n \leq 0) = undefined$	
$\log(n \leq 0) = undefined$	

Box 2.1 Variables and constants

1. There are obvious constants:

   $\pi = 3.14159265$
   $e = 2.718282$
   explicit numbers, such as 3, 18.5, $(7/8)^2$

2. Time (t) is a variable.

   C_p varies as a function of time. (There is one exception where a combination of intravenous bolus and intravenous infusion can result in constant C_p over time.)

3. The first order elimination rate constant (K) is a constant, as the name implies.

4. An expression containing nothing but constants yields a constant:

   $$c = \frac{(a)(b)}{\pi} + 3$$

   where a, b and c are constants

5. An expression containing a single variable yields a variable:

$$x = \frac{ab}{y} + 3$$

where a, b are constants; x, y are variables

$$C_p = (C_p)_0 e^{-Kt}$$

6. A product of two variables will be a variable. The *exception* is when the two variables are inversely proportional.

$$z = (a)(x)(y) \quad \text{for } x \neq \frac{b}{y}$$

$$c = (a)(x)(y) \quad \text{for } x = \frac{b}{y}$$

where a, b and c are constants and x, y and z are variables

7. A quotient of two variables will be a variable. The *exception* is when the two variables are directly proportional.

$$z = \frac{(a)(x)}{y} \quad \text{for } x \neq (b)(y)$$

$$c = \frac{(a)(x)}{y} \quad \text{for } x = (b)(y)$$

where a, b and c are constants and x, y and z are variables

Box 2.2 expands on the subject of pharmacokinetic parameters.

2.6 Significant figures

In performing pharmacokinetic calculations, we must take care to get the most precise answer that can be supported by the data we have. Conversely, we do not want to express our answer with greater precision than we are justified in claiming. The rules of significant figures will help us with this task. These are listed in Box 2.3.

2.7 Units and their manipulation

Box 2.4 shows some typical units used in pharmacokinetics as well as the mathematical rules which apply to units.

Throughout the text, various equivalent units will be mentioned at intervals so that the student will become adept at recognizing them. For example, $1.23 \, \mu g \, mL^{-1}$ can also be expressed as $1.23 \, mcg \, mL^{-1}$ or $1.23 \, mg \, L^{-1}$. Micrograms can be expressed as μg or mcg (not an S.I. unit but commonly used to avoid any confusion

between the letter "m" and the Greek letter "μ" in milligrams [mg] and micrograms [μg] in dosages), and liters can be shortened to "lit" and either a capital or lower case letter L used.

2.8 Slopes, rates and derivatives

A straight line has a slope which is constant. This constant slope, $\Delta y / \Delta x$, is the change in y divided by the change in x. By contrast, in a curved line, there is an instantaneous slope at each point along the curve (calculated by finding the slope of the tangent to that particular point). This instantaneous slope also goes by the name of the derivative dy/dx. We will now demonstrate the concept of slope as it arises in pharmacokinetics.

The simplest pharmacokinetic model (as we shall see in subsequent chapters, this is an intravenous injection of a one-compartment drug eliminated by a first-order process) is described by a single-term exponential equation:

$$C_p = (C_p)_0 e^{-Kt} \tag{2.1}$$

where C_p is the plasma drug concentration at time t; $(C_p)_0$ is the plasma drug concentration

---

Box 2.2   Parameters

1. When is a variable not a variable? *Answer:* when it is a *parameter*.
2. When is a constant not a constant? *Answer:* when it is a *parameter*.

The answers to these questions suggest that a parameter is something between a variable and a constant. This is approximately true; but the very specific meaning of "parameter" in pharmacokinetics is:

> A parameter is a number that is characteristic (and *constant*) for a specific patient receiving a specific drug.

A couple of examples of pharmacokinetic parameters are **elimination half life** (the time it takes for a plasma drug concentration to drop to half its original value) and **apparent volume of distribution** (the volume to which a given dose of drug would have to be diluted in order to have a concentration equal to that concentration detected in the blood).

Now, the value of one person's volume of distribution (in liters) for a drug (e.g. theophylline) is most probably not the same as that of another person. In other words, the parameter volume of distribution will vary between subjects who receive the same drug. That is, it can be a variable, rather than a constant, when two different people receive the drug. Similarly, one person's elimination half life (in time) for one drug (e.g. theophylline) will most probably not be the same as that for another drug (e.g. digoxin). Even though it is the same person, it is a case of two different drugs; and the parameter elimination half life becomes a variable. A parameter is a constant only for the same person on the same drug.

The power of using parameters is that, once the value of a parameter for a given patient receiving a given drug has been identified, this value is *constant* and can be used in pharmacokinetic equations to individualize therapy for this patient. The outcome of using a dosing regimen based on a patient's characteristic parameters and therefore "tailored" for this individual patient is greater ability to give a dose of drug that will *maximize therapeutic efficacy* while *minimizing adverse effects* of the drug.

Box 2.3   Significant figures

There are two kinds of numbers: *absolute* numbers and *denominate* numbers.

An example of an **absolute number** would be seen in a problem in which you are asked to calculate plasma drug level at a time two elimination half lives after a dose is given. In this case the number is exactly 2.0000000000... to an infinite number of decimal points.

However, when things are *measured*, such as doses or plasma drug levels, there is some degree of uncertainty in the measurement and it is necessary to indicate to what degree of precision the value of the number is known. This is called a **denominate number**. Precision is indicated in these numbers by reporting them to a certain number of **significant figures**. Significant figures may be defined as the digits in a number showing how precisely we know the value of the number. Significant figures are *not* to be confused with the number of digits to the right of the decimal place. Some digits in a number simply serve as placeholders to show how far away the rest of the digits are from the decimal point.

For example, each of the following numbers has *three significant figures*. This can be more readily appreciated by expressing them in scientific notation.

Number	Scientific notation	Remark
102.	1.02×10^2	The zero between non-zero integers is significant
10.0	1.00×10^1	If a trailing zero after a decimal point is expressed, it is *intended* to be significant

1.23	1.23×10^0	Non-zero integers are significant
0.123	1.23×10^{-1}	Zero before the decimal point is not significant
0.00123	1.23×10^{-3}	Leading zeros after the decimal point are merely placeholders, and not significant

Occasionally, it is unclear how many significant figures a number possesses. For example, the number 100 could be represented in scientific notation by 1×10^2, 1.0×10^2 or 1.00×10^2. The only unambiguous way to express this number is by the use of scientific notation.

A calculator performs its calculations with a great degree of precision, although it may not *show* a large number of significant figures in its default (two decimal point) mode. The student is likely to run into trouble when transferring an excessively rounded off value from the calculator to paper. Based on the precision of numbers encountered in pharmacokinetic calculations, a good rule of thumb for pharmacokinetic calculations is as follows:

Be careful to retain at least 3 significant figures throughout all pharmacokinetic calculations and also to report numerical answers to 3 significant figures

Rounding off data or intermediate answers to fewer significant figures can waste precision and cause the answer to be incorrect.

immediately after the intravenous injection; and K is the first-order elimination rate constant. When graphed on rectilinear co-ordinates, this equation produces an exponentially declining curve with y-axis intercept $(C_p)_0$ (Fig. 2.1a). The instantaneous slopes of three separate points are shown.

Using the rules of Table 2.3, we can take the ln of each side of Eq. 2.1, which yields:

$$\ln C_p = (C_p)_0 - Kt \qquad (2.2)$$

This corresponds to taking the ln of each plasma drug concentration in the data set and plotting it versus its corresponding time. Equation 2.2 conforms to the equation of a straight line $y = mx + b$. This is evident in Fig. 2.1b. In this case the slope equals -1 times the rate constant K and the y-axis intercept equals $\ln (C_p)_0$.

By the rules of logarithms and exponents, Eq. 2.1 is identical to:

$$C_p = (C_p)_0 10^{-\frac{Kt}{2.303}} \qquad (2.3)$$

Taking the log of each side of Eq. 2.3 yields:

$$\log C_p = \log (C_p)_0 - \frac{Kt}{2.303} \qquad (2.4)$$

This corresponds to taking the log of each plasma drug concentration in the data set and plotting it versus its corresponding time. Equation 2.4 also conforms to the equation of a straight line, as can be seen in Fig. 2.1c. In this case the slope equals $-K/2.303$ and the y-axis intercept equals $\log(C_p)_0$.

Finally, one can plot plasma drug concentrations versus time on semilogarithmic paper. This has the effect of linearizing Eq. 2.4. The slope equals $-K/2.303$, but the y-axis intercept now equals $(C_p)_0$, since C_p, rather than $\log C_p$ values were plotted (Fig. 2.1d).

2.9 Time expressions

Any kinetic process concerns itself with changes occurring over time. Therefore, it is essential to have a clear idea about the meaning of time expressions in pharmacokinetics. These are summarized in Table 2.4.

2.10 Construction of pharmacokinetic sketches (profiles)

Relationships between pharmacokinetic terms can be demonstrated by the construction of

---

Box 2.4 Units

A pharmacokinetic calculation is not complete unless both the number and the unit have been determined. If the unit that is determined is not the unit expected, this situation can even alert you to a mistake in the calculation. For example, in a problem where a dose of drug is being calculated and the unit comes out to be something other than mass units, you would be well advised to perform the calculation again with particular care.

Typical units used in pharmacokinetics

Dimension	Examples of units
Volume	mL; L (or l); quarts
Mass	g; kg; pounds
Concentration	$mg\,L^{-1}$; g/100 mL (% w/v); $mol\,L^{-1}$
Flow rate (including clearance)	$mL\,min^{-1}$; L/h
Rate of elimination	$mg\,h^{-1}$; µg/min
Time	h; min; s
Reciprocal time	h^{-1};/min; s^{-1}
Area under C_p versus time curve	(µg/mL)·h; $µg\,mL^{-1}\,h$

Mathematical rules for units

1. Retain units throughout the whole calculation and present them with the numerical answer.
2. Some quantities are unitless (e.g. fraction of drug absorbed, *F*). Unitless numbers generally arise from the fact that units of ratios cancel. For example, *F* is the ratio: $(AUC)_{oral}/(AUC)_{IV}$.
3. Add or subtract only those numbers with the same units, or which can be reduced to the same units. For example:

   $1\,mg + 1\,mg = 2\,mg$
   $1\,h^{-1} + 2\,h^{-1} = 3\,h^{-1}$
   $1\,h + 10\,min = 60\,min + 10\,min = 70\,min$ (interconvertible units of time)

4. Exponentiate (raise to a power of *e*) unitless numbers only. For example, for $K = 1\,h^{-1}$ and $t = 2\,h$,

   $e^{-Kt} = e^{-(1\,h^{-1})(2\,h)} = e^{-2} = 0.135$
   (units cancel)

5. Multiply and divide units as for numbers. For example:

   $$\left(\frac{1}{cm}\right)\left(\frac{2\,g}{cm}\right)(3\,cm^{-1}) = 6\,g/cm^3$$

---

sketches (profiles). Rules for the construction of sketches and examples of the most common sketch types that arise in pharmacokinetics are shown in Box 2.5. Facility in the use of sketches will help to provide the student with intuition about the way that variables and parameters interact with each other in pharmacokinetics; additionally, sketches can help to facilitate the solution of complicated or multistep dosing problems.

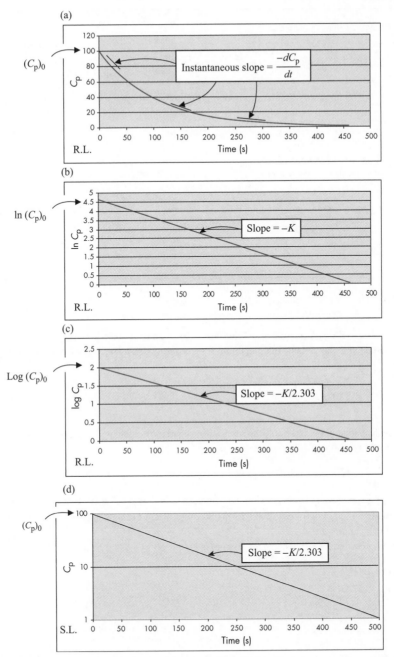

Figure 2.1   Slopes and y-axis intercepts for plots of an intravenous bolus of a one-compartment drug. $(C_p)_0$, plasma concentration at time zero; K, rate constant.

Table 2.4   Time expressions in pharmacokinetics

Symbol	Symbol represents	Units	Variable or constant over time?	Example
t	Continuous time	Time	*Variable* (proceeds at 1 s/s)	t on the x-axis of a graph
t	For a given calculation, if we specify a *point in time* (whose value is t time units which have elapsed since a reference time t_0), then t is a constant	Time	*Constant*	$t = 3$ h since the beginning of an intravenous infusion
Δt	A finite-sized slice of time	Time	*Constant*	Break the time axis up into many Δt values, each having 1 min duration
dt	An infinitesimal slice of time	Time	*Constant*	Δt approaching zero

---

Box 2.5   Method for creating profiles (sketches)

1. You will be asked to sketch A versus B (A as a function of B). When presented in this form, the convention is that A is the y-axis variable the dependent variable) and B is the x-axis variable (the independent variable). For example:

$$\text{Sketch}: \underset{\underset{y}{\uparrow}}{\tau} \quad \text{vs} \quad \underset{\underset{x}{\uparrow}}{(\overline{C}_p)_\infty}$$

2. Next, you will need to (find) and apply the appropriate equation containing the y and x variables you have been asked to sketch. For this example, the equation is:

$$(\overline{C}_p)_\infty = \frac{SFD_0}{VK\tau}$$

Note that we do not have to know the pharmacokinetic interpretation of the symbols at this point. All we need to know is that τ and $(\overline{C}_p)_\infty$ are variables and, for the purposes of constructing the sketch, all the other symbols will be considered to be constants.

3. Next, rearrange the equation to isolate the y variable on the left side of the equal sign. For example:

$$(\overline{C}_p)_\infty VK\tau = SFD_0$$

$$\underset{\underset{y}{\uparrow}}{\tau} = \underset{\underset{x}{\uparrow}}{\frac{SFD_0}{(\overline{C}_p)_\infty VK}}$$

4. The equation is now in the form where y is a function of x. This means that the value of the y variable depends on the value of the x variable and on some constants. (Note that even *time* should be considered constant for the purpose of the sketch if it is not the x variable for the sketch.) Next, rewrite the equation grouping all the individual constants together as a single constant called CON. In this example:

$$\underset{\underset{y}{\uparrow}}{\tau} = CON/\underset{\underset{x}{\uparrow}}{(\overline{C}_p)_\infty}, \text{ where } CON = SFD_0/VK$$

5. Now determine which of the four basic sketch types this equation represents. You may need to do some more rearranging of the equation in order to recognize which family it belongs to. Here are the four basic sketch types and their general equations:

Category	Equation	Sketches
A Linear on rectilinear graph paper	$y = m(x) + b$ ↑ ↑ slope y − intercept $t_{1/2}$ e.g. $t_{1/2} = \frac{0.693}{K}$ Sketch $t_{1/2}$ versus $1/K$ ↑ ↑ y x (In this example, notice that the y-intercept, $b = 0$; so it would conform to sketch A1)	 1. RL 2. RL 3. RL 4. RL
B y = constant (independent of x)	$y = b = \text{CON}$ (notice that this is a subtype of A; with slope = 0) e.g. Sketch $t_{1/2}$ versus t	 RL Also: SL
C Inverse (reciprocal)	$y = \dfrac{CON}{x} = CON\left(\dfrac{1}{x}\right)$ e.g. Sketch $t_{1/2}$ versus K ↑ ↑ y x	

(Continued)

Box 2.5   (Continued)

D   Mono-exponential $y = CON(e^{-Kx})$
e.g. $C_p = (C_p)_0 e^{-Kt}$
$\uparrow \qquad\qquad \uparrow$
$y \qquad\qquad x$

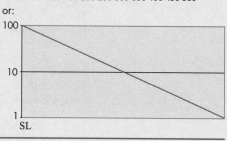

or:

Now we can see that our example equation $\tau = CON/(\overline{C}_p)_\infty$ falls into category C (inverse) and should be sketched as follows:

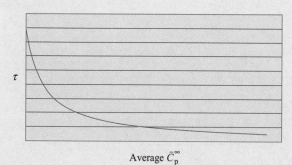

Average $\overline{C}_p^{\infty}$

3

Intravenous bolus administration (one-compartment model)

Objectives

Upon completion of this chapter, you will have the ability to:

- describe the pharmacokinetic parameters apparent volume of distribution, elimination half life, first-order elimination rate constant and clearance
- determine pharmacokinetic parameters from either plasma or urinary data
- state the equation for plasma drug concentration as a function of time after administration of an intravenous bolus of a drug that exhibits one-compartment model characteristics
- calculate plasma drug concentration at time t after the administration of an intravenous bolus dose of a drug
- calculate the intravenous bolus dose of a drug that will result in a target (desired) plasma drug concentration at time t for a patient whose pharmacokinetic parameters have been determined, or for a patient whose pharmacokinetic parameters are estimated by the use of average values of the parameters reported in the literature.

3.1 Introduction

A drug is administered as an injection of a sterile solution formulation. The volume and the concentration of the administered solution must be known in order to calculate the administered dose. For example, five milliliters (5 mL) of a 2% w/v solution will contain 100 mg of a drug (dose). There are several important points to note.

1. This route of administration ensures that the entire administered dose reaches the general circulation.

2. The desired drug concentration in the blood is promptly attained.

3. One must be extremely careful in calculating doses or measuring solutions because of the danger of adverse or toxic effects.

How the fundamental pharmacokinetic parameters of a drug are obtained following the intravenous bolus administration of a drug will be discussed below. These parameters, in turn, form a basis for making rational decisions about the dosing of drugs in therapeutics. The following assumptions are made in these discussions (Fig. 3.1):

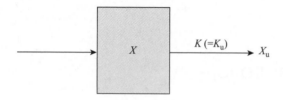

$$X \xrightarrow{K (=K_u)} X_u$$

Figure 3.1 Scheme and setup of one-compartment intravenous bolus model. X, mass (amount) of drug in the blood/body at time, t; X_u, mass (amount) of unchanged drug in the urine at time, t; K, first-order elimination rate constant.

• one-compartment model, first-order process and passive diffusion are operative
• no metabolism takes place (elimination is 100% via renal excretion)
• the drug is being monitored in blood (plasma/serum) and urine.

From Chapter 1, we know the differential equation for a first-order process:

$$\frac{-dY}{dt} = KY \qquad (3.1)$$

where $-dY/dt$ is the negative rate of change of a substance over time. Applying this equation to the elimination of drug (mass X) in the body, gives:

$$\frac{-dX}{dt} = KX \qquad (3.2)$$

The integrated form of Eq. 3.2 is:

$$X = X_0\, e^{-Kt} \qquad (3.3)$$

or

$$\ln (X) = \ln (X_0) - Kt \qquad (3.4)$$

or

$$\log (X) = \log (X_0) - Kt/2.303 \qquad (3.5)$$

where X_0 is the mass (amount) of unchanged drug in the body at time zero ($t=0$). Please note that X_0 is the administered intravenous bolus dose (e.g. µg, mg kg^{-1}) of the drug. Figure 3.2 plots the amount of drug remaining in blood over time.

When drugs are monitored in plasma or serum, it is concentration (not mass or amount) that is measured.

$$\text{Concentration}(C_p \text{ or } C_s)$$
$$= \frac{\text{mass (amount) of drug(mg, µg, etc.)}}{\text{unit volume(V), (mL, L, etc.)}}$$

$$C_p \text{ or } C_s = X/V \qquad (3.6)$$

From Eq. 3.3:

$$X = X_0 e^{-Kt}$$

Dividing Eq. 3.3 by the volume term, V, yields

$$\frac{X}{V} = \frac{X_0}{V} e^{-Kt} \qquad (3.7)$$

and, since $X/V = C_p$ (Eq. 3.6), Eq. 3.7 takes the following form:

$$C_p = (C_p)_0 e^{-Kt} \qquad (3.8)$$

or

$$\ln C_p = \ln (C_p)_0 - Kt \qquad (3.9)$$

or

$$\log C_p = \log (C_p)_0 - Kt/2.303 \qquad (3.10)$$

This can be plotted as in Fig. 3.3.

Of course, the best way to plot the concentration versus time data is by the use of semilogarithmic co-ordinates (S.L. paper or S.L. plot) (Fig. 3.4).

3.2 Useful pharmacokinetic parameters

The following are some of the most useful and fundamental pharmacokinetic parameters of a drug. The knowledge of these parameters is,

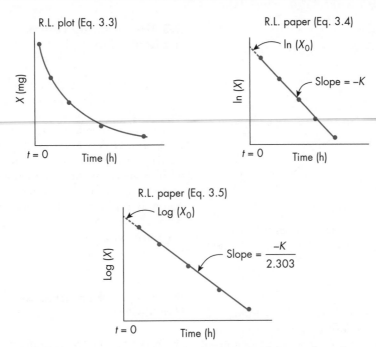

Figure 3.2 Plots of the amount of drug remaining in the blood against time, following the intravenous administration of a drug, according to Eqs 3.3, 3.4 and 3.5. X, concentration of drug; K, rate constant.

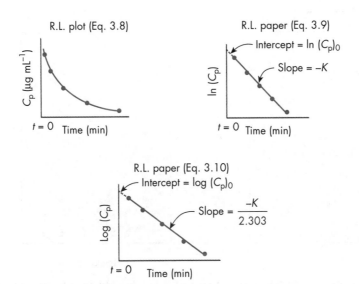

Figure 3.3 Plots of plasma or serum concentrations (C_p) of a drug against time, following the administration of a drug intravenously, according to Eqs 3.8, 3.9 and 3.10. K, rate constant.

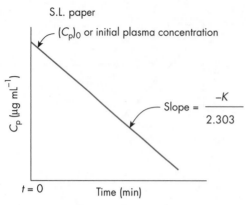

Figure 3.4   A semilogarithmic plot of plasma or serum concentrations (C_p) of a drug against time, following the administration of a drug intravenously. K, rate constant.

therefore, essential and useful for a number of reasons. At this time, however, the objectives are to understand and utilize the methods employed in obtaining these parameters, achieve conceptual understanding of these parameters, and understand the practical and theoretical significance of these parameters in pharmacokinetics.

- apparent volume of distribution (V)
- elimination half life ($t_{1/2}$)
- elimination rate constant (K or K_{el})
- systemic clearance (Cl)$_s$.

3.3 The apparent volume of distribution (V)

Concentrations (mass per unit volume or amount per unit volume), not masses (mg or μg), are usually measured in plasma or serum (more often than blood). Therefore, a term is needed to relate the measured concentration (C_p) at a time to the mass of drug (X) at that time. This term is defined as the apparent volume of distribution (V). Please note that the apparent volume of distribution (V) is simply a proportionality constant whose sole purpose is to relate the plasma concentration (C_p) and the mass of drug (X) in the body at a time. It is not a physiological volume.

The concept of the apparent volume of distribution

Figure 3.5 is a depiction of the concept of apparent volume of distribution.

1. Beakers A and B contain equal but unknown volumes of water.
2. Only beaker B contains a small quantity of charcoal (an adsorbing agent).
3. Let us assume that we add 1 g of potassium iodide (KI), which is soluble in water, to each beaker.

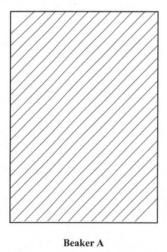

Beaker A

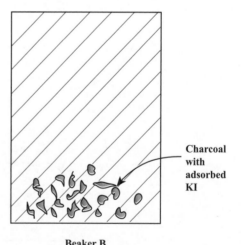

Charcoal with adsorbed KI

Beaker B

Figure 3.5   Illustration of the concept of the apparent volume of drug distribution. Two beakers contain identical but unknown volumes of water. Only one beaker contains a small amount of charcoal. Potassium iodide (KI), which is soluble in water, is added to each beaker.

4. Using a suitable analytical procedure, the concentration ($\mu g\,mL^{-1}$) of potassium iodide in each beaker is determined.

Let us assume that the potassium iodide concentration ($\mu g\,mL^{-1}$) in beakers A and B is determined to be 100 and $50\,\mu g\,mL^{-1}$, respectively. (Please note the difference in the potassium iodide concentration in each beaker, even though the volume of water in each beaker and potassium iodide added to each beaker is identical.)

Point for consideration and discussion:

Why do we have different concentration of potassium iodide in each beaker when the volume of water in each beaker is identical and amount of potassium iodide added to each beaker is identical?

Using the concentration values, knowing the amount of potassium iodide added to each beaker and performing the following calculations, we determine the volume of water present in each beaker as follows:

Beaker A:

$100\,\mu g$ (or 0.1 mg) KI in 1 mL of water

1 g or 1000 mg KI in X mL water(?)

So there will be $(1000\,mg \times 1\,mL)/0.1\,mg$ water in beaker A: 10 000 mL or 10 L.

Beaker B:

$50\,\mu g$ (or 0.05 mg) KI in 1 mL of water

1 g or 1000 mg of KI in X mL water(?)

So there will be $(1000\,mg \times 1\,mL)/0.05\,mg$ water in beaker B: 20 000 mL or 20 L.

It was stated at the outset that each beaker contains an identical but unknown volume of water. Why do we get a different volume of water in each beaker? The presence of a small amount of charcoal (adsorbing agent) is reducing the potassium iodide concentration in the available identical volume of water in beaker B.

If one applies this concept to the animal or human body, one will observe similar outcomes. In this example, one may visualize that the beaker is like a human body, 1 g potassium iodide as the administered dose of a drug, water is equivalent to

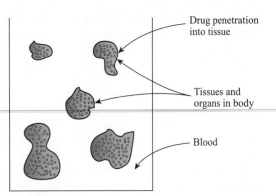

Figure 3.6 Illustration of the concepts of the apparent volume of drug distribution. Application of the beaker concept to the human body, which contains organs and tissues with lipophilic barriers.

the biological fluids and charcoal is equivalent to the organs and tissues that are present in the body (Fig. 3.6).

The penetration of drug molecules into these organs and tissues play an important role in drug distribution and in the assessment and determination of its extent. The more the drug molecules penetrate into tissues and organs following the administration of the dose of a drug, the smaller will be the plasma and/or serum drug concentration and, therefore the higher is the hypothetical volume into which the drug is distributed. The hydrophilic/lipophilic nature of the drug determines the extent to which the drug molecules penetrate into the tissues or the extent of drug distribution. The chemical structure of a compound, in turn, determines the lipophilicity of a drug.

In theory, although each drug will have its own volume of distribution and it will be constant for that drug, it is possible for two different drugs to exhibit identical apparent volumes of distribution.

The apparent volume of distribution in the body

Plasma or serum samples, collected immediately following the administration of an equal dose (i.e. X_0) of two different drugs, may exhibit large differences in the drug concentrations. There may be different initial plasma concentrations [$(C_p)_0$] of these drugs and, even if the elimination half life is the same, there may be different concentrations of these drugs at any given time. This occurs despite the fact that essentially the same amount of each drug is in the body as a whole at any given time. The cause of this difference in concentration is a difference in the volumes of distribution of the two drugs, since distribution of a drug in the body is largely a function of its physicochemical properties and, therefore, of its chemical structure.

As discussed in the definition of volume of distribution, the sole purpose of this parameter is to relate the amount and the concentration of drug in the body at a given time. Therefore, it is important to recognize that the knowledge of this parameter is essential in determining the dose of a drug required to attain the desired initial plasma concentration. It is called an apparent volume because it is not a true volume; however, it does have the appearance of being the actual volume into which a given amount of drug would be diluted in order to produce the observed concentration.

In order to determine this parameter, following the administration of a drug as an intravenous bolus, in theory, we would have to know the amount of drug in the body at a time and the corresponding plasma concentration. However, practically, it is easier to determine the apparent volume of distribution from the knowledge of *initial* plasma concentration ($\mu g\, mL^{-1}$) and the administered dose (mg or $mg\, kg^{-1}$).

The apparent volume of distribution is usually a property of a drug rather than of a biological system. It describes the extent to which a particular drug is distributed in the body tissues. The magnitude of the apparent volume of distribution usually does not correspond to plasma volume, extracellular or total body volume space but may vary from a few liters (7 to 10 L) to several hundred liters (200 L and higher) in a 70 kg subject. The higher the value of the apparent volume of distribution, the greater is the extent to which the drug is distributed in the body tissues and or organs. Furthermore, body tissues, biological membranes and organs being lipophilic in nature, the value of the apparent volume of distribution also reflects the lipophilicity of a drug, which, in turn, reflects its chemical structure. The more lipophilic the nature of the drug, greater

will be the value of the apparent volume of distribution and the smaller will be the initial plasma concentration (assuming that the administered doses of drug are identical). Conversely, if the drug is hydrophilic, the drug will penetrate to a lesser extent into tissue and, consequently, its plasma concentration will be higher and its volume of distribution will be smaller. It is, therefore, accurate to state that the value of the apparent volume of drug distribution is influenced by the lipophilicity of the drug.

Though the apparent of volume of distribution is constant for a drug and remains uninfluenced by the dose administered, certain disease states or pathological conditions may bring about changes in the apparent volume of distribution. Furthermore, since the apparent volume of distribution reflects the extent to which a drug will penetrate into tissues, alteration in the permeability characteristics of tissues will alter the apparent volume of distribution of a drug. It is also important to note that the apparent volume of distribution of a drug may vary with age groups: infants, adults and the geriatric population.

Many acidic drugs, including salicylates, sulfonamides, penicillins and anticoagulants, are either highly bound to plasma proteins or too water soluble to enter into cellular fluid and to penetrate into tissues to a significant degree. These drugs, therefore, have low volumes of distribution and low tissue to plasma concentration ratios. A given dose of these drugs will yield a relatively high plasma concentration. It is tacitly assumed here that the analytical problems in the determination of drug concentration are minimized or do not exist. Basic drugs, including tricyclic antidepressants and antihistamines, are extensively bound to extracellular tissues and are also taken up by adipose tissues. The apparent volumes of distribution of these drugs are large, often larger than the total body space; for example, the apparent volume of distribution of amphetamine is approximately 200 L ($3\, L\, kg^{-1}$). The relatively small doses and large volumes of distribution together produce low plasma concentrations, making quantitative detection in plasma a difficult task.

Please note that the expression $X_0/(C_p)_0$ is applicable for the determination of the apparent volume of drug distribution only when the drug is administered as an intravenous bolus and exhibits the characteristics of a one-compartment model. If the administered drug exhibits the characteristics of a two-compartment model (i.e. slow distribution), then that drug will have more than two apparent volumes of distributions. (We will discuss this in detail later in the text.)

Theoretical limits for apparent volume of distribution will be as low as 7 to 10 L (equivalent to the volume of the body fluid if the drug totally fails to penetrate the tissues or the drug is extremely hydrophilic) to as high as 500 L or even greater. The most commonly reported number, though, is as low as 7 to 10 L and as high as 200 L.

The pharmacokinetic parameters–elimination half life, elimination rate constant, the apparent volume of distribution and the systemic, renal and metabolic clearances (Cl_s, Cl_r, and Cl_m, respectively) for a drug are always independent of the dose administered as long as the drug follows a first-order elimination process and passive diffusion.

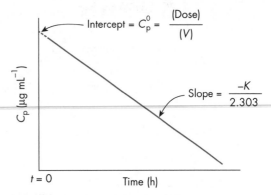

Figure 3.7 Semilogarithmic plot of plasma concentration (C_p) versus time following the administration of a drug as an intravenous bolus. The y-axis intercept yields the initial plasma concentration value (C_p)$_0$. K, rate constant.

How to obtain the apparent volume of distribution

Please note that, in order to determine the apparent volume of distribution of a drug, it is necessary to have plasma/serum concentration versus time data. Once such data are obtained following the administration of a single dose of a drug intravenously, one may prepare a plasma concentration (C_p) versus time plot on semilogarithmic paper, as shown in Fig. 3.7.

Equation 3.6 gave $X = VC_p$ or $C_p = X/V$ or

$$V = \frac{(X)_t}{(C_p)_t}$$

where $(X)_t$ is the mass or amount of drug (mg, μg, etc.) at time, t; V is the apparent volume of distribution (e.g. mL); and $(C_p)_t$ is the plasma concentration (e.g. μg mL^{-1}) at time, t.

Rearranging Eq. 3.6 and expressing it for the conditions at $t = 0$ (immediately after injection of the intravenous bolus) gives:

$$V = \frac{X_0}{(C_p)_0} \qquad (3.11)$$

where X_0 is the administered dose (e.g. ng) of a drug (for a drug injected intravenously, it is also the mass or amount of drug in the body at time $t = 0$) and $(C_p)_0$ is the plasma concentration (e.g. μg mL^{-1}) at time $t = 0$ (i.e. the initial plasma concentration of drug).

Equation 3.11 permits the determination of the apparent volume of distribution of a drug from the knowledge of the initial plasma or serum concentration [i.e. $(C_p)_0$] and the administered dose. In theory, please note, one could use the plasma or serum drug concentration at any time and the corresponding amount of drug; however, for practical considerations, it is a common practice to use the initial concentration and the dose administered to obtain the apparent volume of drug distribution. The word apparent signifies that the volume determined has the appearance of being true but it is not a true volume.

Apparent volumes of distribution are given in units of volume (e.g. mL) or units of volume on a body weight basis (L kg^{-1} body weight). Furthermore, it is important to note that the apparent volume of distribution is a constant for a given drug and is independent of the administered dose and route of drug administration.

Figure 3.8 depicts the plasma concentration against time plot (semilogarithmic paper) following the administration of three different intravenous bolus doses of drug to a subject.

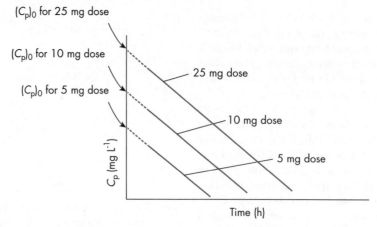

Figure 3.8 Semilogarithmic plot of plasma concentration (C_p) versus time following three different doses of drug as an intravenous bolus. Please note the difference in the intercepts, which are the initial plasma concentrations, (C_p)$_0$.

The values of (C_p)$_0$ (y-axis intercept) are directly proportional to the administered dose of a drug (5, 10 and 25 mg dose); however the ratio of dose (X_0) over the initial plasma concentration, (C_p)$_0$ (Eq. 3.11), remains unchanged:

$$V = \frac{X_0}{(C_p)_0}$$

Equation 3.11 explains why the apparent volume of distribution is independent of the administered dose.

The theoretical limits for the apparent volume of distribution can be as low as approximately 3.5 L (i.e. the volume of plasma water) to as high as greater than 200–300 L. As mentioned above, the ability of the drug to penetrate the lipophilic tissues will determine the value of the apparent volume of drug distribution. If the drug is very hydrophilic and fails to penetrate the tissues, the plasma concentration will be higher; consequently, the apparent volume of drug distribution will be very low. By comparison, if the drug is highly lipophilic and, therefore, penetrates to a greater degree into the tissues, the plasma concentration can be very low and, therefore, the apparent volume of drug distribution can be very high. Figure 3.9 provides the values of the apparent volume of distribution, reported in the literature, for selected drugs.

We know from Eqs 3.8 and 3.11 that

$$C_p = (C_p)_0 e^{-Kt}$$

and

$$V = \frac{\text{Dose}}{(C_p)_0}$$

Therefore, (C_p)$_0 \times V = $ Dose.

Dimensional analysis may be performed as follows: $\mu g/mL \times mL = $ dose (μg); $\mu g/mL \times mL\,kg^{-1}$ = dose ($\mu g\,kg^{-1}$).

3.4 The elimination half life ($t_{1/2}$)

The elimination half life is sometimes called "biological half-life" of a drug.

At a time after administering a dose when equilibrium has been established, the elimination half life may be defined as the time (h, min, day, etc.) at which the mass (or amount) of unchanged drug becomes half (or 50%) of the initial mass of drug.

Determination of the elimination half life

Equation 3.8 expresses the concentration of drug remaining in the plasma at a given time:

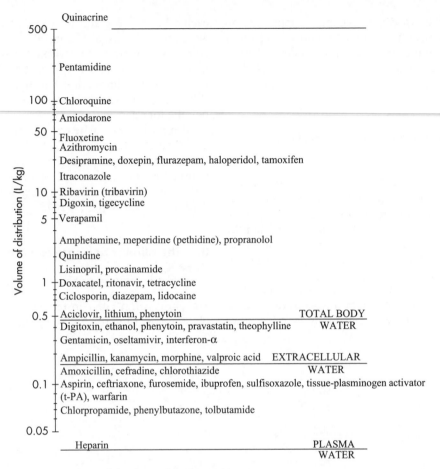

Figure 3.9   The apparent volume of distribution for selected drugs.

$$C_p = (C_p)_0 e^{-Kt}$$

Rearranging this equation gives $C_p/(C_p)_0 = e^{-Kt}$.

By definition, when $C_p = (1/2)(C_p)_0$, time $(t) = t_{1/2}$, hence

$$0.5(C_p)_0/(C_p)_0 = e^{-Kt}$$

$$0.5 = e^{-Kt}$$

or

$$\ln 0.5 = -Kt_{1/2}$$

Converting from natural to common logarithms,

$$\ln 0.5 = 2.303 \times \log 0.5$$
$$\text{(i.e. } \ln a = 2.303 \times \log a)$$

where a stands for any number

$$\ln 0.5 = 2.303 \times (-0.3010)$$

Since $\ln 0.5 = -0.693$,

$$-0.693 = -Kt_{1/2}$$

or

$$Kt_{1/2} = 0.693$$

$$t_{1/2} = 0.693/K \qquad (3.12)$$

The elimination half life has units of time.

As is the case for the parameter apparent volume of distribution, the elimination half life is also a constant for a drug and is independent of the administered dose and the route of drug administration.

Graphical determination of the elimination half life

The elimination half life of a drug may be determined by employing Eq. 3.12, provided that the value of the elimination rate constant is known or provided. Alternatively, the elimination half life may be obtained from the semilogarithmic plot of plasma concentration versus time data, as described in Fig. 3.10.

Please note that you may choose any two concentration values (read off the y-axis of the concentration versus time plot) that are one half of

each other (i.e. 200 and $100\,\mu g\,mL^{-1}$; or 100 and $50\,\mu g\,mL^{-1}$; or 25 and $12.5\,\mu g\,mL^{-1}$, etc.) and the corresponding time values (from the x-axis of the plot). The difference between the two time values represents the elimination half life of the drug. Table 3.1 provides the values of the elimination half life for selected drugs.

Also please note, when an administered drug manifests the characteristics of a first-order elimination process and passive diffusion, the elimination half life (as is the apparent volume of distribution) is constant for a drug and independent of the dose administered.

3.5 The elimination rate constant (K or K_{el})

The elimination rate constant of a drug may be obtained by using the following three steps.

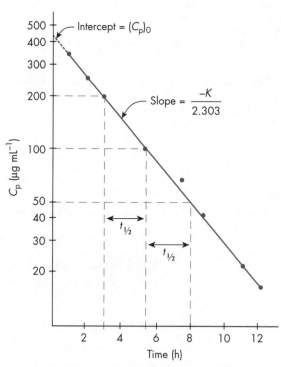

Figure 3.10 Semilogarithmic plot of plasma concentration (C_p) versus time following administration of the drug prednisolone by intravenous bolus injection. Such a plot permits the determination of the elimination half life $(t_{1/2})$ and the elimination rate constant (K). $(C_p)_0$, initial plasma concentration.

Table 3.1   The elimination half life for selected drugs

Selected drugs	Elimination half life ($t_{1/2}$ [h])
Dobutamine	0.04 h (2.4 min)
Acetylsalicylic acid	0.25
Penicillin V	0.6
Ampicillin	1.3
Lidocaine	1.8 (in patient without cirrhosis or chronic heart failure)
Morphine	1.9
Gentamicin	2 to 3
Procainamide	3.0
Salicylate	4.0 (dose dependent)
Vancomycin	5.6
Sulfisoxazole (sulfafurazole)	6.6 (in normal renal function)
Theophylline	9 (in non-smoker)
Sulfadiazine	9.9
Valproic acid	14 (in adults)
Griseofulvin	20
Methadone	35
Digoxin	39 (in normal renal function; no chronic heart failure)
Diazepam	43
Sulfadimethoxine	69
Phenobarbital	100 (in normal adults)
Digitoxin	160
Chloroquine	984 h (41 days)

First, Eq. 3.10 shows:

$$\log C_p = \log (C_p)_0 - Kt/2.303$$

Rearranging this equation gives

$$Kt/2.303 = \log (C_p)_0/C_p = \log (C_p)_0 - \log C_p$$

and

$$K = \frac{2.303 \log \left(\frac{(C_p)_0}{C_p} \right)}{t - t_0} \tag{3.13}$$

Second, from the semilogarithmic plot of plasma concentration versus time, $-K = (\text{slope}) \times 2.303$, so

$$\text{Slope} = \frac{\log y_2 - \log y_1}{t_2 - t_1}$$

Finally, from $t_{1/2} = 0.693/K$, previously derived as Eq. 3.12:

$$K = 0.693/t_{1/2}$$

The first-order rate constant (K) has a unit of reciprocal of time (e.g. h^{-1}) and, for very small time segments, it approximates the fraction of drug removed per unit time ($1 - e^{-Kt}$). Therefore, if $K = 0.1 \text{ min}^{-1}$, it means that approximately 10% of the remaining amount is removed per minute. Since drug is continuously removed from the body, the remaining amount is continuously changing.

The elimination rate constant represents overall drug elimination from the body, which includes renal excretion of unchanged drug (u) and/or the formation of metabolites (m). Hence,

$$K = K_u + K_m$$

or, if there are two metabolites

$$K = K_u + K_{m1} + K_{m2}$$

where K_u and K_m are excretion and metabolic rate constants, respectively.

However, when the drug is removed in unchanged form only (i.e. no metabolite[s]), then $K = K_u$; conversely, $K = K_m$ if the drug is completely metabolized.

Calculating the excretion (K_u) and metabolic (K_m) rate constants

Let us assume that the administered dose is 250 mg and the amount of drug excreted is 125 mg. The amounts of drug removed as metabolites 1 and 2 are 75 and 50 mg, respectively, and the elimination half life of the drug is 4 h. Then

$$K = 0.693/4 \text{ h} = 0.173 \text{ h}^{-1}$$

The percentage excreted is

$$(125\,\text{mg}/250\,\text{mg}) \times 100 = 50\%$$

The percentage removed as metabolite 1 is

$$(75\,\text{mg}/250\,\text{mg}) \times 100 = 30\%$$

The percentage removed as metabolite 2 is

$$(50\,\text{mg}/250\,\text{mg}) \times 100 = 20\%$$

The excretion rate constant (K_u) is given by the percentage excreted $\times K$:

$$K_u = 0.173 \times 0.5 = 0.0866\,\text{h}^{-1}$$

The rate constant for metabolite 1 (K_{m1}) is the percentage metabolite 1 removed $\times K$:

$$K_{m1} = 0.173 \times 0.30 = 0.051\,\text{h}^{-1}$$

The rate constant for metabolite 2 (K_{m2}) is the percentage metabolite 2 removed $\times K$:

$$K_{m2} = 0.173 \times 0.2 = 0.0345\,\text{h}^{-1}$$

and

$$K = K_u + K_{m1} + K_{m2}$$

Table 3.2 Plasma concentration profile after a single 600 mg intravenous dose of ampicillin to an adult; data are plotted in Fig. 3.11

Time (h)	Concentration (C_p [μg mL^{-1}])
1.0	37.0
2.0	21.5
3.0	12.5
5.0	4.5

3.6 Plotting drug concentration versus time

A semilogarithmic plot of plasma concentration against time can be used to obtain important pharmacokinetics parameters such as the elimination half life, the elimination rate constant and the apparent volume of drug distribution. Table 3.2 gives a set of such data; Fig. 3.11 shows the data plotted on rectilinear co-ordinates and

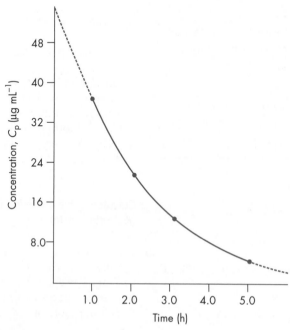

Figure 3.11   Rectilinear plot of data in Table 3.2 for plasma drug concentration (C_p) versus time following administration of the drug by intravenous bolus injection.

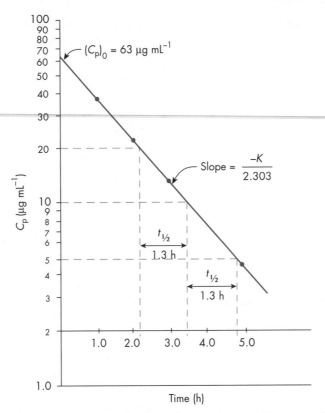

Figure 3.12 Semilogarithmic plot of data in Table 3.2 for plasma drug concentration (C_p) versus time following administration of the drug by intravenous bolus injection. $t_{1/2}$, elimination half life; K, elimination rate constant; $(C_p)_0$, initial plasma concentration.

Fig. 3.12 shows the plot using semilogarithmic co-ordinates.

Determination of the elimination half life and the initial plasma concentration

From the semilogarithmic plot (Fig. 3.12), the elimination half life and the initial plasma concentration can be obtained): 1.3 h and 63 µg mL^{-1}, respectively.

Determination of the apparent volume of distribution

Equation 3.11 gives the relationship of the apparent volume of distribution with dose and plasma concentration:

$$V = \frac{X_0}{(C_p)_0}$$

In the example given in Table 3.2, X_0 is the initial dose of 600 mg (or 600 000 µg) and $(C_p)_0$ was obtained from Fig. 3.12 as 63 µg mL^{-1}. Therefore,

$$V = (600\,000\,\mu g/63\,\mu g\,mL^{-1}) = 9523.8\,mL$$
$$= 9.523\,L$$

Determination of the overall elimination rate constant

Equation 3.12 gives the relationship of the overall elimination rate constant with the half life:

$$K = 0.693/t_{1/2}$$

From the data in Table 3.2, $K = 0.693/1.3\,h = 0.533\,h^{-1}$.

The slope of $\log(C_p)$ against time is $-K/2.303$. So,

$$\text{Slope} = \frac{\log\,(C_p)_2 - \log\,(C_p)_1}{t_2 - t_1}$$

$$\text{Slope} = \frac{\log\,12.5 - \log\,37}{3 - 1\,\text{h}}$$

$$\text{Slope} = \frac{1.0969 - 1.5682}{2.0\,\text{h}}$$

$$\text{Slope} = \frac{-0.4713}{2\,\text{h}} = -0.2357\,\text{h}^{-1}$$

So $(-0.2357\,\text{h}^{-1}) \times 2.303 = -K$.
Then $-K = 0.542\,\text{h}^{-1}$ or $K = 0.542\,\text{h}^{-1}$.

3.7 Intravenous bolus administration of drugs: summary

The following protocol is required.

1. Administer a known dose of a drug.
2. Collect the blood samples for at least $4.32 \times t_{1/2}$ of the drug.
3. Blood samples must also be collected during the early period following the administration of a drug.
4. Plasma or serum samples are analyzed by a suitable method to obtain plasma (C_p) or serum (C_s) concentrations at various times.
5. The plasma (C_p) or serum (C_s) concentration is plotted against time on suitable semilogarithmic paper.
6. From the plot, the various pharmacokinetic parameters [$t_{1/2}$, K or K_u, $(C_p)_0$ and V] can be obtained.

Why collect blood samples up to 4.32 elimination half lives? This is because it always takes $4.32 \times t_{1/2}$ of a drug for 95% of the drug to disappear from the body (blood).

Let us assume that a drug has $t_{1/2} = 1\,\text{h}$. The elimination rate constant K is $0.693/1\,\text{h} = 0.693\,\text{h}^{-1}$. Equation 3.8 is

$$C_p = (C_p)_0 \times e^{-Kt}$$

and $C_p/(C_p)_0 = e^{-Kt}$, which is the fraction drug remaining at time, t.

If $(C_p)_0 = 100\%$ of an intravenous bolus dose and $C_p = 5\%$ of dose. Then

$$\ln \frac{C_p}{(C_p)_0} = -Kt$$

and $\ln\,(5/100) = -(0.693\,\text{h}^{-1} \times t_{5\%})$.
Then

$$\frac{-2.995}{-0.693\,\text{h}^{-1}} = t_{5\%}$$

and

$$4.32\,\text{h} = t_{5\%} = 4.32\,t_{1/2} \qquad (3.14)$$

In this example, since 1 h is equal to one half life ($t_{1/2}$) of the drug, 4.32 h is equal to 4.32 half lives.

Equation 3.8 is applicable when a drug is administered as an intravenous bolus and exhibits the characteristics of a one-compartment model (i.e. rapid distribution) and first-order elimination. This equation may be employed to determine the plasma concentration of drug in the blood at a time provided we know the initial concentration and the elimination half life and/or elimination rate constant (K or K_{el}). This equation also permits the determination of the initial plasma concentration provided we know the concentration value at a time t and the elimination half life and/or elimination rate constant.

Equation 3.8 also permits determination of the elimination rate constant and/or the elimination half life; this, however, will require the knowledge of two plasma concentration values and the corresponding time values. One may also employ this equation to determine the time at which a particular plasma concentration value occurs. This is possible if the initial plasma concentration and the elimination half life and/or rate constant are known.

3.8 Intravenous bolus administration: monitoring drug in urine

The following points should be noted.

1. Urine collection is a non-invasive technique.

SCHEME

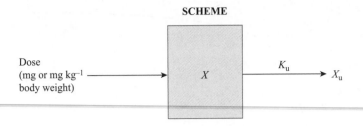

SETUP

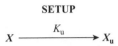

Figure 3.13   Scheme and setup of one-compartment intravenous bolus model eliminated exclusively by urinary excretion. X, mass (amount) of drug in the blood/body at time t; X_u, mass (amount) of unchanged drug in the urine at time t; K_u, first-order excretion rate constant.

2. It is, perhaps, a more convenient method of sample collection, and sample size is generally not a problem. The sampling time, however, reflects drug in urine collected over a period of time, rather than a drug concentration at a discrete time.
3. Urinary data allows direct measurement of bioavailability, both absolute and relative, without the need of fitting the data to a mathematical model.

Figure 3.13 shows a scheme and setup for a one-compartment intravenous bolus model eliminated exclusively by urinary excretion.

The following differential equation describes the setup:

$$\frac{dX_u}{dt} = K_u X \qquad (3.15)$$

Integration of Eq. 3.15 gives:

$$(X_u)_t = X_0(1 - e^{-K_u t}) \qquad (3.16)$$

where X_u is the cumulative mass (amount) of drug excreted into urine at time t; X_0 is the administered dose of drug (e.g. mg); and K_u is the excretion/elimination rate constant (e.g. h^{-1})

If the administered drug is totally removed in the urine in unchanged (unmetabolized) form, then the excretion and elimination processes are synonymous; then, the excretion rate

constant (K_u) equals the elimination rate constant (K). And *only* under this condition, Eq. 3.16 may be written as

$$(X_u)_t = X_0(1 - e^{-Kt}) \qquad (3.17)$$

Equations 3.16 and 3.17 clearly suggest that the cumulative mass of drug excreted and/or eliminated into urine increases asymptotically with time, as illustrated in Fig. 3.14.

Equation 3.16 states:

$$(X_u)_t = X_0(1 - e^{-K_u t})$$

When $t = \infty$; $e^{-K_u t_\infty} = 0$.; therefore,

$$(X_u)_\infty = X_0(1 - 0) \qquad (3.18)$$

or $(X_u)_\infty = X_0 =$ administered dose.

Note that this is applicable when the drug is removed in urine only in the unchanged form (i.e. there is no metabolite in the urine), as is assumed in this situation and illustrated in Fig. 3.15.

At any time, t:

$$(X)_t + (X_u)_t = \text{Dose (or } X_0)$$

where $(X)_t$ is the mass (amount) of drug in the body and $(X_u)_t$ is the cumulative mass of drug in urine.

Another situation applies when the administered dose (X_0) of a drug is not totally

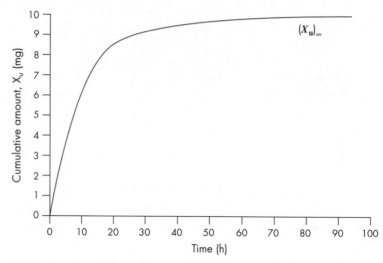

Figure 3.14 A typical plot (rectilinear) of cumulative amount of drug excreted/eliminated in the urine (X_u) against time following the administration of a drug as an intravenous bolus.

removed in the urine in unchanged form: that is, $(X_u)_\infty$ is not equal to the dose administered, which is to say that the excretion rate constant (K_u) is not equal to the elimination rate constant (K) and metabolite of drug is present in the urine (Fig. 3.16).

In this case, at any time t:

$$(X)_t + (X_u)_t + (X_m)_t + (X_{mu})_t = \text{Dose (or } X_0)$$

where $(X)_t$ the mass (amount) of drug in the body; $(X_u)_t$ is the mass of unchanged or excreted drug in urine; $(X_m)_t$ is the mass or amount of metabolite in the body; and $(X_{mu})_t$ is the mass or amount of metabolite in the urine.

Of course, for correct mass balance, the mass of metabolite may need to be adjusted for any difference in molecular weight from that of the parent drug.

3.9 Use of urinary excretion data

There are two methods that permit us to compute some pharmacokinetic parameters from urinary excretion data.

- the "amount remaining to be excreted" method (ARE); also known as the sigma-minus method
- the rate of excretion method.

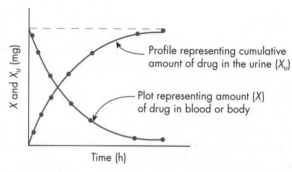

Figure 3.15 Rectilinear plot illustrating the amount of drug remaining in the blood and the amount of drug eliminated in the urine with time following the administration of a drug as an intravenous bolus.

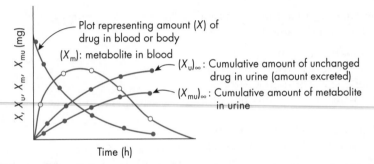

Figure 3.16   Rectilinear plot illustrating the amount of drug and of metabolite remaining in the blood, and the amount of unmetabolized drug and metabolite eliminated in the urine over time following the administration of a drug as an intravenous bolus: the mass of drug in the body (X), plus the mass of unchanged or excreted drug in urine (X_u), equals the dose, $(X)_0$.

The "amount remaining to be excreted" or sigma minus method: theoretical considerations

We know from earlier discussion (Eqs 3.16 and 3.18) that Eq. 3.16

$$(X_u)_t = X_0(1 - e^{-K_u t})$$

or

$$(X_u)_t = X_0 - X_0(e^{-K_u t})$$

and when $t = \infty$

$$(X_u)_\infty = X_0 = \text{Dose} \qquad (3.19)$$

Subtraction of Eq. 3.16 from Eq. 3.19 yields Eq. 3.20

$$(X_u)_\infty = X_0$$
$$(X_u)_t = X_0 - X_0 e^{-K_u t}$$
$$(X_u)_\infty - (X_u)_t = X_0 e^{-K_u t} \qquad (3.20)$$

where $[(X_u)_\infty - (X_u)_t]$ is the amount of drug remaining to be excreted, which is X, the amount of drug in the body at time t.

A plot of $[(X_u)_\infty - (X_u)_t]$ (i.e. the amount of drug remaining to be excreted, which also equals the amount of drug remaining in the blood) against time (Eq. 3.20) should provide a straight line on semilogarithmic paper, as illustrated in Fig. 3.17.

In Fig. 3.17, note that the intercept of the graph represents $(X_u)_\infty$, which equals administered dose because of the assumption made that the drug is being completely removed in unchanged form. The slope of the graph permits the determination of the excretion rate constant,

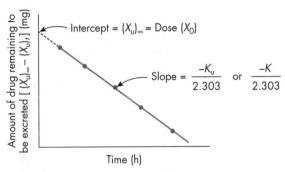

Figure 3.17   A semilogarithmic plot of amount of drug remaining to be excreted against time following the administration of a drug as an intravenous bolus (Equation 3.20). K_u, first-order renal excretion rate constant; K, elimination rate constant.

which is congruent (i.e. equal) to the elimination rate constant because of the assumption made.

1. Obtain the elimination half life ($t_{1/2}$) and the elimination rate constant K (which in this case equals the excretion rate constant K_u) from the graph by employing the methods described previously.
2. Please note that one cannot obtain the apparent volume of distribution (V) from urinary excretion data.
3. Also note that on the semilogarithmic plot shown above, the intercept is $(X_u)_\infty$ or (X_0). This is true only when there is an absence of metabolite(s), as in this case. The slope of the graph permits the determination of the excretion rate constant (K_u), which, in this example, is also equal to the elimination rate constant (K).

Limitations of the "amount remaining to be excreted" (ARE) method

1. Urine samples must be collected until such time that, practically, no additional drug appears in the urine (i.e. $t = 7t_{1/2}$)
2. No urine samples can be lost, or urine from any samples used in the determination of X_u (the exact volume of urine at each time interval must be known)
3. This is a time-consuming method for a drug with a long elimination half life ($t_{1/2}$)
4. There is a cumulative build up of error.

When the administered dose of a drug is not completely removed in unchanged form

Figure 3.18 shows the condition when the administered dose of a drug is not completely removed in unchanged form (i.e. $K \neq K_u$ and $(X_u)_\infty \neq (X_0)$.

$$K = K_u + K_m$$

Equation 3.15 gives:

$$\frac{dX_u}{dt} = K_u X$$

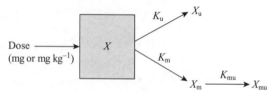

Figure 3.18 Scheme of one-compartment intravenous bolus model of drug eliminated by both urinary excretion and metabolism. X, mass (amount) of drug in the blood/body at time, t; X_u, mass of unchanged drug in the urine at time t; X_m, mass of metabolite in the blood/body at time t; X_{mu}, mass of metabolite in the urine at time t; K_u, first-order renal excretion rate constant (time^{-1}); K_m, first-order metabolite formation rate constant (time^{-1}); K_{mu}, first-order metabolite excretion rate constant (time^{-1}).

Using Laplace transform techniques, this equation can be integrated as:

$$(X_u)_t = \frac{K_u X_0}{K}(1 - e^{-Kt}) \qquad (3.21)$$

where, X_0 is the administered dose (e.g. mg); K is the elimination rate constant (e.g. h^{-1}); K_u is the excretion rate constant (e.g. h^{-1}); and $(X_u)_t$ is the cumulative amount (e.g. mg) of drug excreted in the urine at time t.

Equation 3.21 permits the determination of the cumulative amount of drug excreted in the urine at a specific time. When $t = \infty$, $(X_u) = (X_u)_\infty$ and e^{-Kt} progresses to 0; therefore, Eq. 3.21 reduces to:

$$(X_u)_\infty = \frac{K_u X_0}{K} \qquad (3.22)$$

Substituting $(X_u)_\infty$ for the term $(K_u X_0)/K$ in Eq. 3.21 gives

$$(X_u)t = (X_u)_\infty(1 - e^{-Kt})$$

$$(X_u)_t = (X_u)_\infty - (X_u)_\infty e^{-Kt}$$

$$(X_u)_\infty - (X_u)_t = (X_u)_\infty e^{-Kt} \qquad (3.23)$$

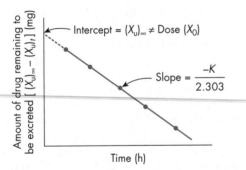

Figure 3.19 A semilogarithmic plot of amount of drug remaining to be excreted against time following the administration of a drug as an intravenous bolus (Equation 3.23). K, elimination constant.

Taking the logarithmic form of the equation yields

$$\log\left[(X_{u})_{\infty} - (X_{u})_{t}\right] = \log(X_{u})_{\infty} - \frac{Kt}{2.303}$$

(3.24)

A plot of $[(X_{u})_{\infty} - (X_{u})_{t}]$, that is the amount of drug remain to be excreted or amount of drug remaining in the blood, against time (Eq. 3.23) on semilogarithmic co-ordinates should provide a straight line. The slope of the line permits the determination of the elimination rate constant (K) and the intercept represents the cumulative amount of drug excreted in the urine at time

infinity, $(X_{u})_{\infty}$, which in this case is not equal to the administered dose. Figure 3.19 represents the semilogarithmic plot of $[(X_{u})_{\infty} - (X_{u})_{t}]$ against time for Eq. 3.23. It also represents the rectilinear plot of Eq. 3.24.

Example of pharmacokinetic analysis of urinary excretion data

An intravenous bolus dose of 80.0 mg of a drug was administered. The drug is one that is eliminated entirely by urinary excretion of unchanged drug following one-compartment model distribution and first-order elimination.

Assumptions:

- one-compartment open model with the entire dose eliminated as unchanged drug
- first-order process and passive diffusion
- intravenous bolus dose (80 mg); in other words, $K = K_{u}$, and $(X_{u})_{\infty} =$ dose administered.

Table 3.3 provides the urinary data in a tabulated form.

The information necessary for the urinary analysis, employing either ARE or rate of excretion method, is presented in nine columns in the table.

Column 1 represents the time interval (h) at which urine samples were collected.
Column 2 represents the volume (mL) of urine samples collected at each time interval.

Table 3.3 Information required for the urinary analysis of an intravenous bolus dose of 80.0 mg of drug in the text example

Time interval of urine collection (h)	Volume urine collected (mL)	Drug concentration in urine (mg mL^{-1})	Mass drug in urine (X_u [mg])	Cumulative mass drug excreted (X_u [mg])	Time (t [h])	ARE (mg)	Average time ($\bar{t}$ [h])	$\left(\dfrac{\Delta X_u}{\Delta t}\right)\bar{t}$
0–1	200	0.200	40.0	40.00	1.00	40.00	0.5	40
1–2	50	0.400	20.0	60.00	2.00	20.00	1.5	20
2–3	50	0.200	10.0	70.00	3.00	10.00	2.5	10
3–4	100	0.050	5.0	75.00	4.00	5.00	3.5	5
4–5	25	0.100	2.5	77.50	5.00	2.50	4.5	2.5
5–6	125	0.010	1.25	78.75	6.00	1.25	5.5	1.25
6–12	250	0.005	1.25	80.0^a	12.0	0.00	9.0	0.21

ARE, amount remaining to be excreted.
^{a} This equals the bolus dose administered: $(X_u)_{\infty} = X_0$.

Column 3 provides the drug concentration ($\mathrm{mg\,mL^{-1}}$) in the urine collected at each time interval.

Column 4 provides the amount (mg) of drug excreted/eliminated in the urine at each time interval. This is obtained by multiplication of the numbers in column 2 and 3 for each time interval.

Column 5 provides the values of the cumulative amount (mg) of drug excreted at each time interval. This is computed by simply adding the amount of drug excreted at each time interval.

Column 6 provides time (h) values to be used when the ARE method is employed to determine the pharmacokinetic parameters.

Column 7 provides the values for the amount (mg) of drug remaining to be excreted (i.e. ARE or $[(X_u)_\infty - (X_u)_t]$) at each time interval. These values are obtained by subtracting the cumulative amount (mg) of drug excreted at each time interval (numbers reported in column 5) from the value of the cumulative amount of drug in the urine at time infinity (80 mg at 12 h or, in this example, the dose administered). It is important to note that the cumulative amount of drug (mg) excreted in urine (i.e. values reported in column 5)

increases asymptotically with time (Figs 3.14 and 3.20). The amount (mg) of drug remaining to be excreted in the urine (i.e. the ARE values reported in column 7), however, decreases with time (Fig. 3.21).

Column 8 provides the values for the average time (h) intervals for the urine samples collection

Column 9 provides the values of the rate of excretion (dX_u/dt; $\mathrm{mg\,h^{-1}}$) of drug corresponding to the average time (h) interval reported in column 8. Calculations of the rate of excretion values, reported in column 9, are presented in Table 3.3.

ARE method calculations

The data reported in column 7 (i.e. ARE or $[(X_u)_\infty - (X_u)_t]$) is plotted against time (data in column 6 of the table) on semilogarithmic paper (Fig. 3.21). The slope of the graph should permit the determination of the elimination rate constant; and the intercept on the y-axis represents the value for $(X_u)_\infty$, which, in this example, is equal to the administered dose. Note that, since the drug is assumed to be totally removed in an unchanged form, the elimination rate constant is equal to the excretion rate constant, and the cumulative amount of drug excreted in the urine at time infinity, $(X_u)_\infty$, is equal to the administered dose.

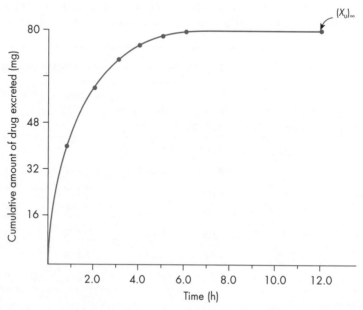

Figure 3.20 Rectilinear plot of cumulative amount of drug excreted in the urine (X_u) versus time for data given in columns 5 and 6 of Table 3.3.

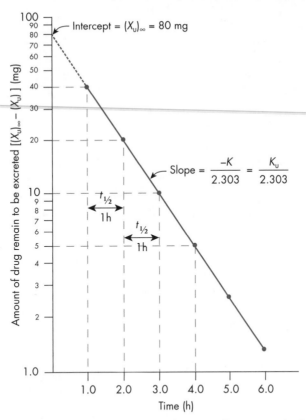

Figure 3.21   Semilogarithmic plot of amount of drug remaining to be excreted (X_u) (ARE method) versus time for data given in columns 6 and 7 of Table 3.3. K, elimination rate constant; $t_{1/2}$, elimination half life.

Rate of excretion method: drug exclusively removed in unchanged form by renal excretion

Theory: we know from an earlier differential equation (Eq. 3.15)

$$\frac{dX_u}{dt} = K_u X$$

Equation 3.3 gives $X = X_0 e^{-Kt}$. For $K = K_u$, this yields

$$X = X_0\, e^{-K_u t}$$

Therefore, substituting X from the above equation into Eq. 3.15 gives:

$$\frac{dX_u}{dt} = K_u X_0 e^{-K_u t} \tag{3.25}$$

In practice, Eq. 3.25 becomes

$$\frac{(dX_u)_{\bar{t}}}{dt} = K_u X_0 e^{-K_u \bar{t}} \tag{3.26}$$

where $\frac{(dX_u)_{\bar{t}}}{dt}$ is the average rate of excretion (e.g. $mg\,h^{-1}$); $\bar{t}$ is the average time between urine collection; K_u is the excretion rate constant (e.g. h^{-1}); and X_0 is the dose (e.g. mg).

Both Eqs 3.25 and 3.26 suggest that the rate of excretion of a drug declines mono-exponentially with time, as shown in Fig. 3.22.

Determine the elimination half life $(t_{1/2})$ and elimination/excretion rate constant (K_u) from semilogarithmic plot of the rate of excretion versus average time $\bar{t}$.

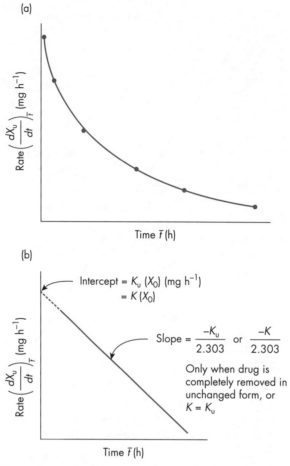

(a)

(b)

Intercept = $K_u (X_0)$ (mg h^{-1})
= $K (X_0)$

Slope = $\dfrac{-K_u}{2.303}$ or $\dfrac{-K}{2.303}$

Only when drug is completely removed in unchanged form, or $K = K_u$

Figure 3.22 A typical rectilinear (a) or semilogarithmic (b) plot of rate of excretion against average time ($\bar{t}$) following the administration of a drug as an intravenous bolus (Equations 3.25). K_u, first-order renal excretion rate constant; X_0, drug at time zero; K, elimination rate constant.

Computation of rate of excretion

The rate of excretion and the average time values reported in columns 9 and 8, respectively, of Table 3.3 are computed as follows.

first sample:

$$\frac{(dX_u)_{\bar{t}}}{dt} = \frac{(X_u)_1 - (X_u)_0}{t_1 - t_0} = \frac{40\,\text{mg} - 0\,\text{mg}}{1\,\text{h} - 0\,\text{h}}$$

$$= 40\,\text{mg h}^{-1}$$

$$\text{average time}\,\bar{t} = \frac{1\text{h} + 0}{2} = 0.5\,\text{h}$$

second sample:

$$\frac{(dX_u)_{\bar{t}}}{dt} = \frac{(X_u)_2 - (X_u)_1}{t_2 - t_1} = \frac{60\,\text{mg} - 40\,\text{mg}}{2\,\text{h} - 1\,\text{h}}$$

$$= 20\,\text{mg h}^{-1}$$

$$\text{average time}\,\bar{t} = \frac{2\text{h} + 1\text{h}}{2} = 1.5\text{h}$$

third sample:

$$\frac{(dX_u)_{\bar{t}}}{dt} = \frac{(X_u)_3 - (X_u)_2}{t_3 - t_2} = \frac{70\,\text{mg} - 60\,\text{mg}}{3\,\text{h} - 2\,\text{h}}$$

$$= 10\,\text{mg h}^{-1}$$

$$\text{average time } \bar{t} = \frac{3\,\text{h} + 2\,\text{h}}{2} = 2.5\,\text{h}$$

last sample:

$$\frac{(dX_u)_{\bar{t}}}{dt} = \frac{(X_u)_{12} - (X_u)_6}{t_{12} - t_6} = \frac{80\,\text{mg} - 78.75\,\text{mg}}{12\,\text{h} - 6\,\text{h}}$$

$$= 0.208\,\text{mg h}^{-1}$$

$$\text{average time } \bar{t} = \frac{12\,\text{h} + 6\,\text{h}}{2} = 9.0\,\text{h}$$

Calculation of excretion rate constant

The data reported in column 9 (i.e. dX_u/dt; mg h^{-1}) of Table 3.3 is plotted against the average time (data in column 8 of the table) on semilogarithmic paper (Fig. 3.23). The slope of the graph should permit the determination of the elimination or excretion rate constant; and the y-axis intercept represents the initial rate of excretion value which, in this example, is equal to the initial rate of elimination. Please note that the drug is assumed to be totally removed in an unchanged form. Consequently, the elimination rate constant is equal to the excretion rate constant, and the intravenous bolus dose equals the cumulative amount of drug excreted in the urine at time infinity [i.e. $(X_u)_\infty$].

The *elimination half life* ($t_{1/2}$) is 1 h (from the plot of rate of excretion versus time in Fig. 3.23).

The *elimination/excretion rate constant* K_u is $0.693/t_{1/2} = 0.693/1\,\text{h} = 0.693\,\text{h}^{-1}$.

At the intercept on the y-axis, $K_u(X_0) = 56\,\text{mg h}^{-1}$.

Intercept$/K_u = X_0$ (the administered dose). So

$$56\,\text{mg h}^{-1}/0.693\,\text{h}^{-1}$$
$$= X_0(\text{the administered dose})$$
$$80.8\,\text{mg} = X_0 = \text{Dose(slight overestimate because of the averaging technique)}.$$

Intercept$/X_u = K_u$. So

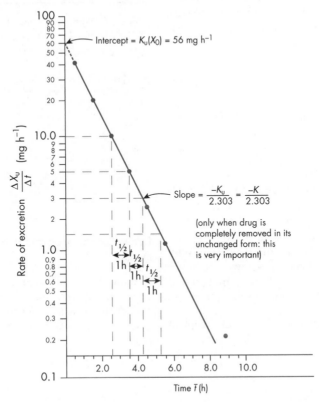

Figure 3.23 Semilogarithmic plot of rate of excretion versus average time ($\bar{t}$). DX_u/Dt represents the mass of drug excreted in urine over a small time period.

$56 \, \text{mg h}^{-1}/80 \, \text{mg} = 0.70 \, \text{h}^{-1} = K_\text{u}.$
Intercept $= K_\text{u} X_0$
Intercept $= 0.693 \, \text{h}^{-1} \times 80 \, \text{mg}$
Intercept $= 55.44 \, \text{mg h}^{-1}.$

Rate of excretion method: drug not exclusively removed in unchanged form by renal excretion

When the administered dose of a drug is not exclusively removed in an unchanged form (i.e. $K \neq K_\text{u}$; $(X_\text{u})_\infty \neq X_0$; and both unchanged drug and metabolite are present in the urine), Eq. 3.15 gives:

$$\frac{dX_\text{u}}{dt} = K_\text{u} X$$

where dX_u/dt is the the rate of excretion (mg h^{-1}); X is the mass (amount) of drug in the body (mg); and K_u is the excretion rate constant (h^{-1}).

However, according to Eq. 3.3, $X = X_0 e^{-kt}$ (when drug is monitored in the blood). Substitute X from Eq. 3.3 for the term X in the rate equation (Eq. 3.15), gives:

$$\frac{dX_\text{u}}{dt} = K_\text{u} X_0 e^{-Kt} \qquad (3.27)$$

The logarithmic form of the equation becomes:

$$\log \frac{dX_\text{u}}{dt} = \log (K_\text{u} X_0) - \frac{Kt}{2.303} \qquad (3.28)$$

If the rate of excretion is plotted (Fig. 3.24) against the average time, on semilogarithmic paper, the slope will permit the determination of the elimination rate constant (K); and the intercept will represent the initial rate of excretion. Please note that from the knowledge of the intercept value (mg h^{-1}) and the administered dose (mg), one can determine the excretion rate constant (K_u).

Please note the difference in the intercept of Figs 3.21 and 3.24.

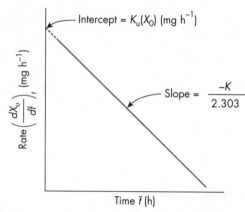

Figure 3.24 A typical semilogarithmic plot of rate of excretion against average time ($\bar{t}$) when the administered intravenous bolus dose of a drug is not totally removed in an unchanged form following administration. $dX_\text{u}/d\bar{t}$ represents the mass of drug excreted in urine over a small time period.

Table 3.4 The more frequent the urine sample collection, the smaller is the error involved in estimating pharmacokinetic parameters

No. half lives	Overestimate (%)
3.00	190.0
2.00	80.00
1.00	20.00
0.50	6.00
0.25	0.03

General comment on rate of excretion method

The method tends to give overestimate of intercept. The overestimation can be minimized by collecting urine samples more frequently (which is not always easy from practical consideration) (Table 3.4).

4

Clearance concepts

Objectives

Upon completion of this chapter, you will have the ability to:

- define the concept of drug *clearance* and distinguish it from the elimination rate and the elimination rate constant
- define the term *extraction ratio* and explain how this parameter is related to clearance
- explain the term *intrinsic clearance*
- explain the dependence of elimination half life on apparent volume of distribution and clearance
- calculate area under the plasma drug concentration versus time curve by use of the trapezoidal rule and by other methods
- calculate a patient's creatinine clearance using the appropriate equation
- calculate dosing adjustments of a renally excreted drug in patients with various degrees of renal impairment (dysfunction).

4.1 Introduction

Clearance is a parameter that has, perhaps, the greatest potential of any pharmacokinetic parameter for clinical applications. Furthermore, it is the most useful parameter available for the evaluation of the elimination mechanism and of the eliminating organs (kidney and liver). The utility of the clearance measurement lies in its intrinsic model independence.

Drugs are eliminated from the body by metabolism and excretion. The liver is the major site of drug metabolism; however, other tissues also contain drug-metabolizing enzymes and, therefore, contribute to the biotransformation of selected drugs. The kidneys are involved in the elimination of many drugs and virtually all drug metabolites.

Some drugs, such as gentamicin and cephalexin (cefalexin), are eliminated from the body almost solely by renal excretion. Many drugs are eliminated in part by the kidneys and even when drug elimination from the body involves biotransformation, the corresponding drug metabolites are usually cleared by the kidneys. Therefore, kidneys play an important role in removal of unchanged drug and/or the metabolites from the body. Some drugs are excreted in the bile and may be eliminated in the feces.

The concept of clearance was developed by renal physiologists in the early 1930s as an empiric measure of kidney function. The pharmacokinetic basis of the term was defined at about the same time, with the recognition that the concept could be more generally applied to other organs and elimination pathways.

This chapter will describe some aspects of the current understanding and applications of clearance with emphasis placed upon the renal excretion of drugs.

Renal physiology

Renal excretion of drugs is a complex phenomenon involving one or more of the following processes:

- glomerular filtration
- active tubular secretion
- passive reabsorption.

These processes occur in the nephron of the kidney (Fig. 4.1).

Depending upon which one of these processes is dominant, renal clearance can be an important, or a negligible, component of drug elimination.

The kidneys receive approximately 25% of the cardiac output, or 1.2–1.5 L of blood per minute.

Approximately 10% of this volume (i.e. 120–150 mL) is removed every minute as it passes through the glomeruli of the kidneys. The types of solute present in this filtrate are normally limited by the size of the solute molecule; however, the pores of the glomerular capillaries are sufficiently large to permit the passage of most drug molecules. In addition, since the glomeruli effectively restrict the passage of blood cells and plasma proteins, only free drug (i.e. drug that is not bound to plasma proteins) can be filtered.

In addition to glomerular filtration, certain drugs can also be secreted into kidney tubules. This secretion process is normally considered to be active and, consequently, involves the movement of drug molecules against a concentration gradient. Active secretion is believed to occur primarily in the proximal tubules of the kidney and does not appear to be influenced by plasma protein binding.

The total amount of drug removed from the blood by either glomerular filtration or active

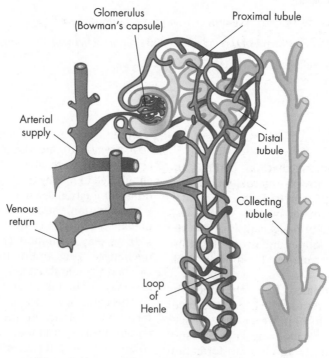

Figure 4.1   The structure of the kidney nephron, where drugs are removed from the blood. From, Smith HW (1951), "The Functional Nephron," Plate I (opp. p. 8), in: *The Kidney: Structure and Function in Health and Disease,* Oxford: University Press. Used with permission.

secretion will, if the drug is highly polar, pass through the loop of Henle and distal tubules into the collecting ducts, which empty into bladder, and eventually be eliminated from the body in the urine. Because of the enormous capacity of the kidneys to reabsorb water from the lumen of these tubules (only about 1–2 mL of the 125 mL of the filtrate reaches the bladder), there is a gradual concentration of the drug filtrate as it passes through the tubules. Hence, a concentration gradient develops that will increase drug concentration the further down the tubules that the solute passes, and this will favor the reabsorption of drug molecules from the luminal fluid into the blood.

Although reabsorption by simple diffusion is theoretically possible for all drugs, it is most significant for non-polar drugs. Therefore, the reabsorption of weakly acidic and basic drugs may be highly dependent on urine pH, since the relative amounts of the ionized and non-ionized form of drug would vary significantly with changes in the urine pH. Consequently, it is important, when studying the pharmacokinetics of weak acids and bases to consider the pH of urine. An additional factor that may influence the extent of reabsorption of a drug from the distal tubule is the urine flow rate. To date, however, insufficient studies have been conducted to evaluate the possible influence of this factor on the renal drug elimination.

It is, therefore, clear that a drug eliminated in urine may undergo one, all or any combination of the processes of glomerular filtration, tubular secretion or reabsorption. However, these mechanisms usually produce the net effect of removing a constant fraction of a drug presented to the kidneys through renal arterial blood.

4.2 Clearance definitions

The most general definition of clearance is that it is "a proportionality constant describing the relationship between a substance's rate of elimination (amount per unit time) at a given time and its corresponding concentration in an appropriate fluid at that time."

Clearance can also be defined as "the hypothetical volume of blood (plasma or serum) or other biological fluids from which the drug is totally and irreversibly removed per unit time."

The abbreviation "Cl" is used for clearance in mathematical manipulations.

The larger the hypothetical value, the more efficient is the eliminating organ (kidney and liver). One limiting factor is the volume of the blood that is presented to the eliminating organ per unit time. For kidney, the upper limit of blood flow is $19 \, mL \, min^{-1} \, kg^{-1}$. For liver, the upper limit of blood flow is approximately $1.5 \, L \, min^{-1}$.

Another limiting factor is the extraction ratio of the organ for the drug being eliminated.

There are a number of subsets to clearance.

- *Systemic (Cl_s) or total body clearance (TBC)*. This is the sum of all individual organ clearances that contribute to the overall elimination of drugs. However, the organ clearance that can be routinely determined independently in humans is renal clearance because this is the only organ for which we can easily determine an elimination rate. The process of drug removal is called elimination, which may include both excretion and metabolism for a particular drug.
- *Renal clearance, (Cl_r)*. The clearance of drug (a fraction of total clearance) for a drug that is removed from the blood (plasma/serum) by the process of renal excretion.
- *Metabolic clearance, (Cl_m)*. The clearance of drug (a fraction of total clearance) for a drug that is removed from the blood (plasma/serum) by the process of metabolism, from whatever metabolic organ.
- *Hepatic clearance, (Cl_H)*. The clearance of drug (a fraction of total clearance) for a drug that is removed from the blood (plasma/serum) by the process of hepatic metabolism; the liver is the organ responsible for most metabolism of drugs.

It can be shown that the total body clearance, or systemic clearance, of a drug is the summation of all the organ clearances. Hence, systemic clearance is often partitioned into renal (Cl_r) and non-renal (Cl_{nr}) clearance.

$$Cl_s = Cl_{nr} + Cl_r \qquad (4.1)$$

Although there may be many sites of drug elimination besides kidney and liver, these two organs are quantitatively the most important and, therefore, have been most thoroughly studied. Nonrenal clearance for many drugs may be considered to be equivalent to hepatic clearance.

The unit for all clearances is a unit of volume per unit time: $mL\,min^{-1}$ or $L\,h^{-1}$. This can also be given on a body weight basis ($mL\,min^{-1}\,kg^{-1}$ or $L\,h^{-1}\,kg^{-1}$) or a body surface area basis ($mL\,min^{-1}/1.73\,m^2$).

4.3 Clearance: rate and concentration

In the same way that the parameter V, the apparent volume of distribution, is necessary in order to relate plasma or serum concentration (C_p or C_s) to mass of drug in the body at a given time (X), there is also a need to have a parameter that relates the plasma or serum concentration (C_p or C_s) to the rate of drug excretion ($dX_u dt$) or of elimination ($-dX/dt$) at any given time. Systemic clearance (Cl_s), or more simply clearance (Cl), is this proportionality constant.

Rate of renal excretion = Renal clearance
$$\times \text{ Plasma (or serum)}$$
$$\text{concentration}$$

or

$$\left(\frac{dX_u}{dt}\right)_t = (Cl_r)(C_p)_t$$
$$= (mL\,h^{-1})(\mu g\,mL^{-1})$$
$$= \mu g\,h^{-1} \qquad (4.2)$$

Rearrangement of Eq. 4.2 yields:

$$Cl_r = \frac{\left(\frac{dX_u}{dt}\right)_t}{(C_p)_t} = \frac{\mu g\,h^{-1}}{\mu g\,mL^{-1}} = mL\,h^{-1} \qquad (4.3)$$

Rate of elimination = Systemic clearance
$$\times \text{ Plasma (or serum)}$$
$$\text{concentration}$$

or

$$\left(\frac{-dX}{dt}\right)_t = Cl(C_p)_t \qquad (4.4)$$

where X is mass of drug in the body at time t.

Rearrangement of Eq. 4.4 yields:

$$Cl = \frac{\left(\frac{-dX}{dt}\right)_t}{(C_p)_t} = \frac{\mu g\,h^{-1}}{\mu g\,mL^{-1}} = mL\,h^{-1} \qquad (4.5)$$

For example, if the rate of elimination and average plasma concentration are $1\,mg\,h^{-1}$ and $1\,mg\,L^{-1}$, respectively; then

$$Cl = 1\,mg\,h^{-1}/1\,mg\,L^{-1} = 1\,L\,h^{-1}.$$

When elimination is exclusively by the renal excretion of unchanged (parent) drug, $Cl = Cl_r$, and Equations 4.3 and 4.5 may be used interchangeably.

Another equation for systemic clearance is:

$$Cl = KV \qquad (4.6)$$

The mathematically equivalent expression $K = Cl/V$ is often used in order to emphasize that, when various physiological factors change, clearance and volume of distribution may vary independently of each other, and that K is more correctly viewed as being dependent upon the values of Cl and V.

For a given rate of excretion, the type of clearance depends upon the site of drug measurement (blood, plasma, serum).

Generally, when a first-order process and passive diffusion are applicable, as the concentration of drug in the body (serum, plasma) increases, so does its rate of elimination; clearance, however, remains independent of the dose administered.

4.4 Clearance: tank and faucet analogy

Figure 4.2 is an attempt to clarify the concept of drug clearance by means of a simple model of a tank filled with drug solution. On the left half of the figure (labeled "At first"), the initial conditions (at $t = t_1$) are shown: drug solution is at concentration C_{p1} (drawn dark). The right-hand side of the figure shows conditions after Δt time units have elapsed ("Some time later"). At this time,

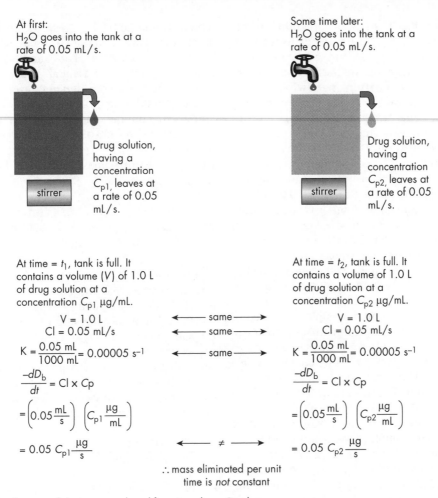

At first:
H$_2$O goes into the tank at a
rate of 0.05 mL/s.

Some time later:
H$_2$O goes into the tank at a
rate of 0.05 mL/s.

stirrer

Drug solution,
having a
concentration
C_{p1}, leaves at
a rate of 0.05
mL/s.

stirrer

Drug solution,
having a
concentration
C_{p2}, leaves at
a rate of 0.05
mL/s.

At time = t_1, tank is full. It
contains a volume (V) of 1.0 L
of drug solution at a
concentration C_{p1} µg/mL.

$$V = 1.0\ L$$
$$Cl = 0.05\ mL/s$$
$$K = \frac{0.05\ mL}{1000\ mL} = 0.00005\ s^{-1}$$
$$\frac{-dD_b}{dt} = Cl \times Cp$$
$$= \left(0.05\,\frac{mL}{s}\right)\left(C_{p1}\,\frac{\mu g}{mL}\right)$$
$$= 0.05\ C_{p1}\,\frac{\mu g}{s}$$

←——— same ———→
←——— same ———→
←——— same ———→

At time = t_2, tank is full. It
contains a volume of 1.0 L
of drug solution at a
concentration C_{p2} µg/mL.

$$V = 1.0\ L$$
$$Cl = 0.05\ mL/s$$
$$K = \frac{0.05\ mL}{1000\ mL} = 0.00005\ s^{-1}$$
$$\frac{-dD_b}{dt} = Cl \times Cp$$
$$= \left(0.05\,\frac{mL}{s}\right)\left(C_{p2}\,\frac{\mu g}{mL}\right)$$
$$= 0.05\ C_{p2}\,\frac{\mu g}{s}$$

←——— $\neq$ ———→

∴ mass eliminated per unit
time is *not* constant

Figure 4.2   Concept of clearance: tank and faucet analogy. D_b, drug mass.

drug concentration (C_{p2}) has been considerably diluted and is drawn visibly lighter.

Looking on both sides, we observe that each tank has a stirrer underneath. This happens to be a very efficient stirrer, causing immediate mixing of the contents of the tank. This will become significant for showing the first-order elimination required for our clearance model. Also, each side has a leaky faucet, delivering pure water to the tank at a rate of 1 USP drop (0.05 mL) every second. The other thing we notice in the picture is that each tank is full. The sequence of events is that a drop of water goes into a tank, this water is immediately

mixed with the contents of the tank, and then one drop of (slightly diluted) drug solution is displaced from the tank and thus removed.

Many repetitions of this sequence have occurred in order to go from the situation shown on the left side of the figure to the situation on the right side, which shows a tank with a visibly dilute solution of drug.

The volume of the tank is constant (1 L). Since the tank is always full of drug solution, the volume of drug solution is always 1 L as well. It is not too large a conceptual jump to see how this volume is a model for the volume of distribution (V) for an actual drug-dosing situation.

Let us consider 1 s to be a nearly infinitesimal length of time. Let us also attempt to see what happens in the very first second in our tank model of clearance. Remember, we start at drug concentration C_{p1}. One way of thinking of what happens during the first second is that 0.05 mL of drug solution (at concentration C_{p1}) is replaced with 0.05 mL of water (having zero concentration of drug). In other words, 0.05 mL of drug solution at concentration C_{p1} is completely cleared of drug. This is where the word "clearance" comes from. In this example the clearance is 0.05 mL s^{-1}. A constant volume of 0.05 mL is cleared of drug every second, from the first second to the last second. The trick is that the concentration of drug is not constant; the drug concentration after 1 s has passed is less than it was before the second has passed. Drug concentration is decreasing over time (and doing so in an exponential fashion).

Knowing that 0.05 mL is completely cleared of drug every second, and knowing that the total volume of the tank is 1 L, we might be tempted to calculate that the tank would be completely free of drug in 20 000 s. This would not be correct. In fact, it would only be correct if the 0.05 mL of drug solution cleared each second always had concentration C_{p1}. The continuous mixing of the drug solution in our example prevents this possibility.

(If, however, we froze the drug solution when it was at concentration C_{p1} and then chipped away a 0.05 mL volume of this ice, containing drug at concentration C_{p1}, every second, we would, in fact, get rid of all the drug in 20 000 s. This would be a zero-order situation.)

But, getting back to our first-order situation as depicted in the figure, it would take until time infinity to get rid of 100% of the drug in our tank. This first-order situation is common for the elimination of many drugs in therapeutic concentrations. This is the kinetics that occurs when the elimination rate is driven by the amount of drug present.

Now, what other analogies to real kinetics can we find in our tank model? If we agree that 1 s is a nearly infinitesimal slice of time, we can closely estimate the amount of drug eliminated over the time interval from our initial time t_1 to t_1 plus 1 s. A volume of 0.05 mL (that is, 0.00005 L) times the initial concentration C_{p1} (mg L^{-1}) yields a mass of drug eliminated over the first second equal to $0.00005 \times C_{p1}$ (mg),

which is equal to $0.05 \times C_{p1} \, \mu g$. Thus, the initial elimination rate equals $0.05 \times C_{p1} \, \mu g \, s^{-1}$. This would not be constant. For example, at t_2, the elimination rate would equal $0.05 \times C_{p2} \, \mu g \, s^{-1}$, which would be a considerably lower rate.

There is still one more analogy to pharmacokinetics that our tank model affords. It was stated above that a mass of $0.05 \times C_{p1} \, \mu g$ of drug is eliminated over the first second. This can be compared with D_1, the entire mass of drug in the tank at time t_1. Now:

$$D_1(\mu g) = C_{p1}(\mu g \, mL^{-1}) \times V(mL)$$
$$D_1(\mu g) = C_{p1}(\mu g \, mL^{-1}) \times 1000(mL)$$
$$= 1000 \times C_{p1}(\mu g)$$

Therefore, at t_1 the fraction of all the drug initially present that will be eliminated over 1 s is $(0.05 \times C_{p1} \, \mu g)/(1000 \times C_{p1} \, \mu g)$, which is 0.00005. A similar calculation for time t_2 gives the same value for this fraction. Since t_2 is an appreciable time later than t_1, we can conclude that this fraction is constant over time. It turns out that 0.00005 s^{-1} is the value of the first-order elimination rate constant, K, for this problem. This can be confirmed by dividing clearance by V:

$$\frac{Cl}{V} = \frac{0.05 \, mL \, s^{-1}}{1000 \, mL} = 0.00005 \, s^{-1}$$

For small time slices, $K \times dt$ is a good approximation of the fraction of total drug in the body eliminated over that time period. (In our example, this equals $(0.00005 \, s^{-1}) \times (1 \, s) = 0.00005$.) Of course, for longer slices of time, we run up against the fact that the mass of drug in the body is changing over this time period, and $K \times dt$ is no longer a good estimate of fraction drug eliminated. However, the real use of K is in our equations containing the term e^{-Kt}. An equation that always is an exact estimate of the fraction of drug eliminated over time (even over long time periods) is:

$$1 - e^{-Kt}$$

4.5 Organ clearance

Consider the situation outlined in Fig. 4.3. Following the administration of a drug, there is

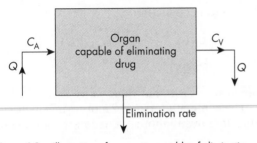

Figure 4.3 Illustration of an organ capable of eliminating a drug from the body. Q, blood flow through the organ; C_A, drug concentration in the arterial blood entering the organ; C_V, drug concentration in the venous blood leaving the organ.

a well-perfused organ (kidney or liver) that is capable of eliminating the drug.

If the organ eliminates or metabolizes some or all of the drug entering the organ, then the drug concentration (e.g. $\mu g\,mL^{-1}$) in the venous blood leaving the organ (C_V) is lower than the drug concentration (e.g. $\mu g\,mL^{-1}$) in the arterial blood entering the organ (C_A). If Q is the blood flow through an eliminating organ (e.g. $mL\,min^{-1}$), then

$C_A \times Q$ = the rate at which drug enters the
$\qquad\qquad$ organ ($\mu g\,min^{-1}$)
$C_V \times Q$ = the rate at which drug leaves the
$\qquad\qquad$ organ ($\mu g\,min^{-1}$)

Based on steady-state and mass-balance considerations, the instantaneous rate of organ elimination is equal to the difference between the rate at which drug enters an organ and the rate at which it leaves an organ. This is equal to the product of the blood flow rate (Q) and the arterial–venous concentration difference ($C_A - C_V$).

Rate of elimination = Blood flow rate
$\qquad\qquad\qquad\qquad$ concentration difference
$= Q(C_A - C_V) = QC_A - QC_V$

Clearance is equal to the rate of elimination divided by the (arterial) drug concentration before drug passes through the organ of elimination (C_a):

$$Cl_{organ} = \frac{Q(C_A - C_V)}{C_A} \qquad (4.7)$$

The ratio of the rate of elimination to the rate at which drug enters an organ is a dimensionless term that is called the *extraction ratio* (E).

$$E = \frac{\text{rate of elimination}}{\text{rate in}} = \frac{Q(C_A - C_V)}{Q(C_A)}$$

$$E = \frac{C_A - C_V}{C_A} \qquad (4.8)$$

The extraction ratio quantifies the efficiency of an organ with respect to drug elimination. If an organ is incapable of eliminating the drug, C_A will be equal to C_V, and the extraction ratio will be zero. If, however, the organ is so efficient in metabolizing or eliminating the drug that $C_V \approx 0$, then the extraction ratio approaches unity. The extraction ratio of a drug will be a number between 0 and 1.0.

The extraction ratio can also be considered as an index of how efficiently the organ clears drug from the blood flowing through it. For example, an extraction ratio of 0.8 indicates that 80% of the blood flowing through the organ will be completely cleared of drug. Following this line of reasoning, organ clearance of a drug can be defined as the product of the extraction ratio (E) and the flow rate (Q).

Organ clearance = blood flow rate
$\qquad\qquad\qquad\qquad$ × extraction ratio

$$Cl = Q \times E \qquad (4.9)$$

It is, in theory, possible to estimate clearance by direct determination of the parameters in this equation. However, the practical difficulty involved in applying this approach usually precludes its use. First, an accurate estimation of organ flow rate (Q) is difficult to obtain. Moreover, the total flow may not necessarily be constant over the study period. Also, measuring the concentration of drug in arteries (C_A) and veins (C_V) is not very easy experimentally, particularly, in humans.

4.6 Physiological approach to clearance

Earlier in this chapter, the concept of an extraction ratio (E) was introduced. Equation 4.8 shows that extraction ratio across an organ of elimination is equal to $(C_A - C_V)/C_A$, where C_A is the plasma drug concentration approaching the organ and C_V is the concentration exiting the organ. Furthermore, Eq. 4.9 introduced another definition for clearance: $Cl = Q \times E$, where Q is plasma flow to the organ.

To provide further appreciation for the hepatic extraction ratio and its interrelationship with other pharmacokinetic parameters, we introduce the following physiological approach.

Picture 10 molecules of drug presented to an organ of elimination over the course of 1 s. Plasma flow to this organ (e.g. the liver) equals plasma flow exiting this organ. (Of course, it is really whole blood, comprising plasma plus formed elements, flowing to and from the organs of the body. We use the equivalent plasma flow rate because our pharmacokinetic equations employ C_p, the drug concentration in the plasma.)

Let $Q_{IN} = Q_{OUT} = 0.0125 \, L \, s^{-1}$.

From this we can calculate the plasma drug concentration entering the liver (C_p):

$$10 \, mol \, s^{-1}/0.0125 \, L \, s^{-1} = 800 \, mol \, L$$

If we are given the total mass of drug in the body $X = 1 \times 10^4 \, mol$, we can find:

$$V = \frac{X}{C_{p_{in}}} = \frac{1 \times 10^4 \, mol}{800 \, mol \, L^{-1}} = 12.5 \, L$$

If we are also told that, of the 10 molecules of drug presented to the liver in 1 s, 2 are metabolized and the other 8 escape metabolism, we can calculate that:

$$E = 2/10 = 0.2$$

Clearance can be defined as the product of liver plasma flow and the hepatic extraction ratio. For this example,

$$Cl = (Q)(E) = \left(\frac{0.0125 \, L}{s}\right)(0.2)$$
$$= 0.0025 \, L \, s^{-1}$$

and

$$K = \frac{Fraction \; drug \; metabolized}{s}$$
$$= \frac{2 \, mol/(1 \times 10^{-4} \, mol)}{s} = \frac{2 \times 10^{-4}}{s}$$

By another equation,

$$Cl = (K)(V) = \left(\frac{2 \times 10^{-4}}{s}\right)(12.5 \, L)$$
$$= 0.0025 \, L \, s^{-1}$$

which agrees with our value above.

The elimination rate is $2 \, mol \, s^{-1}$ metabolized. Therefore, by still another equation, we can obtain:

$$Cl = \frac{\frac{-dX}{dt}}{C_{p_{in}}} = \frac{2 \, mol \, s^{-1}}{800 \, mol \, L^{-1}} = 0.0025 \, L \, s^{-1}$$

our familiar result for clearance.

Figure 4.4, based on the previous calculations, attempts to show a snapshot in time (1 s.) of a drug eliminated (cleared) exclusively by the liver. The cardiac output (CO) is seen to branch into (1) a non-clearance pathway and (2) the plasma flow rate to the liver (Q_H). Q_H must also be the plasma flow exiting the liver. The 10 molecules of drug presented to the liver are shown branching into a pathway where all molecules going through are metabolized (2 molecules) and into another pathway where all molecules that go through escape metabolism (8 molecules). Q_H from the liver adds to $(CO - Q_H)$ from the non-metabolic pathways to produce the venous return to the heart (VRH).

In the scenario described, an hour elapses. We can then calculate $C_{p_{in}}$ at $t = 1 \, h$ and see whether it has changed from the original value. Since K is constant, we have:

$$(C_{p_{in}})_{t=1h} = ((C_{p_{in}})_{t=1 \, h})(e^{-(0.002 \, s^{-1})(3600 \, s)})$$
$$= \left(\frac{800 \, mol}{L}\right)(0.4868)$$
$$= 389.4 \, mol \, L^{-1}$$

which represents a decrease.

Next, let us determine the fraction of original drug that has been eliminated after 1 h has gone by? Also, would K be a good approximation of this value?

The fraction eliminated is $1 - e^{-kt} = 1 - 0.4868 = 0.5132$. That is, 5132 mol (molecules) of the original 10 000 have been eliminated by metabolism. Since $K = 0.720 \, h^{-1}$, it is a poor estimate of the actual fraction drug eliminated over 1 h, namely 0.5132. (K will approximate fraction drug eliminated only for very small time periods.)

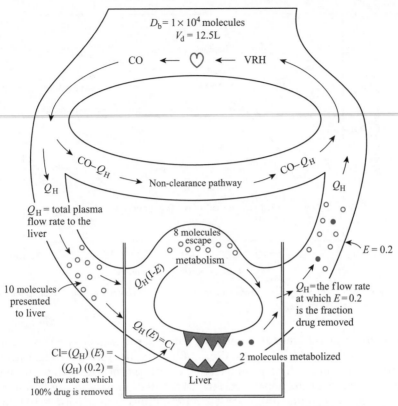

Figure 4.4 Physiological approach to understanding clearance. CO, cardiac output; VRH, venous return to the heart. Q, blood flow rate through the organ; E, extraction ratio; D_b, mass of drug in the body at a given time.

Recalling that V is constant, we can calculate X at $t = 1$ h:

$$(X)_{t=1\,h} = (C_p)_{t=1\,h}(V)$$
$$= (389.4 \text{ mol L}^{-1})(12.5 \text{ L})$$
$$= 4868 \text{ mol}$$

Next, we want to see whether the elimination rate $-dX/dt$ will be the same as it was at $t = 0$. In other words, is the elimination rate constant over time? We calculate:

$$\left(\frac{-dX}{dt}\right)_{t=1\,h} = (Cl)(C_{p_{in}})_{t=1\,h}$$
$$= \left(\frac{0.0025 \text{ L}}{s}\right)\left(\frac{389.4 \text{ mol}}{L}\right)$$
$$= 0.9735 \frac{\text{mol}}{s}$$

Therefore, the elimination rate is lower than the initial elimination rate at $t = 0$. This makes sense when you consider that $C_{p_{in}}$ (the driving force for elimination) is also lower at $t = 1$ h.

Next, let us find out whether the rate drug in at $t = 1$ h is constant (i.e. whether it is the same as it was at $t = 0$ h). Liver blood flow is time invariant for this calculation.

$$(\text{Rate drug in})_{t=1\,h} = [(C_{p_{in}})_{t=1\,h}(Q_H)]$$
$$= \left(\frac{389.4 \text{ mol}}{L}\right)\left(\frac{0.0125 \text{ L}}{s}\right)$$
$$= 4.868 \frac{\text{mol}}{s}$$

Therefore, rate drug in at $t = 1$ h is smaller than its value at $t = 0$ h, when it was 10 mol s^{-1}.

Finally, let's calculate the hepatic extraction ratio E at $t = 1$ h to see whether it is constant:

$$E = \frac{(\text{drug elimination rate})_{t=1\,h}(1\text{ s})}{(\text{rate drug in})_{t=1\,h}(1\text{ s})}$$
$$t = \frac{0.9735 \text{ mol}}{4.868 \text{ mol}} = 0.200$$

So, E is the same at $t = 0$ as at $t = 1$ h; that is, E is constant.

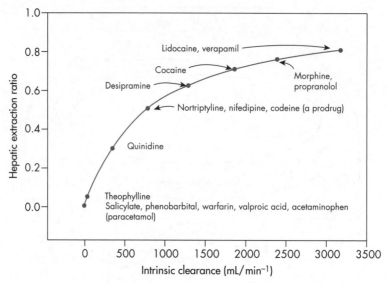

Figure 4.5 Hepatic extraction ratio (*E*) and intrinsic clearance (Cl$_{int}$) of some common drugs. The hepatic extraction ratio is a hyperbolic function of intrinsic clearance.

We next need to consider clearance parameters that are unaffected by hepatic blood flow and/or drug plasma protein binding. These parameters reflect the inherent ability of the hepatocytes to metabolize either total or unbound drug once it is presented to the liver.

Intrinsic clearance (Cl$_{int}$)

Intrinsic clearance (Cl$_{int}$) is defined as the hepatic clearance a drug would have if it was not restricted by hepatic blood (or, more exactly plasma) flow rate. Mathematically, this means that:

$$Q_H \gg Cl_{int}$$

This situation could have two causes: very large Q_H or very small Cl$_{int}$. The former is theoretical since Q_H has an upper physiological limit of 0.8 L min^{-1}. The latter (very small Cl$_{int}$) does occur for many drugs where the liver has little inherent ability to metabolize them. In this case, hepatic clearance can approximately equal the drug's intrinsic clearance. The proof follows.

First, we recognize that the hepatic extraction ratio, *E*, is a (hyperbolic) function of Cl$_{int}$, as seen in Fig. 4.5. As a drug's intrinsic clearance increases, so does its hepatic extraction ratio, but (as seen in Fig. 4.5) not in a linear fashion.

The hepatic extraction ratio of a drug is, in fact, a hyperbolic function of its intrinsic clearance. Several common drugs have been plotted in Fig. 4.5 based on data in the literature. By convention, drugs with hepatic extraction ratios < 0.3 are considered to have low values for intrinsic clearance, while values > 0.7 are considered to be high values. The region between 0.3 and 0.7 contains drugs with intermediate hepatic extraction ratios.

Specifically:

$$E = (Cl_{int})/(Q_H + Cl_{int}) \qquad (4.10)$$

For small Cl$_{int}$ relative to Q_H, $E \approx (Cl_{int})/(Q_H)$. In this case, *E* will be a small number since Cl$_{int}$ itself is small.

Since hepatic clearance, Cl$_H = Q_H E$, we obtain, for the present case:

$$Cl_H \approx (Q_H)(Cl_{int})/(Q_H)$$

Therefore, Cl$_H \approx$ Cl$_{int}$.

If, additionally, there is no plasma protein binding of drug, then:

Cl$_H \approx$ Cl$'_{int}$, the intrinsic free (unbound) clearance of drug (see below).

Other possible cases are summarized in Table 4.1.

Table 4.1　Dependence of hepatic clearance on intrinsic clearance (Cl_{int}) and blood flow to the liver (Q_H)

Case I	Case II
$Q_H \gg Cl_{int}$ $E = Cl_{int}/Q_H$ = small; $Cl_H \cong Cl_{int}$	$Cl_{int} \gg Q_H$ $E \cong 1$ (largest possible); $Cl_H \cong Q_H$
A (definitional only) $Q\uparrow\uparrow$ (much greater than maximum physiological value) E is small because drug is whisked by quickly during a single pass through the liver, but $Cl_H \cong Cl_{int}$, which we have not restricted in size; so Cl_H can be very large	**A physiological** $Q\downarrow\downarrow$ (e.g. hepatic cirrhosis) E is large (approaching 1) because it is easier to extract drug at a gentle flow rate; but $Cl_H \cong Q_H$ and is small
B physiological $Cl_{int}\downarrow\downarrow$ (poorly metabolized drug) ($Q_H = 0.8\,L\,min^{-1}$) E is small because of low Cl_{int} $Cl_H \cong Cl_{int}$ = small	**B physiological** $Cl_{int}\uparrow\uparrow$ (well-metabolized drug) ($Q_H = 0.8\,L\,min^{-1}$) E is large because of high Cl_{int} $Cl_H \cong Q_H = 0.8\,L\,min^{-1}$ (largest possible clearance, since I-A is not physiologically possible)

E, extraction ratio.

Two factors (non-linearly) affect Cl_H: $(Q_H\uparrow) \rightarrow (Cl_H\uparrow)$ and $(Cl_{int}\uparrow) \rightarrow (Cl_H\uparrow)$.

Two factors (non-linearly) affect E: $(Q_H\uparrow) \rightarrow (E\downarrow)$ and $(Cl_{int}\uparrow) \rightarrow (E\uparrow)$.

Intrinsic free (unbound) clearance

Intrinsic free (unbound) clearance (Cl'_{int}) is the intrinsic clearance a drug would have in the absence of plasma protein binding. It is defined as:

$$Cl'_{int} = (Cl_{int})/f_{up} \tag{4.11}$$

where f_{up} is the fraction drug unbound in the plasma.

By this equation, Cl'_{int} becomes a number greater than Cl_{int} when there is any degree of plasma protein binding (i.e. when f_{up} is a number <1). For highly bound drugs, f_{up} is small, and Cl'_{int} can become a very large number.

Parameters affecting hepatic clearance

Combining Eqs 4.9 and 4.10 yields:

$$Cl_H = (Q_H)\frac{Cl_{int}}{Q_H + Cl_{int}} \tag{4.12}$$

Inserting the expression for Cl'_{int} from Eq. 4.11 into Eq. 4.12 yields:

$$Cl_H = (Q_H)\frac{f_{up}Cl'_{int}}{Q_H + f_{up}Cl'_{int}} \tag{4.13}$$

This equation shows the independent parameters responsible for the magnitude of hepatic clearance for a given patient receiving a given drug.

Parameters affecting elimination half life

In order to build an equation showing the effect of independent parameters on elimination half life, we recognize that:

$$t_{1/2} = \frac{0.693}{K} = \frac{(0.693)V}{Cl_{total}} = \frac{(0.693)V}{Cl_R + Cl_H}$$

$$= \frac{(0.693)V}{Cl_R + (Q_H)\frac{f_{up}Cl'_{int}}{Q_H + f_{up}Cl'_{int}}} \tag{4.14}$$

where Cl_R is renal clearance and V is volume of distribution.

One equation relating volume of distribution to its independent parameters is:

$$V = 7 + 8f_{up} + V_T \frac{f_{up}}{f_{ut}} \quad (4.15)$$

where f_{up} is fraction drug unbound in the plasma; f_{ut} is fraction drug unbound in the tissue; and V_T is tissue volume (total body water minus volume of the circulation; approximately $0.40\,L\,kg^{-1}$ body weight).

Inserting Eq. 4.15 for V into Eq. 4.14 yields:

$$t_{1/2} = \frac{(0.693)\left(7 + 8f_{up} + V_T \frac{f_{up}}{f_{ut}}\right)}{Cl_R + (Q_H)\frac{f_{up}Cl'_{int}}{Q_H + f_{up}Cl'_{int}}} \quad (4.16)$$

Inspection of this equation shows that changes in volume of distribution are caused by a set of parameters (namely, f_{up}, f_{ut} and V_T), which is different from the set of parameters affecting total body clearance (namely, Cl_R, f_{up}, Cl'_{int} and Q_H). Thus, volume of distribution and clearance can vary independently of each other.

4.7 Estimation of systemic clearance

Total clearance (Cl_s) can be derived as follows. From an earlier definition, we know that:

$$Cl = \frac{\text{Rate of elimination}}{\text{Plasma drug concentration}}$$

$$= \frac{\left(\frac{-dX}{dt}\right)_t}{(C_p)_t}$$

Integrating the right-hand side of Eq. 4.4 from $t=0$ to $t=\infty$, gives:

$$Cl = \frac{\int_0^\infty \left(\frac{-dX}{dt}\right)_t dt}{\int_0^\infty (C_p)_t dt}$$

Hence, for intravenous bolus administration:

$$Cl_s = \frac{dose}{(AUC)_0^\infty} \quad (4.17)$$

where AUC is the area under the plasma concentration versus time curve.

4.8 Calculating renal clearance (Cl_r) and metabolic clearance (Cl_m)

Renal clearance (Cl_r)

The renal clearance of a drug may be determined by employing any of the following methods.

Method 1

$$Cl_r = K_u V \quad (4.18)$$

Where, K_u is the excretion rate constant (h^{-1}) and V is the apparent volume of distribution (e.g. mL, $L\,kg^{-1}$ body weight).

Method 2

$$Cl_r = \frac{(X_u)_\infty}{(AUC)_0^\infty} \quad (4.19)$$

where $(X_u)_\infty$ is the mass or amount (e.g. mg) of drug excreted (unchanged form only) in urine at $t=\infty$ and AUC here is the area under the plasma concentration versus time curve ($mg\,L^{-1}\,h^{-1}$) from $t=0$ to $t=\infty$.

Method 3

$$Cl_r = \frac{(\%\text{ excreted unchanged}) \times (dose)}{(AUC)_0^\infty} \quad (4.20)$$

Equations 4.19 and 4.20 are equivalent since the product of percentage excreted in unchanged form multiplied by the dose administered (i.e. the numerator of the right-hand side of Eq. 4.20) provides the amount of drug excreted in unchanged form in urine at time infinity ($X_u)_\infty$, the numerator value of the right-hand side of Eq. 4.19).

Method 4: we know that:

$$Cl_r = \frac{\text{Rate of excretion}}{\text{Plasma drug concentration}}$$

$$= \frac{\left(\dfrac{dX_u}{dt}\right)_t}{(C_p)_t}$$

This relationship makes it relatively easy to determine the renal clearance (Cl_r) of any drug that is excreted, to some measurable extent, in unchanged form in the urine:

1. Determine the elimination and/or excretion rate of drug by methods discussed previously.
2. Determine the plasma concentration (C_p) at a point of urine collection interval.

Metabolic clearance (Cl_m)

The metabolic clearance of a drug may be determined by employing any of the following methods.

Method 1

$$Cl_m = K_m V \tag{4.21}$$

Where K_m is metabolite rate constant (e.g. h^{-1}) and V is the apparent volume of distribution (e.g. mL, $L\,kg^{-1}$ body weight).

Method 2

$$Cl_m = K_m V = \frac{(M_u)_\infty}{(AUC)_0^\infty} \tag{4.22}$$

Where $(M_u)_\infty$ is the amount or mass of metabolite in urine at time $t=\infty$ and $(AUC)_0^\infty$ is the area under the plasma concentration versus time curve (e.g. $mg\,L^{-1}\,h^{-1}$) from $t=0$ to $t=\infty$

Method 3

$$Cl_m = K_m V$$
$$= \frac{(\% \text{ of metabolite in the urine}) \times (\text{dose})}{(AUC)_0^\infty}$$
$$\tag{4.23}$$

Equations 4.22 and 4.23 are equivalent since the product of percentage of metabolite in urine multiplied by the dose administered (i.e. the numerator of the right-hand side of Eq. 4.23)

provides the amount of metabolite in urine at time infinity $(M_u)_\infty$ (the numerator value of the right-hand side of Eq. 4.22).

Please note that when the drug is removed completely in unchanged form (i.e. $(X_u)_\infty = X_0$) then renal clearance (Cl_r) is equal to systemic clearance (Cl_s). Analogously, if the drug is completely eliminated as a metabolite (i.e. $(M_u)_\infty = $ Dose or X_0), then metabolic clearance (Cl_m) is equal to systemic clearance (Cl_s).

$$Cl_s = Cl_r + Cl_m \tag{4.24}$$

or

$$Cl_m = Cl_s - Cl_r$$

or

$$Cl_r = Cl_s - Cl_m$$

4.9 Determination of the area under the plasma concentration versus time curve: application of the trapezoidal rule

It is clear from Eqs 4.17 through 4.23 that knowledge of the area under the plasma concentration versus time curve AUC_0^∞ is essential for the determination of the systemic, renal and metabolic clearance of a drug. It was stated in Ch. 1 (Eqs 1.1 and 1.2) that the knowledge of this parameter is also essential for the determination of the amount of the administered dose of a drug that reaches the general circulation. When a dose of a drug is administered intravenously, of course, the entire dose is in general circulation; however, when a drug is administered extravascularly, the entire administered dose may not always reach the general circulation (incomplete absorption). The application and the utility of this parameter will also be abundantly evident in the subsequent chapters of this text. Therefore, the importance of this parameter should not be overlooked. At this stage, however, let us look at the application of the trapezoidal rule as an available method for the determination of the area under the plasma concentration versus time curve.

Application of the trapezoidal rule

In the absence of the knowledge of the intercept of the plasma concentration versus time plot and the rate constant(s) accompanying the data, this method permits the determination the area under the plasma concentration time curve (AUC). The method, however, requires knowledge of plasma concentrations at various times. Furthermore, the method requires the computation of the average plasma concentration from two consecutive concentration values (starting with concentrations at time 0 and time 1, then time 1 and time 2, etc.). These average values are multiplied by the difference between the corresponding time (dt) values. By employing this approach, as illustrated below, one can compute the AUC value for each trapezoid (Fig. 4.6).

For an intravenous bolus of a drug exhibiting the characteristics of a one-compartment model:

$$\int_0^\infty (C_p)_t \, dt = (\text{AUC})_0^\infty$$

$$= (\text{AUC})_0^{t^*} + (\text{AUC})_{t^*}^\infty \qquad (4.25)$$

$(\text{AUC})_0^{t^*}$ can be determined by the application of trapezoidal rule and $(\text{AUC})_{t^*}^\infty$ can be obtained by using an equation.

Illustration of how to use the trapezoidal method

The following expression yields the AUC for the first trapezoid of the concentration versus time plot:

$$\int_{t_0}^{t_1} C_p \, dt = (\text{AUC})_{t_0}^{t_1} = \frac{(C_p)_0 + (C_p)_1}{2} \times (t_1 - t_0)$$

$$= \text{average } C_p \times dt$$

where units of $(\text{AUC})_0^{t_1}$ are $\mu\text{g mL}^{-1} \times \text{h} = \mu\text{g mL}^{-1}\text{h}$.

The AUC for the second trapezoid of the concentration versus time plot is:

$$\int_{t_1}^{t_2} C_p \, dt = (\text{AUC})_{t_1}^{t_2} = \frac{(C_p)_1 + (C_p)_2}{2} \times (t_2 - t_1)$$

$$= \text{average } C_p \times dt$$

This procedure is followed to determine the AUC for each trapezoid until the last observed plasma concentration value $(C_p)^*$.

The sum (addition) of all these individual trapezoidal values will provide the area under the plasma concentration from time 0 to time t^* (i.e. $(\text{AUC})_0^{t^*}$).

$$(\text{AUC})_0^{t^*} = \text{Sum of individual trapezoid values}$$

Determination of the area under the plasma concentration from time t* to time ∞

The following equation gives the AUC from time time t^* to time ∞:

$$(\text{AUC})_{t^*}^\infty = \int_{t^*}^\infty C_p \, dt = \frac{C_p^*}{K} \qquad (4.26)$$

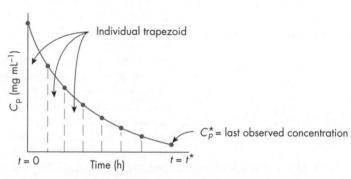

Figure 4.6 Application of the trapezoidal rule to determine the area under the plasma concentration (C_p) versus time curve (AUC). (Rectilinear plot of plasma or serum concentration versus time following the administration of an intravenous bolus of a drug fitting a one-compartment model.)

where C_p^* is the last observed plasma concentration (e.g. $\mu g\,mL^{-1}$) and K is the elimination rate constant (h^{-1}). Therefore, in agreement with what we have seen in Eq. 4.25:

$$\int_0^\infty (C_p)_t dt = (AUC)_0^\infty = (AUC)_0^{t^*} + (AUC)_{t^*}^\infty$$

Example calculation

This example uses data from question 4 in Problem set 1.

$$x\int_{t_0}^{t_1} C_p dt = (AUC)_0^{t_1} = \frac{(C_p)_0 + (C_p)_1}{2} \times (t_1 - t_0)$$
$$= (12.0 + 11.6)/2 \times (0.25 - 0)$$
$$= 11.8\,\mu g\,mL^{-1} \times 0.25\,h$$
$$(AUC)_0^{t_1} = 2.95\,\mu g\,mL^{-1}\,h$$
$$(AUC\ from\ t = 0\ to\ t = 1)$$

$$\int_{t_1}^{t_2} C_p dt = (AUC)_{t_1}^{t_2} = \frac{(C_p)_1 + (C_p)_2}{2} \times (t_2 - t_1)$$
$$= (11.6 + 8.4)/2 \times (0.5 - 0.25)$$
$$= 10.0\,\mu g\,mL^{-1} \times 0.25\,h$$
$$(AUC)_{t_1}^{t_2} = 2.50\,\mu g\,mL^{-1}\,h$$
$$(AUC\ from\ t = 1\ to\ t = 2)$$

$$\int_{t_2}^{t_3} C_p dt = (AUC)_{t_2}^{t_3} = \frac{(C_p)_2 + (C_p)_3}{2} \times (t_3 - t_2)$$
$$= (8.4 + 7.2)/2 \times (0.75 - 0.5)$$
$$= 7.8\,\mu g\,mL^{-1} \times 0.25\,h$$
$$(AUC)_{t_2}^{t_3} = 1.95\,\mu g\,mL^{-1}\,h$$
$$(AUC\ from\ t = 2\ to\ t = 3)$$

This procedure is followed until the last observed serum concentration (i.e. $C_s = 0.09\,\mu g\ mL^{-1}$). The cumulative AUC is determined by adding the individual AUC values up to the last observed concentration (i.e. $C_s = 0.09\,\mu g\,mL^{-1}$ at 8 h).

In this example,

$$\int_0^{8\,h} C_p dt = (AUC)_{t_2}^{t_8} = 19.177\,\mu g\,mL^{-1}\,h$$

$$\int_8^\infty C_p dt = (AUC)_8^\infty = \frac{C_p^*(\mu g\,mL^{-1})}{K(h^{-1})}$$
$$= \frac{0.09\,\mu g\,mL^{-1}}{0.577\,h^{-1}}$$
$$(AUC)_8^\infty = 0.156\,\mu g\,mL^{-1}\,h$$

$$\int_0^\infty C_p dt = (AUC)_0^\infty = (AUC)_0^8 + (AUC)_8^\infty$$
$$(AUC)_0^\infty = 19.177 + 0.156$$
$$(AUC)_0^\infty = 19.333\,\mu g\,mL^{-1}\,h$$

Alternatively, for drugs that are administered as an intravenous bolus dose, Eq. 4.17,

$$Cl_s = \frac{Dose}{(AUC)_0^\infty}$$

Rearrangement of Eq. 4.17, substitution of VK from Eq. 4.6 for Cl_s, and division of numerator and denominator by V produce, in turn:

$$(AUC)_0^\infty = \frac{Dose}{Cl_s} = \frac{Dose}{VK} = \frac{(C_p)_0}{K} \qquad (4.27)$$

4.10 Elimination mechanism

The appearance of drug in the urine is the net result of filtration, secretion and reabsorption processes.

$$\begin{aligned} Rate\ of\ excretion = &\ Rate\ of\ filtration \\ &+ Rate\ of\ secretion \\ &- Rate\ of\ reabsorption \end{aligned}$$

If a drug is only filtered and all the filtered drug is excreted into the urine, then

$$Rate\ of\ excretion = Rate\ of\ filtration$$

and

$$Renal\ clearance(Cl_r) = f_u \times GFR$$

where f_u is the fraction of unbound drug and GFR is the glomerular filtration rate.

Creatinine and inulin (an exogenous polysaccharide) are not bound to plasma proteins nor are they *secreted* into urine. Therefore, renal clearance for each of these substances is a clear measure of

GFR and, consequently, of kidney function. Both are used to assess kidney function.

4.11 Use of creatinine clearance to determine renal function

Creatinine clearance

Creatinine clearance (Cl_{cr}) is renal clearance (Cl_r) applied to endogenous creatinine. It is used to monitor renal function and is a valuable parameter for calculating dosage regimens in elderly patients or those suffering from renal dysfunction.

Normal creatinine clearance (Cl_{cr}) values are:

- adult males: $120 \pm 20 \, mL \, min^{-1}$
- adult females: $108 \pm 20 \, mL \, min^{-1}$.

Normal serum creatinine concentrations vary:

- adult men: 8.0 to $13 \, mg \, L^{-1}$ ($0.8–1.3 \, mg \, dL^{-1}$)
- adult women: 6.0 to $10 \, mg \, L^{-1}$ ($0.6–1.0 \, mg \, dL^{-1}$).

Measuring renal function using creatinine clearance

Creatinine is an end-product of muscle metabolism and appears to be eliminated from the body by the kidneys. The normal range of serum creatinine concentration is between 1 and $2 \, mg \, 100 \, mL^{-1}$. Renal excretion of endogenous creatinine is largely dependent on glomerular filtration and closely approximates the GFR as measured by inulin, both in healthy individuals and individuals with impaired renal function. Since creatinine production bears a direct relation to the muscle mass of an individual, creatinine clearance measurements are, where possible, normalized to a body surface area of $1.73 \, m^2$ in order to obtain a more comparative measurement for different individuals. However, initial dosing calculations and nomograms for renally eliminated drugs, such as the aminoglycosides, rely on the patient's (unnormalized) creatinine clearance value.

Although inulin clearance is generally accepted as the most accurate method for the estimation of glomerular filtration rate, which is approximately $125 \, mL \, min^{-1}$ in healthy indivi-duals, its practical utility for evaluating renal function is limited.

Renal function can be measured in several ways. The most common method involves determining circulatory levels and excretion of creatinine or creatinine clearance. Creatinine is formed from muscle metabolism in the body and circulates in the plasma of individuals with normal renal function at a concentration of approximately 1 mg%. Creatinine is cleared via kidneys by filtration to yield a creatinine clearance of approximately $130 \, mL \, min^{-1}$. This value depends partially on body size, degree of activity, muscle mass and age.

As kidney function declines, for whatever reason, the GFR and, hence, creatinine clearance will also decline. If kidneys are working with only 50% efficiency, the creatinine clearance will fall to $50–60 \, mL \, min^{-1}$ depending on age and other factors. According to the intact nephron hypothesis, other kidney functions will also decline, including tubular secretion. This decline in kidney function leads to the reasonable assumption that, provided a drug is cleared via the kidneys, the systemic clearance of a drug will also be affected to a similar extent as creatinine clearance, even though the compound may also be secreted, and/or reabsorbed.

The use of serum creatinine to determine renal function has been reviewed in considerable detail by Lott *et al.* (1978).

Direct measurement of creatinine clearance

The mass of endogenous creatinine excreted into the urine, collected over a given time interval (Δt), is determined. (For each interval, mass creatinine excreted is the product of urinary creatinine concentration times the volume of urine collected.) The mass excreted per unit time is the rate of creatinine excretion, which is calculated by dividing the mass of creatinine excreted by the time over which it was collected. Next, the mean serum creatinine concentration ($(C_s)_{cr}$) over that interval is calculated from sample determinations; this represents the concentration halfway through the interval. In practice, $\Delta t = 24 \, h$ (1440 min). As $(C_s)_{cr}$ is usually relatively constant, the serum sample is taken at any convenient time.

The directly measured creatinine clearance is then calculated by Eq. 4.28:

$$Cl_{cr} = \frac{\left(\frac{\Delta X_u}{\Delta t}\right)}{(C_s)_{cr}} \tag{4.28}$$

where ΔX_u is the mass of creatinine excreted over time Δt, and $\Delta X_u/\Delta t$ is the rate of creatinine excretion.

If, for example, the rate of excretion of creatinine is $1.3\,mg\,min^{-1}$ and serum creatinine concentration is $0.01\,mg\,mL^{-1}$, then the creatinine clearance is $130\,mL\,min^{-1}$.

Please note that one must obtain both creatinine excretion rate and the average serum creatinine concentration to measure creatinine clearance accurately.

This direct measurement technique is used for patients with low ($<1\,mg\,dl^{-1}$ [$<10\,mg\,l^{-1}$]) values for serum creatinine.

Indirect measurement of creatinine clearance

When only serum creatinine $(C_s)_{cr}$ is available or if it is not be desirable to wait 24 h to measure ΔX_u, the following formulae can be used to predict creatinine clearance.

Adults
For adults (non-obese adults whose serum creatinine is $10\,mg\,L^{-1}$ or higher and stable [neither increasing nor decreasing] and who do not have chronic renal failure), the Cockcroft–Gault equation is used but adjusted for men and women.

For males:

$$Cl_{cr} = \frac{Weight(kg) \times (140 - age)}{72 \times (C_s)_{cr}[mg\%]} \tag{4.29}$$

For females:

$$Cl_{cr} = [0.85]\left[\frac{Weight(kg) \times (140 - age)}{72 \times (C_s)_{cr}[mg\%]}\right] \tag{4.30}$$

The patient's age is expressed in years, body weight in kilograms and serum creatinine con-

centration in mg/100 mL. The factor 0.85 in Eq. 4.30 for female patients causes a 15% reduction in the creatinine clearance estimate.

Children by height
Children are divided into two groups, based on age.

For children aged 0 to 1 year:

$$\text{Normalized } Cl_{cr} \text{ [in mL min}^{-1}/1.73\,m^2]$$
$$= \frac{0.45 \times \text{height [in cm]}}{(C_s)_{cr}[\text{in mg dL}^{-1}]} \tag{4.31}$$

This must be unnormalized for the specific patient by multiplying the above value by the patient's body surface area (m^2).

Children aged 1 to 20 years:

$$\text{Normalized } Cl_{cr}[\text{in mL min}^{-1}/1.73\,m^2]$$
$$= \frac{0.55 \times \text{height [in cm]}}{(C_s)_{cr}[\text{in mg dL}^{-1}]} \tag{4.32}$$

This must be unnormalized for the specific patient by multiplying the above value by the patient's body surface area (m^2).

Again here, it is the use of a different factor (0.45 or 0.55, respectively) that allows differentiation between the clearance in children under 1 year and older children.

Children (by age)
The method of Shull *et al.* (1978) is as follows:

$$\text{Normalized } Cl_{cr} \text{ [in mL/min/1.73 } m^2 \text{ or in mL min}^{-1}/1.73\,m^2]$$
$$= \frac{(35 \times age) + 236}{(C_s)_{cr}} \tag{4.33}$$

Obese patients (>30% above lean body weight)
First, the lean body weight (LBW; in kilograms) of the individual must be calculated.

For males

$$LBW(kg) = 50 + [2.3 \times (\text{height in inches} - 60)]$$
$$LBW(kg) = 50 + [90.55 \times (\text{height in meters} - 1.524)].$$

For females

$$LBW(kg) = 45 + [2.3 \times (\text{height in inches} - 60)]$$
$$LBW(kg) = 45 + [90.55 \times (\text{height in meters} - 1.524)].$$

This will allow estimation of whether the patient's actual weight is >30% above this value.

For obese males:

$$Cl_{cr}(\text{in mL min}^{-1}) = \frac{\{137 - \text{age in years}\} \times \{(0.285)(\text{weight in kg}) + (12.1)(\text{height in m})(\text{height in m})\}}{51 \times (C_s)_{cr}[\text{in mg dL}^{-1}]}$$

(4.34)

For obese females:

$$Cl_{cr}[\text{in mL min}^{-1}] = \frac{\{146 - \text{age in years}\} \times \{(0.287)(\text{weight in kg}) + (9.74)(\text{height in m})(\text{height in m})\}}{60 \times (C_s)_{cr}[\text{in mg dL}^{-1}]}$$

(4.35)

Notice that the value for the factor height (expressed in meters) is multiplied by itself in both of the above equations.

Patients with chronic renal failure or unstable serum creatinine values

The following four-step procedure is used if the patient has chronic renal failure has unstable (changing) serum creatinine values.

Step 1: calculate ER_1 (the nominal excretion rate of creatinine at steady state):

$$ER_1(\text{females}) = LBW(\text{in kg}) \times \{29.3 - (0.203)(\text{age [in years]})\}$$
$$ER_1(\text{males}) = LBW(\text{in kg}) \times \{25.1 - (0.175)(\text{age [in years]})\}$$

where LBW is lean body weight.

Step 2: calculate ER_2 (the excretion rate of creatinine at steady state, corrected for non-renal elimination):

$$ER_2 = ER_1 \times \{1.035 - (0.0337)(C_s)_{av}[\text{in mg dl}^{-1}])\}$$

Step 3: calculate ER_3 (the current excretion rate of creatinine corrected for non-steady-state conditions):

$$ER_3 = \frac{ER_2 - (4)(LBW [\text{in kg}])([(C_s)_{cr}]_1 - [(C_s)_{cr}]_2)}{t_1 - t_2}$$

where $[(C_s)_{cr}]_1$ and $[(C_s)_{cr}]_2$ are the first and second serum creatinine concentrations (in mg dl^{-1}) and where $t_1 - t_2$ is the elapsed time (in days) between the collection times of these two serum samples.

Step 4: finally, an accurate estimate of creatinine clearance can be obtained:

$$Cl_{cr}[\text{mL min}^{-1}] = \frac{ER_3}{(14.4 - (C_s)_{cr}^*[\text{in mg dl}^{-1}])}$$

where $(C_s)_{cr}^* = [(C_s)_{cr}]_2$ if serum concentration is rising; otherwise,

$$(C_s)_{cr}^* = [(C_s)_{cr}]_{ave} = \frac{([(C_s)_{cr}]_1 + [(C_s)_{cr}]_2)}{2}$$

(4.36)

Significance of creatinine clearance

1. Generally, a normal creatinine clearance value indicates that the kidney is functioning normally.
2. In some disease states or pathological conditions, or in elderly population, the creatinine clearance is likely to alter, leading to lower values for creatinine clearance.
3. If creatinine clearance is reduced, dose adjustment for drugs that are eliminated by the kidneys must be considered. Failure to adjust the dose of a drug will result in much higher blood

concentrations (perhaps toxic concentrations) for the same dose of the drug.

4. An alternative to adjusting the dose of a drug is to decrease the frequency at which the normal dose is administered. For example, if a normal is dose is 250 mg four times a day (qid) or one tablet four times a day, then this can be reduced to three times a day or twice a day dosing.

5. A lower creatinine clearance value will affect other so-called "constant" parameters such as the elimination and/or excretion rate constants (K or K_u), the elimination half life ($t_{1/2}$) and, possibly, the apparent volume of distribution. These, in turn, will influence the value of any other pharmacokinetic parameter mathematically related to them. (This example is for a one-compartment model). These parameters include plasma concentration (C_p) at any time t, the area under the concentration versus time curve from $t=0$ to $t=\infty$, and clearance.

Renal clearance of intravenous bolus of drug (one compartment)

An intravenous bolus dose of drug that fits a one-compartment model will obey the following equations:

$$C_p = (C_p)_0 e^{-Kt} \text{ and } (C_p)_0 = X_0/V$$
$$t_{1/2} = 0.693/K \text{ and } Cl = KV$$
$$(AUC)_0^\infty = \frac{\text{Dose}}{Cl_s}$$

as in Eq. 4.27

Figure 4.7 is a semilogarithmic plot of plasma concentration against time following the administration of an identical dose of a drug to three subjects with different degrees of renal impairment.

In Fig. 4.7, please note the differences in the slope of the concentration versus time data, which will be reflected in the elimination rate constant and the elimination half life of the drug. Questions for reflection: Is the initial plasma concentration of the drug also affected by the renal insufficiency? Will the apparent volume of drug distribution be different in three subjects? Will the systemic clearance of this drug be different in each subject? Will the area under the plasma concentration $(AUC)_0^\infty$ be different in each subject?

Renal clearance of an orally administered dose of a drug

As for the intravenous bolus, above, the drug fits a one-compartment model. Figure 4.8 is a semilogarithmic plot of plasma concentration against time following the administration of an identical extravascular dose of a drug to two subjects with different degrees of renal impairment.

Please make observations regarding the pharmacokinetic parameters that are likely to be affected by the renal impairment.

Table 4.2 provides the values of the elimination rate constants for selected drugs in patients

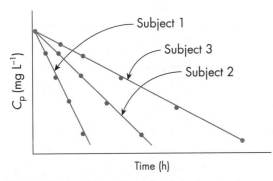

Figure 4.7 A semilogarithmic plot of plasma or serum concentration (C_p) versus time following the administration of an identical dose of drug, as an intravenous bolus, to three subjects with different degrees of renal insufficiency.

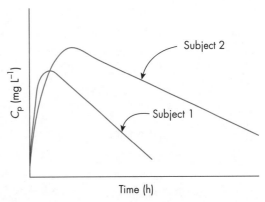

Figure 4.8 A semilogarithmic plot of plasma or serum concentration (C_p) versus time following the administration of an identical dose of drug, by an extravascular route, to two subjects with different degree of renal insufficiency.

Table 4.2 Drugs ranked in order of decreasing percentages of normal elimination occurring in severe renal impairment (K_N/K_{nr}); where K_N and K_{nr} are the elimination rate constants in normal renal function and severe renal impairment, respectively

Group	Drugs[a]	K_N (per h)	K_{nr} (per h)	K_N/K_{nr} (%)
A	Minocycline	0.04	0.04	100.0
	Rifampicin	0.25	0.25	100.0
	Lidocaine	0.39	0.36	92.3
	Digitoxin	0.00475	0.00417	87.7
B	Doxycycline	0.037	0.031	83.8
	Chlortetracycline	0.12	0.095	79.2
C	Clindamycin	0.16	0.12	75.0
	Choramphenicol	0.26	0.19	73.1
	Propranolol	0.22	0.16	72.8
	Erythromycin	0.39	0.28	71.8
D	Trimethoprim	0.054	0.031	57.4
	Isoniazid (fast)	0.53	0.30	56.6
	Isoniazid (slow)	0.23	0.13	56.5
E	Dicloxacillin	1.20	0.60	50.0
	Sulfadiazine	0.069	0.032	46.4
	Sulfmethoxazole	0.084	0.037	44.0
F	Nafcillin	1.26	0.54	42.8
	Chlorpropamide	0.020	0.008	40.0
	Lincomycin	0.15	0.06	40.0
G	Colistimethate	0.154	0.054	35.1
	Oxacillin	1.73	0.58	33.6
	Digoxin	0.021	0.007	33.3
H	Tetracycline	0.120	0.033	27.5
	Cloxacillin	1.21	0.31	25.6
	Oxytetracycline	0.075	0.014	18.7
I	Amoxicillin	0.70	0.10	14.3
	Methicillin	1.40	0.19	13.6
J	Ticarcillin	0.58	0.066	11.4
	Penicillin G	1.24	0.13	10.5
	Ampicillin	0.53	0.05	9.4
	Carbenicillin	0.55	0.05	9.1
K	Cefazolin	0.32	0.02	6.2
	Cephaloridine	0.51	0.03	5.9
	Cephalothin[b]	1.20	0.06	5.0

	Gentamicin	0.30	0.015	5.0
L	Flucytosine	0.18	0.007	3.9
	Kanamycin	0.28	0.01	3.6
	Vancomycin	0.12	0.004	3.3
	Tobramycin	0.32	0.01	3.1
	Cephalexin	1.54	0.032	2.1

[a] Fast and slow indicate acetylator phenotype.
[b] K_{nr} value for cephalothin from repeated dosing.
From Welling and Craig (1976).

with normal renal function (K_N) and in patients with severe renal impairment (K_{nr}), and the percentage of normal elimination in severe renal impairment (ratio K_{nr}/K_N).

Figure 4.9 illustrates the relationship between serum half life and creatinine clearance for two drugs.

In Fig. 4.9, note the influence of creatinine clearance on the serum half life of each drug. When the creatinine clearance decreases, it is clear from the figure that the serum half life of cefazolin increases. Furthermore, it is also obvious from the figure that there is a dramatic increase in the serum half life of cefazolin when the creatinine clearance falls below $40 \, \text{mL} \, \text{min}^{-1}$. The serum half life of minocycline, by comparison, remains unaffected by a decrease in creatinine clearance. This is attributed to the fact that minocycline is eliminated by the liver.

This clearly suggests that when there is a decrease in the creatinine clearance in a subject in renal impairment and if a drug is removed by the kidneys, it is imperative that the dose of the drug be adjusted. Failure to adjust the dose of a drug will result in higher, and perhaps toxic, concentrations of the drug in the body.

The practical application of the use of creatinine clearance for adjusting the dose or dosage regimen of a drug, which is being eliminated by kidneys, is illustrated in Tables 4.3 and 4.4.

Aciclovir (Zovirax) is used in initial and recurrent mucosal and cutaneous infections with herpes simplex viruses 1 and 2 in immunocompromised adults and children and for severe initial clinical episodes of genital herpes. Approximately 62 to 91% of an intravenous dose is excreted renally in unchanged form. Table 4.3 illustrates the relationship between the creatinine clearance, systemic clearance and the elimination half life of the drug.

Ceftazidime (Fortaz, Tazicef, Tazidime) is a cephalosporin antibiotic that is used for infections of, for example, the lower respiratory tract, skin and urinary tract. It is excreted, almost exclusively, by glomerular filtration. Table 4.4 shows the relationship between the creatinine clearance and recommended dose or dosage regimen.

An alternatively approach for decision making on the adjustment of dosage of a drug that is eliminated by the kidneys is the use of a nomogram for the specific drug. Use of such nomograms (Figs 4.10 and 4.11) requires knowledge of the serum creatinine value and/or creatinine clearance value

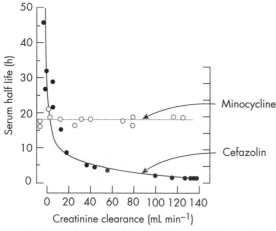

Figure 4.9 The relationship between serum half lives of two drugs and their creatinine clearance: cefazolin and minocycline.

Table 4.3 Illustration of the relationship between creatinine clearance, total body clearance, and the elimination half life of acyclovir (Zovirax)

Creatinine clearance (ml min^{-1} 1.73 m^{-2})	Elimination half life (h)	Total body clearance (ml min^{-1} 1.73 m^{-2})
>80.0	2.5	327.0
50–80	3.0	248.0
15–50	3.5	190.0
0.0 (anuric)	19.5	29.0

Drug Facts and Comparisons, 56 ed. (2002), p.1514, Lippincott, St Louis. Reprinted with permission.

Table 4.4 Recommended maintenance doses in renal insufficiency: relationship between creatinine clearance, recommended dose and the dosing interval for ceftazidine

Creatinine clearance (mL min^{-1})	Recommended dose of ceftazidime	Frequency of dosing or dosing interval (τ)
50–31	1 g	Every 12 h
30–16	1 g	Every 24 h
15–6	500 mg	Every 48 h
<5	500 mg	Every 48 h

Drug Facts and Comparisons, 56 ed. (2002), p.1514, Lippincott, St Louis. Reprinted with permission.

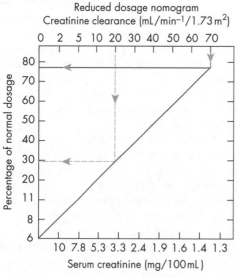

Figure 4.10 Nomogram for tobramycin, an aminoglycoside antibiotic. *Drug Facts and Comparisons*, 56 ed. (2002), p.1408, Lippincott, St Louis. Reprinted with permission.

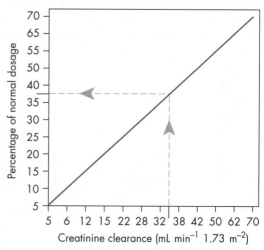

Figure 4.11 Nomogram for netilmicin, an aminoglycoside antibiotic. The adjusted daily dose is the normal daily dose multiplied by the percentage of normal dose recommended by the nomogram. *Drug Facts and Comparisons*, 56 ed. (2002), p.1410, Lippincott, St Louis. Reprinted with permission.

and the recommended daily dose of the drug in normal subject. The value of serum creatinine or creatinine clearance is entered on the *x*-axis and the corresponding recommended percentage of normal dose is read off from the *y*-axis.

For example, if the normalized creatinine clearance (adjusted for body area) in a patient is determined to be $70 \, \text{mL} \, \text{min}^{-1}/1.73 \, \text{m}^2$, then the recommended tobramycin daily dose will be approximately 75% of the normal daily dose (Fig. 4.10). If the creatinine clearance is reported to be $20 \, \text{mL} \, \text{min}^{-1}/1.73 \, \text{m}^2$, the daily dose will be approximately 26% of the normal daily dose. It should be clear from this that if the drug is being eliminated by the kidneys then the greater the decrease in the creatinine clearance value, or greater the degree of renal insufficiency or impairment, the greater is the reduction in the daily dose required. One may also use the following formula to determine the daily recommended dose:

$$\text{Reduced daily dose} = \text{Normal daily dose} \\ \times \% \, \text{normal dose from the nomogram}$$

$$(4.37)$$

Figure 4.11 shows a similar nomogram for netilmicin (Netromycin), an aminogycoside.

Calculation of adjusted daily dose

In general, when a drug is being eliminated exclusively by the kidneys, one may also take the following approach to determine the adjusted daily dose of a drug:

$$\text{Adjusted daily dose} = (X_0)_{\text{NR}} \\ \times \frac{\text{Patient's creatinine clearance}}{\text{Normal creatinine clearance}} \quad (4.38)$$

where $(X_0)_{\text{NR}}$ is the dose for a patient with normal renal function.

Problem set 1

Problems for Chapters 3 and 4

Question 1

Table P1.1 gives plasma drug concentrations (C_p) obtained following an intravenous bolus administration of a 250 mg dose of a drug that exhibited the characteristics of a one-compartment model and was eliminated exclusively by urinary excretion. Plot the data and, using the plot, determine the following.

a. The elimination half life ($t_{1/2}$).
b. The overall elimination rate constant (K).
c. The initial plasma concentration, $(C_p)_0$.
d. The apparent volume of distribution (V).

     Using the answers obtained in parts a–d, to determine the following.

e. The drug plasma concentration at 75 min following the administration of a 2.5 mg kg^{-1} dose to a subject weighing 70 kg.

f. The time at which the plasma concentration of the drug will fall below 20 µg mL^{-1}, following the administration of a 275 mg dose.

Question 2

Cinoxacin (Cinobac) is a synthetic organic antibacterial compound reported to show antibacterial activity against Gram-negative rods responsible for urinary tract infection. Israel *et al.* (1978) reported the serum concentrations in Table P1.2 following intravenous bolus administration of 50 and 100 mg of cinoxacin to healthy male volunteers.

Table P1.1

Time (h)	Plasma concentration (µg mL^{-1})
0.5	68.0
1.0	54.0
2.0	30.0
3.0	18.5
5.0	6.0
7.0	1.8

Table P1.2

Time (h)	Mean serum concentrations (µg mL^{-1} ($\pm$ SD))	
	50 mg dose	100 mg dose
0.25	2.0 $\pm$ 1.1	3.6 $\pm$ 0.2
0.50	1.4 $\pm$ 0.1	2.6 $\pm$ 0.4
0.75	1.1 $\pm$ 0.2	1.8 $\pm$ 0.3
1.00	0.8 $\pm$ 0.2	1.4 $\pm$ 0.5
1.50	0.5 $\pm$ 0.2	0.8 $\pm$ 0.4
2.00	0.3 $\pm$ 0.1	0.6 $\pm$ 0.4
3.00	0.1 $\pm$ 1.1	0.2 $\pm$ 0.06
4.00	0.03 $\pm$ 0.05	0.06 $\pm$ 0.02
6.00	–	0.02 $\pm$ 0.05

Plot the data and, using the plot, determine the following for each dose.

a. The elimination half life ($t_{1/2}$).
b. The elimination rate constant (K or K_{el}).
c. The initial serum concentrations, $(C_s)_0$.
d. The apparent volume of distribution (V).
e. Plot the graph on rectilinear paper of $t_{1/2}$, K and V against the administered doses (i.e. 50 and 100 mg).
f. Following the administration of cinoxacin to a 70 kg healthy subject, the serum concentration at 2.5 h was reported to be 225 $\mu g\,L^{-1}$ (0.225 $mg\,L^{-1}$; 0.225 $\mu g\,mL^{-1}$); calculate the administered dose of cinoxacin.

Question 3

The following cumulative amounts of drug in the urine (X_u) were obtained after an intravenous bolus injection of 500 mg of the drug (X_0), which is eliminated exclusively by urinary excretion (Table P1.3).

Plot the data in as many ways as possible and, by means of your plots determine the following.

a. The elimination half life ($t_{1/2}$).
b. The elimination rate constant (K).
c. The cumulative amount of drug eliminated (X_u) in the urine at 7 h following the administration of a 500 mg dose.

Table P1.3

Time (h)	X_u (mg)
2.0	190.0
4.0	325.0
6.0	385.0
8.0	433.0
10.0	460.0
12.0	474.0
Infinity	500.0

Table P1.4

Time (h)	Mean serum concentrations ($\mu g\,mL^{-1}$ ($\pm$SD))
0.25	11.6 ± 1.3
0.50	8.4 ± 1.0
0.75	7.2 ± 1.1
1.00	6.1 ± 1.1
1.50	4.2 ± 1.0
2.00	3.2 ± 0.9
3.00	1.9 ± 0.7
4.00	1.0 ± 0.4
6.00	0.3 ± 0.2
8.00	0.09 ± 0.1

Question 4

Cinoxacin (Cinobac) is a synthetic organic antibacterial compound used in the urinary tract infection. Israel *et al.* (1978) reported serum concentrations (C_s) following intravenous bolus administration of 250 mg of cinoxacin to nine healthy male volunteers (Table P1.4).

Plot the data and, using the plot, determine the following.

a. The elimination half life ($t_{1/2}$).
b. The elimination rate constant (K).
c. The apparent volume of distribution (V).
d. The systemic clearance, Cl_s.
e. The area under the serum concentration time curve, $(AUC)_0^\infty$, by two different methods.
f. Israel *et al.* (1978) also assayed the urine samples for unchanged drug and a metabolite until 24 h. The percentage of the administered dose recovered in the urine as unchanged drug was 50.1%. Determine the renal clearance (Cl_r), metabolic clearance (Cl_m), the excretion rate constant (K_u), and the metabolite rate constant (K_m).

Question 5

Israel *et al.* (1978) reported urinary excretion data for cinoxacin following intravenous bolus

Table P1.5

Time interval (h)	Mass cinoxacin recovered in urine (mg (±SD))
0–2	88.0 ± 34
2–4	25.0 ± 13
4–6	10.0 ± 4
6–8	3.0 ± 3
8–24	0.4 ± 0.5

administration of 250 mg of drug to nine healthy male volunteers (Table P1.5).

Plot the data in suitable manners and, by means of your plot, determine the following.

a. The elimination rate constant (K).
b. A comparison of the elimination rate constant obtained by both methods.
c. A comparison of the elimination rate constant obtained by these methods with that obtained in question 4.
d. The excretion (K_u) and metabolite rate (K_m) constants.

Problem-solving exercise

Procainamide is used for the treatment of ventricular tachyarrhythmia. Its therapeutic range is 4–8 μg mL^{-1} and it is administered intravenously as well as by extravascular routes. The elimination half life and the apparent volume of distribution of procainamide are reported to be 3 h and 2 L kg^{-1}, respectively.

A patient (75 kg) is rushed to the hospital and a decision is made to administer an intravenous dose so that the plasma procainamide concentration of 7 μg mL^{-1} is attained immediately.

1. Determine the dose (X_0) required to attain concentration [$(C_p)_0$] 7 μg mL^{-1} immediately.
2. For how long will the procainamide plasma concentration remain within the therapeutic range?
3. Administration of 10.715 mg kg^{-1} procainamide hydrochloride dose to a subject yielded the initial plasma concentration of 5.3575

μg mL^{-1}. Determine the apparent volume of distribution.
4. Following the administration of a dose, the initial plasma concentration and the plasma concentration at 5 h are reported to be 5.3575 μg mL^{-1} and 1.6879 μg mL^{-1}, respectively. Determine the elimination half life ($t_{1/2}$) and the plasma concentration at 8 h following the administration of a 10 mg kg^{-1} dose.
5. It is also reported that 65% of the administered dose (750 mg) is excreted in the urine as procainamide and the remaining 35% of the dose appears in the urine as a metabolite (N-acetylprocainamide). Determine the amount of procainamide (i.e. amount excreted) in urine at 4 h, the amount of N-acetylprocainamide (i.e. amount of metabolite) in urine at 4 h and the total amount of drug eliminated at 4 h, following the administration of a 450 mg dose.
6. Determine the rate of elimination and the rate of excretion, at 3 h, following the administration of a 500 mg dose.
7. Determine systemic clearance, renal clearance and metabolic clearance for the drug from the available information.
8. Determine the area under the plasma concentration time curve $(AUC)_0^\infty$, by as many ways as possible, for 750 mg intravenous dose. What other information can be calculated from knowledge of the $(AUC)_0^\infty$?
9. What will be the effect of renal impairment?

Answers

This problem set will provide you with the plasma concentration versus time data (questions 1, 2 and 4) as well as urinary data (questions 3 and 5), following the intravenous bolus administration of a drug that follows the first-order process and exhibits the characteristics of a one-compartment model. The following are our answers to these five questions. Please note that your answers may differ from these owing to the techniques employed in obtaining the best fitting straight line for the data provided. These differences will, therefore, be reflected in the subsequent answers.

Question 1 answer

We plotted plasma concentration versus time data on a two-cycle semilogarithmic graph paper and then determined the following:

a. $t_{1/2} = 1.275\,h$.
b. $K = 0.543\,h^{-1}$.
c. $(C_p)_0 = 90\,\mu g\,mL^{-1}$. The initial plasma concentration is obtained from the intercept of the semilogarithmic plot of concentration versus time data. Please note that one can also determine initial plasma concentration by employing an equation:

$$C_p = (C_p)_0 e^{-Kt}$$

d. $V = Dose/(C_p)_0 = 2.77\,L$.
e. Plasma concentration at 75 min is 31.956 $\mu g\,mL^{-1}$. Use of the following equation permits the determination of the plasma concentration at any time t,

$$C_p = (C_p)_0 e^{-Kt}$$

where $(C_p)_0 = Dose/V = 175\,mg/2.77\ L = 63.176\,\mu g\,mL^{-1}; K = 0.543\,h^{-1}$; time is $75\,min = 1.25\,h$

f. The time at which the plasma concentration of the drug will fall below $20\,\mu g\,mL^{-1}$ is 2.94 h. Once again, the following equation can be used to determine the answer:

$$C_p = (C_p)_0 e^{-Kt}$$

where $(C_p)_0 = Dose/V = 275\,000\,\mu g/2770\,mL = 99.277\,\mu g\,mL^{-1};\quad K = 0.543\,h^{-1};\quad C_p = 20\,\mu g\,mL^{-1}$.

Question 2 answer

In this question, plasma concentration versus time data is provided following the administration of two different doses of a drug (cinoxacin; Cinobac). Because of the assumption of the first-order process and passive diffusion, one would expect the plasma concentration of a drug at any time to be directly proportional to the dose administered; however, the fundamental pharmacokinetic *parameters* of a drug will remain unaffected by the administered dose. We plotted plasma concentration versus time data on semi-logarithmic graph paper.

a. 50 mg dose: $t_{1/2} = 0.60\,h$
   100 mg dose: $t_{1/2} = 0.60\,h$

   (do not worry if you observe small differences in the elimination half life for each dose of the drug).

b. 50 mg dose: $K = 1.155\,h^{-1}$
   100 mg dose: $K = 1.155\,h^{-1}$

   (once again, do not be concerned about a small difference observed in the elimination rate constants).

c. Intercept of the semilogarithmic plot of the concentration versus time data for each dose will provide the initial plasma concentration for each dose

   50 mg dose: $(C_p)_0 = 2.55\,\mu g\,mL^{-1}$
   100 mg dose: $(C_p)_0 = 5.10\,\mu g\,mL^{-1}$.

Please note that one can also determine initial plasma concentration by employing an equation:

$$C_p = (C_p)_0 e^{-Kt}.$$

d. $V = Dose/(C_p)_0 = 19.60\,L$ for each dose.
e. You should find that the elimination half life, elimination rate constant and the apparent volume of distribution do not change with a change in dose.
f. Administered dose of cinoxacin is 79 159.93 μg, which is 79.159 mg or $1.130\,mg\,kg^{-1}$ for a 70 kg person; first determine the initial plasma concentration by employing the equation $C_p = (C_p)_0 e^{-Kt}$ using,

C_p at $2.5\,h = 225\,\mu g\,L^{-1}$
$K = 1.155\,h^{-1}$
$t = 2.5\,h$.

Once the initial plasma concentration $(C_p)_0$ is determined, one can calculate the administered dose from:

$$Dose = V \times (C_p)_0, \text{ where } V = 19.60\,L.$$

Question 3 answer

This question provides urinary data following the administration of an intravenous bolus dose

(500 mg) of a drug. Note that the drug is totally eliminated in urine by excretion (i.e. $K = K_u$ and $(X_u)_\infty =$ Dose administered). In addition, the cumulative amount of drug excreted and/or eliminated, at each time, is provided for you.

These data can be treated by two different methods to obtain some of the pharmacokinetic parameters of a drug; the ARE (amount of drug remained to be excreted) method and the rate of excretion method. The former requires determination of ARE at each time and then a plot of these values (mg) against time on appropriate semilogarithmic graph paper. The rate of excretion method requires determination of the rate of excretion (dX/dt) at each time and then a plot of the rate of excretion against average time on an appropriate semilogarithmic paper. From such plots, the following can be determined:

a. $t_{1/2} = 2.8$ h.
b. $K = 0.2475$ h^{-1}.
c. At 7 h, $X_u = X_0(1 - e^{-Kt})$, where X_0 is the administered dose (375 mg); therefore, $X_u = 308.45$ mg.

Please note, as time increases, greater amounts of drug will be in the urine and lesser amounts of drug will be in the body (blood). At $t = \infty$, the entire dose will have been excreted in the urine.

Question 4 answer

This question provides the plasma concentration versus time data following the intravenous bolus administration (250 mg dose) of cinoxacin, a drug that is used for urinary tract infections, to nine healthy volunteers.

In this problem, in addition to determining the pharmacokinetic parameters such as the elimination half life, elimination rate constant and the apparent volume of distribution of the drug, the systemic clearance of the drug and the area under the plasma concentration time curve for the administered dose of the drug are required. The plot of plasma concentration versus time data was made on suitable semilogarithmic paper. From the graph, the following can be determined (for healthy subjects):

a. $t_{1/2} = 1.2$ h.
b. $K = 0.577$ h^{-1}.

c. $V = 20.833$ L.
d. $Cl_s = VK = 20.833$ L $\times 0.577$ h$^{-1} = 12.02$ L h^{-1}.
e. AUC can be determined by the trapezoidal method and/or by employing the equation

$(AUC)_0^\infty = X_0/VK$
$(AUC)_0^\infty = 19.177 \,\mu g \,mL^{-1}$ h (trapezoidal rule)
$(AUC)_0^\infty = 20.797 \,\mu g \,mL^{-1}$ h (by equation).

f. Since it is reported that the 50.1% of the administered dose (250 mg) is recovered in urine as unchanged drug, the remaining 49.1% is recovered in urine as a metabolite; this is used to determine the excretion and metabolite rate constants for the drug:

$K_u = K \times \%$ excreted $= 0.577$ h$^{-1} \times 0.501 = 0.289$ h^{-1}
$K_m = K \times \%$ metabolite $= 0.577$ h$^{-1} \times 0.499 = 0.287$ h^{-1}
$Cl_r = K_u V_r = 0.289$ h$^{-1} \times 20.833$ L $= 6.020$ L h^{-1}
$Cl_m = K_m V = 0.287$ h$^{-1} \times 20.833$ L $= 5.979$ L h^{-1}.

Please note that systemic clearance is the sum of the renal and metabolic clearances. Therefore, $Cl_s = Cl_r + Cl_m = 6.020$ L h$^{-1} + 5.979$ L h^{-1} $= 11.999$ L h^{-1}.

Question 5 answer

This question provided urinary data for a drug that is *not totally removed in an unchanged form* (excretion). Furthermore, it is equally important to note that the data provides the amount of drug excreted in the urine at each time (i.e. not the cumulative amount excreted). Therefore, it is absolutely essential to transform the data provided into the cumulative amount excreted. Such transformation will clearly suggest that the cumulative amount excreted at 24 h is not equal to the administered dose of a drug. From the knowledge of the amount excreted at 24 h and the administered dose, it is easy to determine the cumulative amount of metabolite in the urine.

Follow the ARE method (plot of ARE against time on a suitable semilogarithmic graph paper) and rate of excretion method (plot of dX_u/dt against the average time on a suitable semilogarithmic graph paper). From the graph the following are obtained:

a. $K = 0.577$ h^{-1}.

b. The elimination rate constant is identical, regardless of the method employed.

c. The elimination rate constant is identical whether the drug is monitored in plasma (question 4) or urine (question 5).

d. $K_u = 0.295\,h^{-1}$
$K_m = 0.282\,h^{-1}$.

Please note that sum of these rate constant should be equal to the elimination rate constant.

Problem-solving exercise answer

1. Dose (X_0) required to attain concentration $[(C_p)_0]$ 7 $\mu g\,mL^{-1}$ immediately:

$$\frac{Dose}{V} = \frac{X_0}{V} = (C_p)_0$$

$X_0 = (C_p)_0 \times V = 7\,\mu g\,mL^{-1} \times 2000\,mL\,kg^{-1} = 14\,000\,\mu g\,kg^{-1}$. This is $14\,mg\,kg^{-1}$.

Alternatively,

$V = 2000\,mL\,kg^{-1} \times 75\,kg$ (patient's weight) $= 150\,000\,mL$. This is $150\,L$.
$X_0 = (C_p)_0 \times V = 7\,\mu g\,mL^{-1} \times 150\,000\,mL = 1\,050\,000\,\mu g$. This is $1050\,mg$.

2. The time for which the procainamide plasma concentration will remain within the therapeutic range can be calculated from:

$$C_p = (C_p)_0 e^{-Kt}$$

$$\frac{C_p}{(C_p)_0} = e^{-Kt}$$

$$\frac{\ln\left(\frac{C_p}{(C_p)_0}\right)}{-K} = t$$

$(C_p)_0 = 7\,\mu g\,mL^{-1}$; $K = 0.231\,h^{-1}$; $C_p = 4\,\mu g\,mL^{-1}$.

$$t = \frac{\ln\left(\frac{4\,\mu g\,mL^{-1}}{7\,\mu g\,mL^{-1}}\right)}{-0.231\,h^{-1}} = \frac{-0.55961}{-0.231\,h^{-1}} = 2.422\,h.$$

At 2.42 h, following the administration of an intravenous bolus dose, the plasma procainamide concentration will be $4\,\mu g\,mL^{-1}$ and after 2.42 h the procainamide plasma concentration will be *below* the therapeutic range of the drug.

3. The apparent volume of distribution is determined from:

$$\frac{Dose}{V} = (C_p)_0$$

$$\frac{Dose}{(C_p)_0} = V$$

As dose is $10.715\,mg\,kg^{-1}$ and $(C_p)_0$ is 5.3575 $\mu g\,mL^{-1}$,

$$\frac{10\,715\,\mu g\,kg^{-1}}{5.3575\,\mu g\,kg^{-1}} = V = 2000\,mL\,kg^{-1}.$$

4a. The elimination half life $(t_{1/2})$ following the $10\,mg\,kg^{-1}$ dose is given by $0.693/K$ where $-K = (slope \times 2.303)$.

$$Slope = \frac{\log y_2 - \log y_1}{t_2 - t_1}$$

$$Slope = \frac{\log 1.6879 - \log 5.3575}{5.0\,h - 0\,h}$$

$$= \frac{0.2273 - 0.7289}{5.00\,h} = \frac{-0.5016}{5.00\,h}$$

$$Slope = -0.10032\,h^{-1}$$

So $K = (0.10032\,h^{-1} \times 2.303) = 0.2310\,h^{-1}$.
$t_{1/2} = 0.693/K = 0.693/0.231\,h^{-1} = 3\,h$.

b. The plasma concentration (C_p) at 8 h after the dose is given by $(C_p)_0 e^{-Kt}$, where

$$(C_p)_0 = Dose/V = 10\,000\,\mu g\,kg^{-1}/$$
$$2000\,mL\,kg^{-1} = 5\,\mu g\,mL^{-1}$$
$$K = 0.231\,h^{-1}$$
$$t = 8\,h$$
$$C_p = 5\,\mu g/mL \times e^{-(0.231\,h^{-1})(8\,h)}$$

So at 8 h, $C_p = 5\,\mu g\,mL^{-1} \times 0.15755$
$= 0.78775\,\mu g\,mL^{-1}$.

5. Values for the elimination rate constant (K), the excretion rate constant (K_u) and the metabolic rate constant (K_m) are required to calculate the amount of procainamide (unchanged form) excreted in urine at 4 h, the amount of the metabolite N-acetylprocainamide in urine

at 4 h and the total amount of drug eliminated at 4 h:

$$\text{Dose} = 450\,\text{mg}$$
$$K = 0.231\,\text{h}^{-1}$$
$$K_u = K \times \%\ \text{excreted} = 0.231\,\text{h}^{-1} \times 0.65$$
$$= 0.150\,\text{h}^{-1}$$
$$K_m = K \times \%\ \text{metabolite} = 0.231\,\text{h}^{-1} \times 0.35$$
$$= 0.0808\,\text{h}^{-1}.$$

a. Cumulative amount of procainamide (unchanged form) in the urine at 4 h, $(X_u)_4$, can be determined as follows:

$$(X_u)_4 = \frac{K_u \text{Dose}}{K}(1 - e^{-Kt})$$

$$\frac{(0.150\,\text{h}^{-1})(450\,\text{mg})}{0.231\,\text{h}}(1 - e^{-(0.231)(4)}) =$$

$$\frac{(0.150\,\text{h}^{-1})(450\,\text{mg})}{0.231\,\text{h}}(1 - e^{-0.924}) =$$

$$\frac{(0.150\,\text{h}^{-1})(450\,\text{mg})}{0.231\,\text{h}}(1 - 0.3969) =$$

$$(292.21\,\text{mg})(0.6031)$$

$$(X_u)_4 = 292.2077\,\text{mg} \times 0.6031$$
$$= 176.230\,\text{mg}.$$

b. The cumulative amount of N-acetylprocainamide (metabolite) in urine at 4 h $[(X_{mu})_4]$ can be determined as follows:

$$(X_{mu}) = \frac{K_m \text{Dose}}{K}(1 - e^{-Kt}) =$$

$$\frac{(0.0808\,\text{h}^{-1})(450\,\text{mg})}{0.231\,\text{h}}(1 - e^{-(0.231)(4)}) =$$

$$\frac{(0.0808\,\text{h}^{-1})(450\,\text{mg})}{0.231\,\text{h}}(1 - e^{-0.924}) =$$

$$\frac{(0.0808\,\text{h}^{-1})(450\,\text{mg})}{0.231\,\text{h}}(1 - 0.3969) =$$

$$(157.40\,\text{mg})(0.6031)$$

$$(X_{mu})_4 = 157.4025\,\text{mg} \times 0.6031$$
$$= 94.929\,\text{mg}.$$

c. The total amount of drug eliminated from the body at 4 h is the sum of the renal excretion and the metabolic clearance:

$$(X_{el})_4 = (X_u)_4 + (X_{mu})_4$$
$$(X_{el})_4 = 176.230\,\text{mg} + 94.929\,\text{mg} = 271.159\,\text{mg}$$

Alternatively, total amount of drug eliminated $(X_{el})_4$ by time t is:

$$(X_{el})_4 = \text{Dose}\,[1 - e^{-Kt}]$$
$$(X_{el})_4 = 450\,\text{mg}\,[1 - e^{-0.231 \times 4}]$$
$$= 450\,\text{mg}\,[1 - e^{-0.924}]$$
$$(X_{el})_4 = 450\,\text{mg}\,[1 - 0.3969]$$
$$= 450\,\text{mg} \times 0.6031$$
$$= 271.395\,\text{mg}.$$

6a. Rate of elimination (dX_u/dt) at 3 h:

$$\frac{-dX}{dt} = KX_0 e^{-Kt}$$

where X is the amount of drug in the body at time t and X_0 is the administered dose.

$$\frac{-dX}{dt} = (0.231\,\text{h}^{-1})(500\,\text{mg})(e^{-(0.231\,\text{h}^{-1})(3\,\text{h})})$$
$$= 115.5\,\text{mg h}^{-1}(e^{-0.693})$$
$$= 115.5\,\text{mg h}^{-1}(0.500) = 57.75\,\text{mg h}^{-1}.$$

b. Rate of renal excretion of procainamide at 3 h is determined by an analogous approach:

$$\frac{dX_u}{dt} = K_u X_0 e^{-Kt}$$

$$\frac{dX_u}{dt} = (0.150\,\text{h}^{-1})(500\,\text{mg})(e^{-(0.231\,\text{h}^{-1})(3\,\text{h})})$$
$$= 75\,\text{mg h}^{-1}(e^{-0.693})$$
$$= 75\,\text{mg h}^{-1}(0.500)$$
$$= 37.5\,\text{mg h}^{-1}.$$

7a. Systemic clearance $(Cl_s) = VK$:

$$K = 0.693/t_{1/2} = 0.693/3\,\text{h} = 0.231\,\text{h}^{-1}$$
$$Cl_s = VK = 140\,000\,\text{mL} \times 0.231\,\text{h}^{-1}$$
$$\text{or } 2000\,\text{mL kg}^{-1} \times 0.231\,\text{h}^{-1}$$
$$Cl_s = 32\,340\,\text{mL h}^{-1} \text{ or } 32.34\,\text{L h}^{-1}$$
$$\text{or } 462\,\text{mL kg}^{-1}\text{h}^{-1}.$$

b. Renal clearance $Cl_r = K_u V$:

$$K_u = K \times \%\ \text{excreted} = 0.231\,\text{h}^{-1} \times 0.65 =$$
$$0.150\,\text{h}^{-1}$$
$$Cl_r = 0.150\,\text{h}^{-1} \times 140.0\,\text{L} = 21.021\,\text{L h}^{-1}$$
$$(21\,021\,\text{mL h}^{-1})$$
$$Cl_r = 0.150\,\text{h}^{-1} \times 2.0\,\text{L kg}^{-1} = 0.3\,\text{L kg}^{-1}\text{h}^{-1} \text{ on}$$
a body weight basis.

Alternatively,

$Cl_r = Cl_s \times \%$ excreted
$Cl_r = 32.34\,L\,h^{-1} \times 0.65 = 21.021\,L\,h^{-1}$
$(21\,021\,mL\,h^{-1})$.

c. Metabolic clearance Cl_m:

$Cl_m = K_m V$
$K_m = K \times \%$ metabolite $= 0.231\,h^{-1} \times 0.35 = 0.0808\,h^{-1}$
$Cl_m = 0.0808\,h^{-1} \times 140.0\,L = 11.319\,L\,h^{-1}$
$(11\,319\,mL\,h^{-1})$.
$Cl_m = 0.0808\,h^{-1} \times 2.0\,L\,kg^{-1}$
$= 0.1616\,L\,kg^{-1}\,h^{-1}$ on a body weight basis.
Alternatively,
$Cl_m = Cl_s \times \%$ metabolite
$Cl_m = 32.34\,L\,h^{-1} \times 0.35 = 11.319\,L\,h^{-1}$
$(11\,319\,mL\,h^{-1})$.

Important comments on question 7. Total (systemic) clearance is the sum of all the individual clearances:

$Cl_s = Cl_r + Cl_m$
$Cl_s = 21.021\,L\,h^{-1} + 11.319\,L\,h^{-1} = 32.34\,L\,h^{-1}$
$(32\,340\,mL\,h^{-1})$.
$Cl_s = VK$,
so $K = Cl_s/V = 32.34\,L\,h^{-1}/140\,L = 0.231\,h^{-1}$,
and $V = Cl_s/K = 32.34\,L\,h^{-1}/0.231\,h^{-1} = 140\,L$
Analogously for Cl_r:
$Cl_r = K_u V$
$K_u = Cl_r/V = 21.021\,L\,h^{-1}/140\,L = 0.150\,h^{-1}$
and $V = Cl_r/K_u = 21.021\,L\,h^{-1}/0.150\,h^{-1}$
$= 140.14\,L$
Analogously for Cl_m:
$Cl_m = K_m V$
$K_m = Cl_m/V = 11.319\,L\,h^{-1}/140\,L = 0.0808\,h^{-1}$
and $V = Cl_m/K_m = 11.319\,L\,h^{-1}/0.0808\,h^{-1}$
$= 140\,L$.
Percentage excreted can be calculated from:
$K = K_u + K_m$
$K = 0.150\,h^{-1} + 0.0808\,h^{-1} = 0.2308\,h^{-1}$
fraction excreted $= K_u/K = 0.150\,h^{-1}/0.231\,h^{-1}$
$= 0.6493$
% excreted in urine = fraction excreted $\times$ 100 $= 0.6493 \times 100 = 64.93\%$
fraction drug removed as metabolite $= K_m/K$
$= 0.0808\,h^{-1}/0.231\,h^{-1} = 0.3497$
% metabolite = fraction excreted $\times$ 100
$= 0.3497 \times 100\,34.97\%$.

The systemic clearance, renal clearance and metabolic clearance can also be determined from the knowledge of the rate of elimination, the rate of excretion and rate of metabolite formation at a given time for the corresponding plasma concentration. For example, if the rate of elimination and plasma concentration at a specific time are known, the systemic clearance can be determined.

For the 500 mg dose procainamide hydrochloride, the rate of elimination (dX_u/dt) at 3 h was calculated as 57.75 mg h^{-1} (in answer 6a, above) and the plasma concentration at 3 h $[(C_p)_3]$ can be calculated as follows:

$C_p = (C_p)_0\,e^{-Kt}$

where $(C_p)_0 = $ Dose$/V = 3.5714\,\mu g\,mL^{-1}$
So $(C_p)_3 = 3.5714\,e^{-0.231 \times 3} = 3.5714 \times 0.500$
$= 1.785\,\mu g\,mL^{-1}$.
$Cl_s = (dX_u/dt)/C_p$

$$Cl_s = \frac{57.75\,mg\,h^{-1}}{1.785\,\mu g\,mL^{-1}} = \frac{57750\,\mu g\,h^{-1}}{1.785\,\mu g\,mL^{-1}}$$
$$Cl_s = 32352\,mL\,h^{-1}\,(32.35\,L\,h^{-1}).$$

Using a similar approach, the renal clearance of procainamide at 3 h can be determined. The rate of excretion (dX_u/dt) is 37.5 mg h^{-1} (calculated in answer 6b). The $Cl_r = (dX_u/dt)/C_p$

$$Cl_r = \frac{37.50\,mg\,h^{-1}}{1.785\,\mu g\,mL^{-1}} = \frac{37\,500\,\mu g\,h^{-1}}{1.785\,\mu g\,mL^{-1}}$$
$$Cl_r = 21\,008\,mL\,h^{-1}\,(21.008\,L\,h^{-1}).$$

Once the values of the excretion (K_u) and the metabolite (K_m) rate constants are known, the cumulative amount excreted in urine at a given time, the cumulative amount of a metabolite in urine at this time and the total amount of the drug eliminated at this time can be determined. For example, question 5 of this problem-solving exercise asked for determination of the amount of procainamide in urine at 4 h, the amount of N-acetylprocainamide in urine at 4 h and the amount of dose eliminated at 4 h following the administration of a 450 mg dose.

8. Determination of $(AUC)_0^\infty$ for an intravenous dose (750 mg).

$$(AUC)_0^\infty = \frac{Dose}{VK} = \frac{Dose}{Cl_s}$$
$$(AUC)_0^\infty = 750\,000\,\mu g/32\,340\,mL\,h^{-1}$$
$$= 23.1911\,\mu g\,mL^{-1}\,h.$$

Alternatively, as

$$(AUC)_0^\infty = \frac{Dose}{VK} \quad \text{and} \quad \frac{Dose}{VK} = (C_p)_0$$

$(C_p)_0 = Dose/V = 750\,000\,\mu g/140\,000\,mL$
$\quad = 5.3571\,\mu g\,mL^{-1}$
$K = 0.231\,h^{-1}$ (determined above).

Therefore, $(AUC)_0^\infty = (C_p)_0/K = 5.3571$
$\mu g\,mL^{-1}/0.231\,h^{-1} = 23.1911\,\mu g\,mL^{-1}\,h.$

Using the $(AUC)_0^\infty$, one can calculate other parameters such as the amount of drug excreted in urine at time ∞, $(X_u)_\infty$, and the amount of metabolite in urine at time ∞, $(X_{mu})_\infty$.

$$Cl_r = \frac{(X_u)_\infty}{(AUC)_0^\infty}$$

$(X_u)_\infty = Cl_r \times (AUC)_0^\infty$
$(X_u)_\infty = 21\,021\,mL\,h^{-1} \times 23.1911\,\mu g\,mL^{-1}\,h$
$\quad = 487\,500.11\,\mu g\,(487.50\,mg).$

Analogously, metabolite clearance in urine is:

$$Cl_m = \frac{(X_{mu})_\infty}{(AUC)_0^\infty}$$

$(X_{mu})_\infty = Cl_m \times (AUC)_0^\infty = 11\,319\,mL\,h^{-1}$
$\quad \times 23.1911\,\mu g\,mL^{-1}\,h = 262\,500.060\,\mu g$
$(262.50\,mg).$

Alternatively, the amount excreted and amount of metabolite in urine can be calculated as follows.

$$(X_u)_\infty = \frac{K_u Dose}{K}$$

$$(X_u)_\infty = \frac{0.150\,h^{-1} \times 750\,mg}{0.231\,h^{-1}}$$
$$= 487.012\,mg\,procainamide.$$

$$(X_{mu})_\infty = \frac{K_m Dose}{K}$$

$$(X_{mu})_\infty = \frac{0.0808\,h^{-1} \times 750\,mg}{0.231\,h^{-1}}$$
$$= 262.33\,mg\,N\text{-acetylprocainamide.}$$

This can be checked by adding $(Xu)_\infty$ and $(X_{mu})_\infty$, which should be the dose given.

9. In a patient with renal impairment, the elimination half life of procainamide is reported to be 14 h (The range is 9–43 h):

$K = 0.693/t_{1/2} = 0.693/14\,h = 0.0495\,h^{-1}$
$Cl_s = VK$
$Cl_s = 140\,000\,mL \times 0.0495\,h^{-1} = 6930\,mL\,h^{-1}$
$(6.930\,L\,h^{-1}).$ Normal value is $32340\,mL\,h^{-1}.$

5

Drug absorption from the gastrointestinal tract

Objectives

Upon completion of this chapter, you will have the ability to:

- explain both passive and active mechanisms of drug absorption from the gastrointestinal tract
- use Fick's law of diffusion to predict the effect of various factors affecting rate of drug absorption
- use the Henderson–Hasselbalch equation to calculate the fraction ionized of a weakly acidic or a weakly basic drug at a given pH and its significance in drug absorption.

5.1 Gastrointestinal tract

Figures 5.1 and 5.2 provide an overview of the microanatomy of the human stomach (Fig. 5.1) and intestines (Fig. 5.2).

When drug molecules pass through the gastrointestinal tract, they encounter different environments with respect to the pH, enzymes, electrolytes, surface characteristics and viscosity of the gastrointestinal fluids. All these factors can influence drug absorption and interactions. Variations in the pH of various portions of the gastrointestinal tract are depicted in Fig. 5.3.

Important features of the gastrointestinal tract

The following are some of the important features of the human gastrointestinal tract.

1. There is a copious blood supply.
2. The entire tract is lined with mucous membrane through which drugs may be readily transferred into the general circulation.
3. The interior surface of the stomach is relatively smooth.

4. The small intestine presents numerous folds and projections.
5. Approximately 8–10 L per day of fluids are produced or secreted into the gastrointestinal tract and an additional 1–2 L of fluid is obtained via food and fluid intake.
6. The gastrointestinal tract is highly perfused by a capillary network, which allows absorption and distribution of drugs to occur. This immediate circulation drains drug molecules into the portal circulation, where absorbed drugs are carried to the liver and may undergo first-pass effect.

Important features of the stomach

1. The stomach contents are in pH range of 1–3.5; with a pH of 1–2.5 being the most commonly observed.
2. The squeezing action of the stomach produces a mild but thorough agitation of the gastric contents.
3. A dosage form (tablet, capsule, etc.) may remain in the stomach for approximately 0.5–2 h prior to moving to the pylorus and to the duodenum. This transfer of drug may be

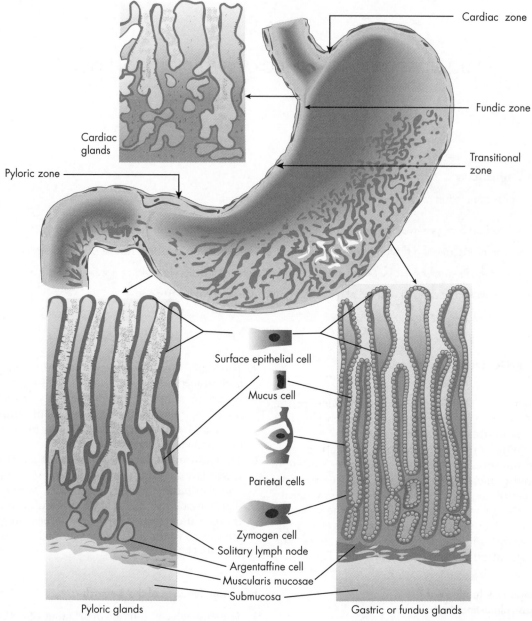

Cardiac zone

Fundic zone

Transitional zone

Cardiac glands

Pyloric zone

Surface epithelial cell

Mucus cell

Parietal cells

Zymogen cell
Solitary lymph node
Argentaffine cell
Muscularis mucosae
Submucosa

Pyloric glands

Gastric or fundus glands

Figure 5.1   Mucous membrane of stomach. (From Netter FH (1959). *The Ciba Collection of Medical Illustrations*: Vol. 3, Part 1, *Upper Digestive Tract*. Ciba Pharmaceutical Co., Basel, Switzerland, p. 52.)

rapid on the fasting stomach or very slow if taken with heavy high fat meal. Furthermore, this gastric emptying of a drug can be influenced by factors such as the type of food, volume of liquid, viscosity and temperature.

Important features of the duodenum

1. In the duodenum, drugs are subjected to a drastic change of pH (pH range 5–7).
2. Drugs will encounter additional enzymes that were not present earlier (in the stomach).

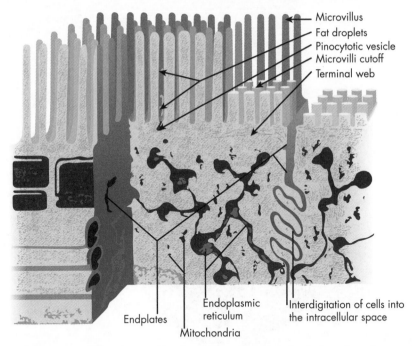

Figure 5.2   Three-dimensional schema of striated border of intestinal epithelial cells (based on ultramicroscopic studies). (From Netter FH (1962). *The Ciba Collection of Medical Illustrations*: Vol 3, Part 2, *Lower Digestive Tract*. Ciba Pharmaceutical Co., Basel, Switzerland, p. 50.)

3. The duodenum, jejunum and upper region of ileum provide the most efficient areas in the gastrointestinal tract for drug absorption.
4. The occurrence of villi presents a large surface area for the transport of drug molecules into the systemic circulation (absorption).
5. The capillary network in the villi and microvilli is the primary pathway by which most drugs reach the circulation.

Some drugs are absorbed better from the stomach than from the intestine and vice versa. Drugs that are ideal for gastric absorption are only partly (10–30%) absorbed from the stomach before reaching the small intestine. This is because of the short residence time (30–120 min) in the stomach and the limited surface area.

For absorption to begin, drugs administered orally should be in a physiologically available form (i.e. solution). The rate of drug absorption, in turn, will affect the onset of action, duration of action, bioavailability and the amount absorbed.

5.2 Mechanism of drug absorption

Following the administration of a drug in a dosage form, drug molecules must somehow gain access to the bloodstream, where the distribution process will take it to the "site of action." For absorption to occur, therefore, the drug molecule must first pass through a membrane.

Membrane physiology: the gastrointestinal barrier

The membrane that separates the lumen of the stomach and the intestine from the systemic circulation and site of drug absorption is a complex structure;

- it is made up of lipids, proteins, lipoproteins and polysaccharide material
- it is semipermeable in nature or selectively permeable (i.e. allowing rapid passage of some chemicals while restricting others).

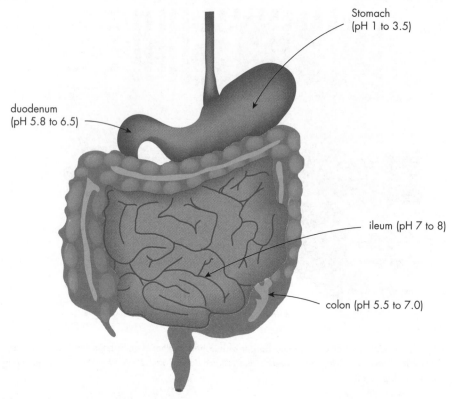

Stomach
(pH 1 to 3.5)

duodenum
(pH 5.8 to 6.5)

ileum (pH 7 to 8)

colon (pH 5.5 to 7.0)

Figure 5.3 Variations in pH along the gastrointestinal tract.

For example: amino acids, sugars and fatty acids will cross the membrane, while virtually no transfer of plasma proteins and certain toxins will occur. Figure 5.4 is a schematic of drug being absorbed across the gastrointestinal membrane.

Active and passive mechanisms of drug absorption

Once the drug is available in solution form, there are two major processes available for drug absorption to occur:

- active transport
- passive diffusion.

Passive diffusion

The membrane plays a passive role in drug absorption during passive diffusion; most drugs pass through membrane by this mechanism. The rate of drug transfer is determined by the physicochemical properties of the drug and the drug concentration gradient across the membrane. The driving force for the movement of drug molecules from the gastrointestinal fluid to the blood is the drug concentration gradient (i.e. the difference between the concentration of drug in the gastrointestinal fluid and that in the bloodstream). The passage of drug molecules through the membrane being a continuous process, there will always be an appreciable concentration gradient between the gastrointestinal tract and the bloodstream (because of volume differences), which, in turn, will yield a continuous drug transfer and maintain a so-called "sink" condition.

Passive diffusion or transfer follows first-order kinetics (i.e. the rate of transfer is directly proportional to the concentration of drug at absorption and/or measurement sites).

Active transport

Chemical carriers in the membrane combine with drug molecules and carry them through the

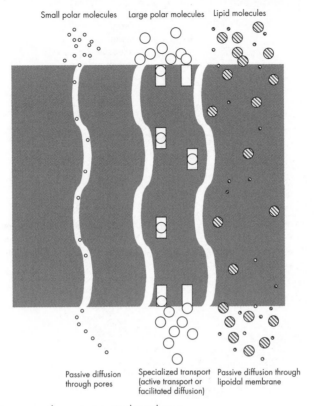

Small polar molecules   Large polar molecules   Lipid molecules

Passive diffusion through pores   Specialized transport (active transport or facilitated diffusion)   Passive diffusion through lipoidal membrane

Figure 5.4   Drug absorption across the gastrointestinal membrane.

membrane to be discharged on the other side. This process is called active transport because the membrane plays an active role. Important features are that chemical energy is needed and that molecules can be transferred from a region of low concentration to one of higher concentration (i.e. against a concentration gradient.) Fig. 5.5 shows a drug in solution being absorbed via active transport.

The striking difference between active and passive transport, however, is that active transport is a saturable process and, therefore, obeys laws of saturation or enzyme kinetics. This means that the rate of absorption, unlike that of passive diffusion, is not directly proportional to the drug concentration in large doses.

The rate of absorption reaches a saturation point, at which time an increase in drug concentration (larger doses) does not result in a directly proportional increase in the rate of absorption. This is because of a limited number of carriers in the membrane.

$$\text{Absorption rate} = \frac{dC_a}{dt} = \frac{V_{max}C_a}{K_m + C_a} \qquad (5.1)$$

where V_{max} is the theoretical maximum rate of the process; K_m is the Michaelis–Menten constant (i.e. the concentration of drug at the absorption site when the absorption rate is half of V_{max}); C_a is the concentration of drug at the absorption site (e.g. in the gastrointestinal tract) at a given time.

At low solute concentration (i.e. at low doses): $K_m \gg C_a$

$$\text{Absorption rate} = \frac{V_{max}C_a}{K_m}$$

However, $V_{max}/K_m = K$; therefore:

$$\text{Rate of absorption} = KC_a \qquad (5.2)$$

This equation, by nature, is a first-order equation. At this condition (i.e. low doses) there are

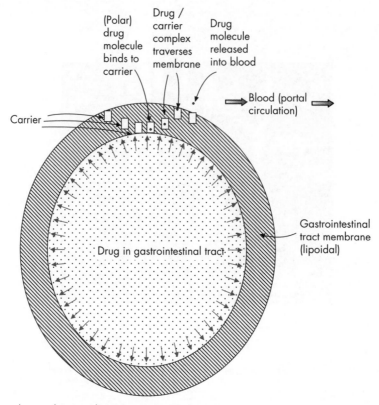

Figure 5.5 Cell membrane, showing absorption via active transport.

sufficient number of carriers available to transport the number of drug molecules presented to the membrane.

At high solute concentration (i.e. high doses): because of a much larger concentration of drug molecules, the number of available carriers are insufficient and $C_a \gg K_m$

Therefore,

$$\text{Absorption rate} = \frac{dC_a}{dt} = \frac{V_{max}C_a}{C_a}$$

or

$$\text{Absorption rate} = V_{max}/K_m = K_0 \qquad (5.3)$$

Because V_{max} is a constant for a given drug, this equation represents a zero-order process.

Drugs that are believed to be transported by this mechanism include phenytoin, methyldopa, nicotinamide, vitamin B_{12}, 5-fluorouracil and thiamine.

5.3 Factors affecting passive drug absorption

Fick's law of diffusion

Passive diffusion involves transfer of drug molecules from a region of high concentration to a region of low concentration, with the driving force being the effective drug concentration on one side of membrane. Fick's law mathematically describes the process. The equation can be written as,

$$dC/dt = K(C_{GIT} - C_{blood}) \qquad (5.4)$$

where K is the specific permeability coefficient, given by

$$K = \frac{K_{m/f}AD}{h}$$

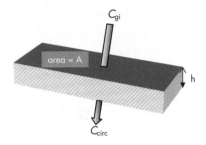

$$\frac{dC_{circ}}{dt} = \frac{DKA}{h}(C_{gi} - C_{circ}) \simeq \frac{DKA}{h}(C_{gi})$$

Figure 5.6 Absorption in terms of Fick's law of diffusion. GIT, gastrointestinal tract; dC/dt, rate of absorption; $K_{m/f}$, partition coefficient of the drug between the membrane (lipid) and the GIT fluid (aqueous); A, the surface area of the membrane; D, diffusion coefficient of the drug; h, membrane thickness; C_{GIT}, drug concentration in GIT fluids; C_B, free drug concentration in blood of membranes; $C_{GIT} - C_B$, concentration gradient across membrane; K, special permeability coefficient.

Fick's law of diffusion states that the rate of absorption (dC/dt) is directly proportional to:

- the surface area (A) of a membrane
- the membrane to fluid partition coefficient ($K_{m/f}$) of a drug
- the diffusion coefficient (D) of the drug.

The rate of absorption (dC/dt) is inversely proportional to:

- the membrane thickness (h).

Figure 5.6 shows the process of absorption in terms of Fick's law of diffusion.

The partition coefficient ($K_{m/f}$, K or P)

Consider a single solute (drug) species that is distributed between two immiscible liquids:

solute in lower phase ↔ solute in upper phase.

At equilibrium, the ratio of concentration of solute (drug) species in two phases is constant:

$K_{m/f} =$

$$\frac{\text{Concentration of drug in upper phase } (C_U)}{\text{Concentration of drug in lower phase } (C_L)}$$

where $K_{m/f}$ is the partition coefficient of a drug (also given by K or P).

Usually one of the two phases is aqueous (a buffer of biological pH or water); the second phase is the organic solvent or oil

$$K_{m/f}(\text{or P, or } K) = \frac{C_{organic}}{C_{aqueous}} \text{ or } \frac{C_{oil}}{C_{water}}$$

where $C_{organic}$ is the concentration of drug in upper or organic phase and $C_{aqueous}$ is the concentration of drug in lower or aqueous phase.

A guide to lipid solubility of a drug is provided by its partition coefficient (P or K) between a water-immiscible organic solvent (such as chloroform, olive oil or octanol) and water or an aqueous buffer.

Octanol and olive oil are believed to represent the lipophilic characteristics of biological membrane better than other organic solvents such as chloroform.

Some drugs may be poorly absorbed following oral administration even though they are present in a largely unionized form. This may be because of the low lipid solubility of the unionized species.

The effect of the partition coefficient and, therefore, of lipid solubility, on the absorption of a series of barbituric acid derivatives is shown in Fig. 5.7.

5.4 pH–partition theory of drug absorption

The dissociation constant, expressed as pK_a, the lipid solubility of a drug, as well as the pH at the

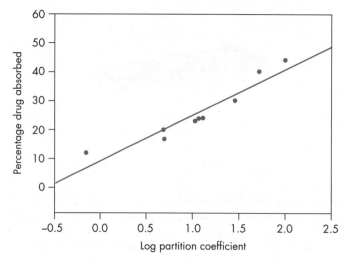

Figure 5.7   The effect of the partition coefficient on the absorption of a series of barbituric acid derivatives.

absorption site often dictate the magnitude of the absorption of a drug following its availability as a solution. The interrelationship among these parameters (pH, pK_a and lipid solubility) is known as the pH–partition theory of drug absorption. This theory is based on the following assumptions:

1. The drug is absorbed by passive transfer
2. The drug is preferentially absorbed in unionized form
3. The drug is sufficiently lipid soluble.

The fraction of drug available in unionized form is a function of both the dissociation constant of the drug and the pH of the solution at the site of administration. The dissociation constant, for both acids and bases, is often expressed as $-\log K_a$, referred to as pK_a.

For weak acids

Ionization of weak acids is described by an adaptation of a classical Henderson–Hasselbalch equation.

$$pH - pK_a = \log \frac{\alpha}{1 - \alpha} \qquad (5.5)$$

where α is the the fraction of ionized species and $(1 - \alpha)$ is the fraction of unionized species. The equation may, therefore, be written as,

$$\frac{\alpha}{1 - \alpha} = 10^{(pH - pK_a)} \qquad (5.6)$$

or

$$\frac{\alpha}{1 - \alpha} = \text{antilog} \ (pH - pK_a)$$

This equation clearly indicates that the ratio of ionized/unionized species, $\alpha/(1 - \alpha)$, is solely dependent upon pH and the pK_a.

For weak acids

- when $pH = pK_a$, $\alpha = 0.5$, or 50% of the drug is in ionized form
- when pH is 1 unit *greater* than pK_a, $\alpha = 0.909$, or ~90% of the drug, is in ionized form
- when pH is 2 units *greater* than pK_a, $\alpha = 0.99$, or 99% of the drug, is in ionized form
- when pH is 1 unit *below* pK_a, $1 - \alpha = 0.9$, or 90% of the drug, is in unionized form
- when pH is 2 unit *below* pK_a, $1 - \alpha = 0.99$, or 99% of the drug, is in unionized form.

As the pH of the solution increases, the degree of ionization (percentage ionized) also increases.

Hence, weak acids are preferentially absorbed at low pH.

For weak bases

For weak bases, the Henderson–Hasselbalch equation takes the following form:

$$pK_a - pH = \log \frac{\alpha}{1-\alpha} \tag{5.7}$$

which is analogous to

$$\frac{\alpha}{1-\alpha} = 10^{(pK_a - pH)}$$

or

$$\frac{\alpha}{1-\alpha} = \text{antilog}\,(pK_a - pH) \tag{5.8}$$

Equations 5.7 and 5.8 suggest that the value of $\alpha/(1-\alpha)$ or the degree of ionized/unionized species is solely dependent upon the pH and pK_a and that the degree of ionization (percentage

ionized) decreases as the pH of the solution increases:

- when $pH = pK_a$, $\alpha = 0.5$, or 50% of the drug is in the ionized form
- when pH is 1 unit *below* pK_a, $\alpha = 0.909$, or ~90% of the drug, is in the ionized form
- when pH is 2 units below pK_a, $\alpha = 0.99$, or 99% of the drug, is in the ionized form
- when pH is 1 unit *above* the pK_a of the drug, $1 - \alpha = 0.909$, or ~90% of the drug, is present in unionized form
- when pH is 2 units *above* pK_a, $1 - \alpha = 0.99$, or 99% of the drug, is present in unionized form.

As the pH of the solution increases, the degree of ionization (percentage ionized) decreases. Therefore, weak basic drugs are preferentially absorbed at higher pH.

Examples:

- aspirin, a weak acid with pK_a of ~3.47–3.50, has a greater fraction ionized in a more alkaline (higher pH) environment
- erythromycin, a weak base with pK_a of 8.7, has a greater fraction ionized in a more acidic (lower pH) environment.

Table 5.1   The effect of pH on the gastric and intestinal absorption of various acidic and basic drugs in the rat

	Drug	pKa	pH and site)					
			1.0 (G)	4.0 (I)	5.0 (I)	7.0 (I)	8.0 (I)	8.0 (G)
Stronger	5-Sulfosalicylic acid	<2.0	0	–	–	–	–	0
↑	5-Nitrosalicylic acid	2.3	52	40	27	0	0	16
ACIDS	Salicylic acid	3.0	61	64	35	30	10	13
↓	Acetylsalicylic acid	3.5	–	41	27	–	–	–
Weaker	Benzoic acid	4.2	–	62	36	35	5	–
	Thiopental	7.6	46	–	–	–	–	34
Weaker	Aniline	4.6	6	40	48	58	61	56
↑	Aminopyridine	5.0	–	21	35	48	52	–
BASES	p-Toluidine	5.3	0	30	42	65	64	47
↓	Quinine	8.4	0	9	11	41	54	18
Stronger	Dextromethorphan	9.2	0	–	–	–	–	16

G, gastric; I, intestinal.

Table 5.1 shows the effect of pH on the gastric and intestinal absorption of various acidic and basic drugs in the rat.

General comments

From the above equations, it is obvious that most weak acidic drugs are predominantly present in the unionized form at the low pH of gastric fluid (pH 1–2.5) and may, therefore, be significantly absorbed from the stomach and to some extent from intestine.

Some very weak acidic drugs (pK_a 7 or higher) such as barbiturates, phenytoin (Dilantin) and theophylline remain, essentially, in unionized form throughout the gastrointestinal tract.

A weak acid such as aspirin (pK_a 3.5) is approximately 99% unionized in the gastric fluid at pH 1.0 but only 0.1% of aspirin is unionized at pH 6.5 (small intestine). Despite this seemingly unfavorable ratio of unionized to ionized molecules, aspirin and most weak acids are absorbed predominantly in the small intestine. This is attributed to a large surface area, a relatively long residence time and limited absorption of the ionized species (factors not considered by the pH–partition theory).

Most weak bases are poorly absorbed, if at all, in the stomach since they are largely ionized at low pH. When a basic drug reaches the small intestine, where pH is in the range 5–8, efficient absorption takes place. This is owing to lipid solubility and the unionized form of the drug molecules.

It should be emphasized that the pH–partition theory does not explain all drug absorption processes or why some drugs are absorbed and other are not. Drug absorption is a relative thing, not an all-or-nothing phenomenon. Most drugs are absorbed to some extent from both stomach and intestine. In fact, most drugs, regardless of their pK_a, are absorbed from the small intestine. Although weakly acidic drugs are absorbed from the stomach, a drug is usually not in the stomach long enough for a large amount to be absorbed; also the surface area of the stomach is relatively small.

6

Extravascular routes of drug administration

Objectives

Upon completion of this chapter, you will have the ability to:

- calculate plasma drug concentration at any given time after the administration of an extravascular dose of a drug, based on known or estimated pharmacokinetic parameters
- interpret the plasma drug concentration versus time curve of a drug administered extravascularly as the sum of an absorption curve and an elimination curve
- employ extrapolation techniques to characterize the absorption phase
- calculate the absorption rate constant and explain factors that influence this constant
- explain possible reasons for the presence of *lag time* in a drug's absorption
- calculate peak plasma drug concentration, $(C_p)_{max}$, and the time, t_{max}, at which this occurs
- explain the factors that influence peak plasma concentration and peak time
- decide when flip-flop kinetics may be a factor in the plasma drug concentration versus time curve of a drug administered extravascularly.

6.1 Introduction

Drugs, through dosage forms, are most frequently administered extravascularly and the majority of them are intended to act systemically; for this reason, absorption is a prerequisite for pharmacological effects. Delays or drug loss during absorption may contribute to variability in drug response and, occasionally, may result in a failure of drug therapy.

The gastrointestinal membrane separates the absorption site from the blood. Therefore, passage of drug across the membrane is a prerequisite for absorption. For this reason, drug must be in a solution form and dissolution becomes very critical for the absorption of a drug. The passage of

drug molecules from the gastrointestinal tract to the general circulation and factors affecting this are shown in Figs 6.1 and 6.2. Any factor influencing dissolution of the drug is likely to affect the absorption of a drug. These factors will be discussed, in detail, later in the text.

Drug, once in solution, must pass through membranes before reaching the general circulation. Hence, the physicochemical properties of the drug molecule (pK_a of the drug, partition coefficient of the drug, drug solubility, etc.), pH at the site of drug administration, nature of the membrane and physiological factors will also influence the absorption of a drug.

The present discussion will deal with general principles that determine the rate and extent of

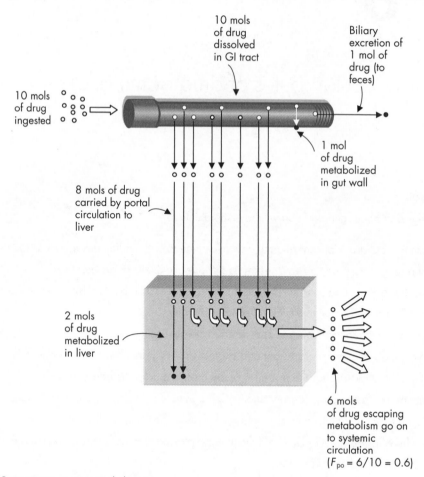

Figure 6.1   Barriers to gastrointestinal absorption.

drug absorption and the methods used to assess these and other pharmacokinetic parameters, from plasma concentration versus time data following oral administration of drugs. Emphasis is placed upon absorption of drugs following oral administration because it illustrates all sources of variability encountered during drug absorption.

Please note that a similar approach may be applied to determine pharmacokinetic parameters of drugs when any other extravascular route is used.

The following assumptions are made:

- drug exhibits the characteristics of one-compartment model
- absorption and elimination of a drug follow the first-order process and passive diffusion is operative at all the time

- drug is eliminated in unchanged form (i.e. no metabolism occurs)
- drug is monitored in the blood

Useful pharmacokinetic parameters

Figure 6.3 outlines the absorption of a drug that fits a one-compartment model with first-order elimination. The following information is useful.

1. Equation for determining the plasma concentration at any time, t
2. Determination of the elimination half life ($t_{1/2}$) and rate constant (K or K_{el})
3. Determination of the absorption half life ($t_{1/2})_{abs}$ and absorption rate constant (K_a)

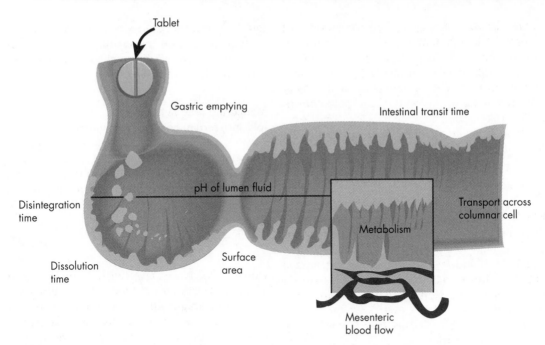

Figure 6.2 Passage of drug in the gastrointestinal tract until transport across the membrane.

4. Lag time (t_0), if any
5. Determination of the apparent volume of distribution (V or V_d) and fraction of drug absorbed (F)
6. Determination of the peak time ($t_{max.}$)
7. Determination of the peak plasma or serum concentration, $(C_p)_{max.}$

6.2 Drug remaining to be absorbed, or drug remaining at the site of administration

Equation 6.1 describes the changes with drug over time at the site of administration.

$$\frac{-dX_a}{dt} = K_a(X_a)_t \qquad (6.1)$$

<u>SCHEME:</u>

X_a K_a (h^{-1}) X (drug in body or blood) K (h^{-1}) X_u
(absorbable drug at absorption site)   absorption   elimination

<u>SETUP:</u>

$$X_a \xrightarrow{K_a} X \xrightarrow{K} X_u$$

Figure 6.3 Absorption of a one-compartment drug with first-order elimination. where X_a is the mass or amount of absorbable drug remaining in the gut, or at the site of administration, at time t (i.e. drug available for absorption at time t); X is the mass or amount of drug in the blood at time, t; X_u is the mass or amount of drug excreted unchanged in the urine at time, t; K_a is the first-order absorption rate constant (h^{-1} or min^{-1}); and K (or K_{el}) is the first-order elimination rate constant (h^{-1} or min^{-1}).

where $-dX/dt$ is the decrease in the amount of absorbable drug present at the site of administration per unit time (e.g. $mg\,h^{-1}$); K_a is the first-order absorption rate constant (h^{-1}; min^{-1}); and $(X_a)_t$ is the mass or amount of absorbable drug at the site of administration (e.g. the gastrointestinal tract) at time t.

Upon integration of Eq. 6.1, we obtain the following:

$$(X_a)_t = (X_a)_{t=0}e^{-K_a t} = FX_0 e^{-K_a t} \tag{6.2}$$

where $(X_a)_{t=0}$ is the mass or amount of absorbable drug at the site of administration at time $t = 0$ (for extravascular administration of drug, $(X_a)_{t=0}$ equals FX_0); and F is the fraction or percentage of the administered dose that is available to reach the general circulation; X_0 is the administered dose of drug.

If $F = 1.0$, that is, if the drug is completely (100%) absorbed, then

$$(X_a)_t = X_0 e^{-K_a t} \tag{6.3}$$

Both Eqs 6.2 and 6.3 and Fig. 6.4 clearly indicate that the mass, or amount, of drug that remains at the absorption site or site of administration (or remains to be absorbed) declines monoexponentially with time.

However, since we cannot measure the amount of drug remaining to be absorbed (X_a) directly, because of practical difficulty, Eqs 6.2 and 6.3, for the time being, become virtually useless for the purpose of determining the absorption rate constant; and, therefore, we go to other alternatives such as monitoring drug in the blood and/or urine to determine the absorption rate constant and the absorption characteristics.

Monitoring drug in the blood (plasma/serum) or site of measurement

The differential equation that follows relates changes in drug concentration in the blood with time to the absorption and the elimination rates

$$\frac{dX}{dt} = K_a X_a - KX \tag{6.4}$$

where dX/dt is the rate ($mg\,h^{-1}$) of change of amount of drug in the blood; X is the mass or amount of drug in the blood or body at time, t; X_a is the mass or amount of absorbable drug at the absorption site at time t; K_a and K are the first-order absorption and elimination rate constants, respectively (e.g. h^{-1}); $K_a X_a$ is the first-order rate of absorption ($mg\,h^{-1}$; $\mu g\,h^{-1}$, etc); and KX is the first-order rate of elimination (e.g. $mg\,h^{-1}$).

Equation 6.4 clearly indicates that rate of change in drug in the blood reflects the difference between the absorption and the elimination rates (i.e. $K_a X_a$ and KX, respectively). Following the administration of a dose of drug, the difference between the absorption and elimination rates (i.e. $K_a X_a - KX$) becomes smaller as time increases; at peak time, the difference becomes zero.

Please note that, most of the time, the absorption rate constant is greater than the elimination

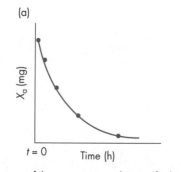
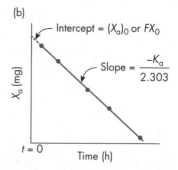

Figure 6.4   Amount of drug remaining at the site of administration against time in a rectilinear plot (a) and a semilogarithmic plot (b). X_a, amount of absorbable drug at the site of administration; $(X_a)_0$, amount of absorbable drug at the site of administration at time $t = 0$; F, fraction of administered dose that is available to reach the general circulation.

rate constant. (The exceptional situation when $K > K_a$, termed "flip-flop kinetics," will be addressed in the last section of this chapter.) Furthermore, immediately following the administration of a dose of drug, the amount of (absorbable) drug present at the site of administration will be greater than the amount of drug in the blood. Consequently, the rate of absorption will be greater than the rate of elimination up to a certain time (prior to peak time); then, exactly at peak time, the rate of absorption will become equal to the rate of elimination. Finally, the rate of absorption will become smaller than the rate of elimination (post peak time). This is simply the result of a continuous change in the amount of absorbable drug remaining at the site of administration and the amount of drug in the blood. Also, please note that rate of absorption and the rate of elimination change with time (consistent with the salient feature of the first-order process), whereas the absorption and the elimination rate constants do not change.

Integration of Eq. 6.4 gives:

$$(X)_t = \frac{K_a (X_a)_{t=0}}{K_a - K} [e^{-Kt} - e^{-K_a t}]$$

$$= \frac{K_a F X_0}{K_a - K} [e^{-Kt} - e^{-K_a t}] \qquad (6.5)$$

where $(X)_t$ is the mass (amount) of drug in the body at time t; X_0 is the mass of drug at the site of administration at $t = 0$ (the administered dose); F is the fraction of drug absorbed; $(X_a)_0 = FD_0$ and is the mass of administered dose that is available

to reach the general circulation, which is the same as the bioavailable fraction times the administered dose.

Equation 6.5 and Fig. 6.5 show that the mass or amount of drug in the body or blood follows a biexponential profile, first rising and then declining.

For orally or extravascularly administered drugs, generally $K_a \gg K$; therefore, the rising portion of the graph denotes the absorption phase.

If $K \gg K_a$ (perhaps indicating a dissolution-rate-limited absorption) the exact opposite will hold true. (Please see the discussion of the flip-flop model at the end of this chapter.)

6.3 Determination of elimination half life ($t_{1/2}$) and elimination rate constant (K or K_{el})

Equation 6.5, when written in concentration (C_p) terms, takes the following form:

$$(C_p)_t = \frac{K_a F X_0}{V(K_a - K)} [e^{-Kt} - e^{-K_a t}] \qquad (6.6)$$

where $\frac{K_a F X_0}{V(K_a - K)}$ is the intercept of plasma drug concentration versus time plot (Fig. 6.6).

When time is large, because of the fact that $K_a \gg K$, $e^{-K_a t}$ approaches zero, and Eq. 6.6 reduces to:

$$(C_p)_t = \frac{K_a F X_0}{V(K_a - K)} [e^{-Kt}] \qquad (6.7)$$

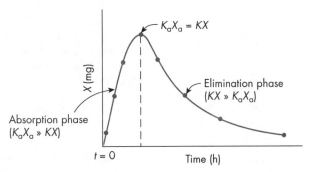

Figure 6.5   A typical rectilinear profile illustrating amount of drug (X) in blood or body against time. X_a, amount of absorbable drug at the absorption site at time t; K_a and K, first-order absorption and elimination rate constants, respectively; $K_a X_a$ and KX, first-order rates of absorption and elimination, respectively.

(a)

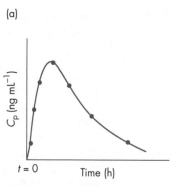

(b)

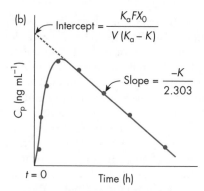

Figure 6.6 A plot of plasma concentration (C_p) against time on rectilinear (a) and semilogarithmic (b) paper. ($(X_a)_0$, amount of absorbable drug at the site of administration at time $t = 0$; F, fraction of administered dose that is available to reach the general circulation; K_a and K, first-order absorption and elimination rate constants, respectively; V, apparent volume of distribution.

The elimination half life and elimination rate constant can be obtained by methods described earlier and illustrated in Figure 6.7.

6.4 Absorption rate constant (K_a)

The absorption rate constant is determined by a method known as "feathering," "method of residuals" or "curve stripping." The method allows the separation of the monoexponential constituents of a biexponential plot of plasma concentration against time. From the plasma concentration

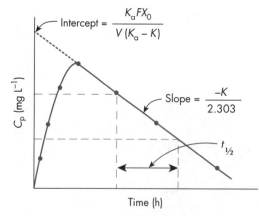

Figure 6.7 Semilogarithmic plot of plasma drug concentration (C_p) versus time of an extravascular dosage form: visualization of elimination half life ($t_{1/2}$). Other abbreviations as in Fig. 6.6.

versus time data obtained or provided to you and the plot of the data (as shown in Fig. 6.8) we can construct a table with headings and columns as in Table 6.1 for the purpose of determining the absorption rate constant.

In column 1 of the table, the time values are recorded that correspond to the observed plasma concentrations. This is done only for the absorption phase. In column 2, the observed plasma concentration values provided only from the absorption phase are recorded (i.e. all values prior to reaching maximum or highest plasma concentration value). In column 3, the plasma concentration values obtained only from the extrapolated portion of the plasma concentration versus time plot are recorded (these values are read from the plasma concentration–time plot); and, in column 4, the differences in the plasma concentrations $(C_p)_{diff}$ between the extrapolated and observed values for each time in the absorption phase are recorded.

The differences in plasma concentrations between the extrapolated and observed values (in column 4 of Table 6.1) should decline monoexponentially according to the following equation:

$$(C_p)_{diff} = \frac{K_a F X_0}{V(K_a - K)}[e^{-K_a t}] \tag{6.8}$$

where $\frac{K_a F X_0}{V(K_a - K)}$ is the intercept of plasma drug concentration versus time plot. A plot of this difference between extrapolated and observed plasma concentrations against time, on semilogarithmic

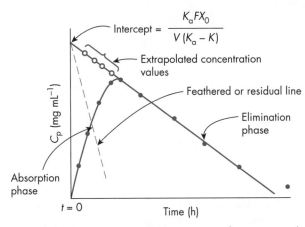

Figure 6.8 Semilogarithmic plot of plasma concentration (C_p) versus time of an extravascular dosage form, showing the method of residuals. Other abbreviations as in Fig. 6.6.

Table 6.1   Illustration of the table created for determination of the first-order absorption rate constant K_a

Time (h)	Observed plasma concentration $(C_p)_{obs}$	Extrapolated plasma concentration $(C_p)_{extrap}$	$(C_p)_{diff} = (C_p)_{extrap} - (C_p)_{obs}$
Time values corresponding to observed plasma concentrations for absorption phase only	Values only from the absorption phase (i.e. all values prior to reaching maximum or highest plasma concentration) (units, e.g. $\mu g\,mL^{-1}$)	Values only from the extrapolated portion of the plot of plasma concentration–time (units, e.g. $(\mu g\,mL^{-1})$)	Differences between extrapolated and observed values for each time in the absorption phase (units, e.g. $\mu g\,mL^{-1}$)

paper (Fig. 6.9), should yield a straight line, which, in turn, should allow determination of:

- the half life of the feathered or residual line (i.e. the $t_{1/2}$ of absorption phase)
- the first-order absorption rate constants, using the equation $K_a = 0.693/(t_{1/2})_{abs}$, or $K_a = -$ (slope) $\times 2.303$.

6.5 Lag time (t_0)

Theoretically, intercepts of the terminal linear portion and the feathered line in Fig. 6.8 should be the same; however, sometimes, these two lines do not have the same intercepts, as seen in Fig. 6.10.

A plot showing a lag time (t_0) indicates that absorption did not start immediately following the administration of drug by the oral or other extravascular route. This delay in absorption may be attributed to some formulation-related problems, such as:

- slow tablet disintegration
- slow and/or poor drug dissolution from the dosage form
- incomplete wetting of drug particles (large contact angle may result in a smaller effective surface area) owing to the hydrophobic nature of the drug or the agglomeration of smaller insoluble drug particles
- poor formulation, affecting any of the above
- a delayed release formulation.

Negative lag time ($-t_0$)

Figure 6.11 shows a plot with an apparent negative lag time.

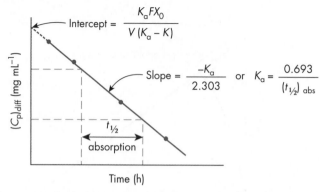

Figure 6.9   Semilogarithmic plots of plasma concentration $(C_p)_{diff}$ between calculated residual concentrations and measured ones versus time, allowing the calculation of the absorption rate constant. ($t_{1/2}$)$_{abs}$, absorption half life; other abbreviations as in Fig. 6.6.

What does negative lag time mean? Does it mean that absorption has begun prior to the administration of a drug? That cannot be possible unless the body is producing the drug! The presence of a negative lag time may be attributed to a paucity of data points in the absorption as well as in the elimination phase. Another possible reason may be that the absorption rate constant is not much greater than the elimination rate constant.

The absorption rate constant obtained by the feathering, or residual, method could be erroneous under the conditions stated above. Should that be the case, it is advisable to employ some other methods (Wagner and Nelson method, statistical moment analysis, Loo–Rigelman method for a two-compartment model, just to mention a few) of determining the absorption rate constant. Though these methods tend to be highly

mathematical and rather complex, they do provide an accurate estimate of the absorption rate constant, which, in turn, permits accurate estimation of other pharmacokinetic parameters such as peak time, peak plasma concentration, as well as the assessment of bioequivalence and comparative and/or relative bioavailability.

6.6 Some important comments on the absorption rate constant

Figure 6.12 indicates that the greater the difference between the absorption and the elimination rate constants (i.e. $K_a \gg K$), the faster is drug absorption and the quicker is the onset of action (in Fig. 6.12, apply the definition of onset of action). Please note the shift in the peak time

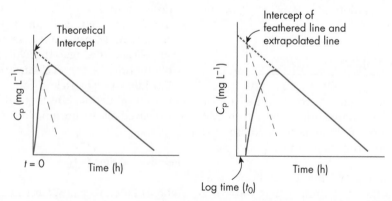

Figure 6.10   Semilogarithmic plots of the extrapolated plasma concentration (C_p) versus time showing the lag time (t_0).

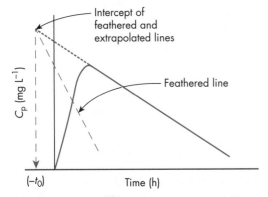

Figure 6.11 Semilogarithmic plot of plasma concentration (C_p) versus time showing a negative value for the lag time (t_0).

and peak plasma concentration values as the difference between absorption rate constant (K_a) and elimination rate constant (K) becomes smaller, as you go from left to right of the figure. If the absorption rate constant (K_a) is equal to the elimination rate constant (K), we need to employ a different pharmacokinetic model to fit the data.

Please note that the absorption rate constant for a given drug can change as a result of changing the formulation, the dosage form (tablet, suspension and capsule) or the extravascular route of drug administration (oral, intramuscular, subcutaneous, etc.). Administration of a drug with or without food will also influence the absorption rate constant for the same drug administered orally through the same formulation of the same dosage form.

6.7 The apparent volume of distribution (V)

For a drug administered by the oral, or any other extravascular, route of administration, the apparent volume of distribution cannot be calculated from plasma drug concentration data alone. The reason is that the value of F (the fraction of administered dose that reaches the general circulation) is not known. From Eqs 6.7 and 6.8:

$$\text{Intercept} = \frac{K_a F X_0}{V(K_a - K)} \tag{6.9}$$

If we can reasonably assume, or if it has been reported in the scientific literature, that $F = 1.0$ (i.e. the entire administered dose has reached the general circulation), only then can we calculate the apparent volume of distribution following the administration of a drug by the oral or any other extravascular route.

In the absence of data for the fraction of administered dose that reaches the general circulation, the best one can do is to obtain the ratio of V/F:

$$\frac{V}{F} = \frac{K_a X_0}{(K_a - K)} \left(\frac{1}{\text{Intercept}}\right) \tag{6.10}$$

6.8 Time of maximum drug concentration, peak time (t_{max})

The peak time (t_{max}) is the time at which the body displays the maximum plasma

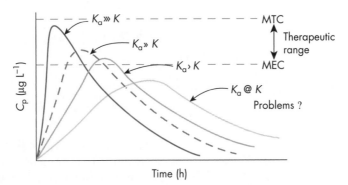

Figure 6.12 Rectilinear plot of plasma concentration (C_p) versus time for various magnitudes of absorption (K_a) and elimination (K) rate constants. MTC, minimum toxic concentration; MEC, minimum effective concentration.

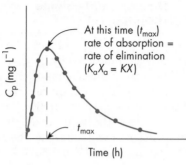
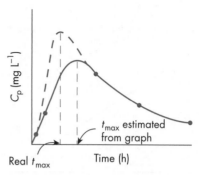

Figure 6.13 Dependency of estimate of the peak time (t_{max}) on the number of data points. K_a, absorption rate constant; K, elimination rate constant; X_a, absorbable mass or amount of drug at the absorption site; X, mass or amount of drug in the blood or body; C_p, plasma concentration.

concentration, $(C_p)_{max}$. It occurs when the rate of absorption is equal to the rate of elimination (i.e. when $K_a X_a = KX$). At the peak time, therefore, $K_a (X_a)_{t_{max}} = K(X)_{t_{max}}$.

The success of estimations of the peak time is governed by the number of data points.

Calculating peak time

According to Eq. 6.4, derived above,

$$\frac{dX}{dt} = K_a X_a - KX$$

When $t = t_{max}$, the rate of absorption ($K_a X_a$) equals the rate of elimination (KX) Hence, Eq. 6.4 becomes:

$$\frac{dX}{dt} = K_a(X_a)_{t_{max}} - K(X)_{t_{max}} = 0$$

or

$$K_a(X_a)_{t_{max}} = K(X)_{t_{max}} \qquad (6.11)$$

We know from earlier equations (Eqs 6.5 and 6.2) that:

$$(X)_t = \frac{K_a F X_0}{K_a - K}[e^{-Kt} - e^{-K_a t}]$$

and

$$(X_a)_t = F X_0 e^{-K_a t}$$

When $t = t_{max}$, Eqs 6.5 and 6.2 become Eqs 6.12 and 6.13, respectively:

$$(X)_{t_{max}} = \frac{K_a F X_0}{K_a - K}[e^{-Kt_{max}} - e^{-K_a t_{max}}] \qquad (6.12)$$

$$(X_a)_{t_{max}} = F X_0 e^{-K_a t_{max}} \qquad (6.13)$$

Equation 6.11 shows that $K_a(X_a)_{t_{max}} = K(X)_{t_{max}}$. Substituting for $(X_a)_{t_{max}}$ (from Eq. 6.13) and $(X)_{t_{max}}$ (from Eq. 6.12) in Eq. 6.11, then rearranging and simplifying, yields:

$$K_a e^{-K_a t_{max}} = K e^{-Kt_{max}} \qquad (6.14)$$

Taking natural logarithms of Eq. 6.14 yields:

$$\ln K_a - K_a \cdot t_{max} = \ln K - K \cdot t_{max}$$

$$\ln K_a - \ln K = K_a \cdot t_{max} - K \cdot t_{max}$$

$$\ln (K_a/K) = t_{max}(K_a/K)$$

or

$$t_{max} = \frac{\ln (K_a/K)}{K_a - K} \qquad (6.15)$$

Equation 6.15 indicates that peak time depends on, or is influenced by, only the absorption and elimination rate constants; therefore, any factor that influences the absorption and the elimination rate constants will influence the

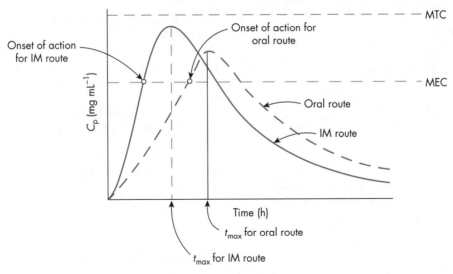

Figure 6.14   Rectilinear plots of plasma concentration (C_p) against time following the administration of an identical dose of a drug via the oral or intramuscular (IM) extravascular routes to show variation in time to peak concentration (t_{max}) and in onset of action. MTC, minimum toxic concentration; MEC, minimum effective concentration.

peak time value; however, the peak time is always independent of the administered dose of a drug.

What is not immediately apparent from Eq. 6.15 is that a small value of either the absorption rate constant (as may occur in a poor oral formulation) or of the elimination rate constant (as may be the case in a renally impaired patient) will have the effect of lengthening the peak time and slowing the onset of action. This may be proved by changing the value of one parameter at a time in Eq. 6.15.

Significance of peak time

The peak time can be used:

- to determine comparative bioavailability and/ or bioequivalence
- to determine the preferred route of drug administration and the desired dosage form for the patient
- to assess the onset of action.

Differences in onset and peak time may be observed as a result of administration of the same drug in different dosage forms (tablet, suspension, capsules, etc.) or the administration of the same drug in same dosage forms but different

formulations (Fig. 6.14). Please note that this is due to changes in K_a and not in K (elimination rate constant).

6.9 Maximum (peak) plasma concentration $(C_p)_{max}$

The peak plasma concentration $(C_p)_{max}$ occurs when time is equal to t_{max}.

Significance of the peak plasma concentration

The peak plasma concentration:

- is one of the parameters used to determine the comparative bioavailability and/or the bioequivalence between two products (same and or different dosage forms) but containing the same chemical entity or therapeutic agent
- may be used to determine the superiority between two different dosage forms or two different routes of administration
- may correlate with the pharmacological effect of a drug.

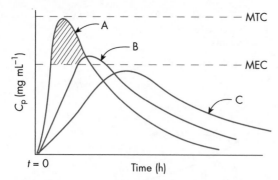

Figure 6.15 Rectilinear plots of plasma concentration (C_p) against time following the administration of an identical dose of a drug via three different formulations (A–C). MTC, minimum toxic concentration; MEC, minimum effective concentration.

Figure 6.15 shows three different formulations (A, B and C) containing identical doses of the same drug in an identical dosage form. (Similar plots would arise when giving an identical dose of the same drug via different extravascular routes or when giving identical doses of a drug by means of different dosage forms.)

Please note the implicit assumption made in all pharmacokinetic studies that the pharmacological effects of drugs depend upon the plasma concentration of that drug in the body. Consequently, the greater the plasma concentration of a drug in the body (within the therapeutic range or the effective concentration range) the better will be the pharmacological effect of the drug.

How to obtain the peak plasma concentration

There are three methods available for determining peak plasma concentration ($(C_p)_{max}$). Two are given here.

Method 1. Peak plasma concentration obtained from the graph of plasma concentration versus time (Fig. 6.16).

Method 2. Peak plasma concentration obtained by using an equation. (Equation 6.6) shows that:

$$(C_p)_t = \frac{K_a F X_0}{V(K_a - K)}[e^{-Kt} - e^{-K_a t}]$$

If t_{max} is substituted for t in Eq. 6.6:

$$(C_p)_{max} = \frac{K_a F X_0}{V(K_a - K)}[e^{-Kt_{max}} - e^{-K_a t_{max}}] \quad (6.16)$$

We also know from Eqs 6.6 and 6.7 that the intercept (I) of the plasma concentration–time plot is given by:

$$I = \frac{K_a F X_0}{V(K_a - K)}$$

Hence, substituting for the term $\frac{K_a F X_0}{V(K_a - K)}$ in Eq. 6.16 with I will yield Eq. 6.17:

$$(C_p)_{max} = I[e^{-Kt_{max}} - e^{-K_a t_{max}}] \quad (6.17)$$

Figure 6.17 shows this relationship.

The peak plasma concentration, like any other concentration parameter, is directly proportional

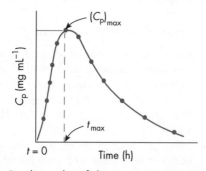
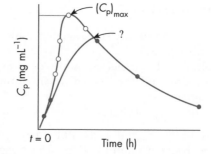

Figure 6.16 Rectilinear plots of plasma concentration (C_p) against time following the administration of a drug via extravascular route. The accuracy of the estimation of the peak plasma concentration ($(C_p)_{max}$) depends upon having sufficient data points (full points) to identify the time of peak concentration (t_{max}).

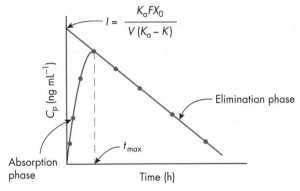

Figure 6.17 Semilogarithmic plot of plasma concentration (C_p) against time following the administration of a drug via the extravascular route, showing the intercept (I) and the time of peak concentration (t_{max}). Other abbreviations as in Fig. 6.6.

to the mass of drug reaching the general circulation or to the administered dose. This occurs when the first-order process and passive diffusion are operative (another example of linear pharmacokinetics).

6.10 Some general comments

1. The elimination rate constant, the elimination half life and the apparent volume of distribution are constant for a particular drug administered to a particular patient, regardless of the route of administration and the dose administered.
2. Therefore, it is a common practice to use values of the elimination rate constant, the elimination half life and the apparent volume of distribution obtained from intravenous bolus or infusion data to compute parameters associated with extravascular administration of a drug.
3. The absorption rate constant is a constant for a given drug formulation, dosage form and route of administration. That is, the same drug

is likely to have a different absorption rate constant if it is reformulated, if the dosage form is changed and/or if administered by a different extravascular route.
4. The fraction absorbed, like the absorption rate constant, is a constant for a given drug formulation, a dosage form and the route of administration. The change in any one of these may yield a different fraction absorbed for the same drug.
5. Therefore, if the same dose of the same drug is given to the same subject via different dosage forms, different routes of administration or different formulations, it may yield different peak times, peak plasma concentrations and the area under the plasma concentration–time curve (AUC). Peak time and the area under the plasma concentration time curve characterize the rate of drug absorption and the extent of drug absorption, respectively. Peak plasma concentration, however, may reflect either or both of these factors.

Tables 6.2 to 6.4 (Source: Facts and Comparison) and Fig. 6.18 illustrate the differences in the rate

Table 6.2 Lincomycin, an antibiotic used when patient is allergic to penicillin or when penicillin is inappropriate

Route of administration	Fraction absorbed	Mean peak serum concentration ($\mu g\ mL^{-1}$)	Peak time (h)
Oral	0.30	2.6	2 to 4
Intramuscular	Not available	9.5	0.5
Intravenous	1.00	19.0	0.0

Table 6.3   Haloperidol (Haldol), a drug used for psychotic disorder management

Route of administration	Percentage absorbed	Peak time (h)	Half life (h [range])
Oral	60	2 to 6	24 (12–38)
Intramuscular	75	0.33	21 (13–36)
Intravenous	100	Immediate	14 (10–19)

Table 6.4   Ranitidine HCl (Zantac)

Route and dose	Fraction absorbed	Mean peak levels (ng mL^{-1})	Peak time (h)
Oral (150 mg)	0.5–0.6	440–545	1–3
Intramuscular or intravenous (50 mg)	0.9–1.0	576	0.25

and extent of absorption of selected drugs when administered as different salts or via different routes. Please note the differences in the fraction absorbed, peak time and peak plasma concentration, but not in the fundamental pharmacokinetic parameters (half life and elimination rate constant) of the drug.

6.11 Example for extravascular route of drug administration

Concentration versus time data for administration of 500 mg dose of drug are given in Table 6.5 and plotted on rectilinear and semilogarithmic paper

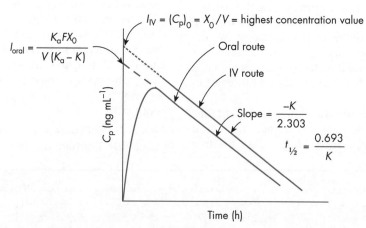

Figure 6.18   Administration of a drug by intravascular (IV) and extravascular (oral) routes (one-compartment model). Even for administration of the same dose, the value of plasma concentration (C_p) at time zero [$(C_p)_0$] for the intravenous bolus may be higher than the intercept for the extravascular dose. This will be determined by the relative magnitudes of the elimination rate constant (K) and the absorption rate constant (K_a) and by the size of fraction absorbed (F) for the extravascular dosage form. X_0, oral dose of drug; X_0, IV bolus dose of drug.

Table 6.5 Plasma concentration–time data following oral administration of 500 mg dose of a drug that is excreted unchanged and completely absorbed ($F = 1.0$); determine all pharmacokinetic parameters

Time (h)	Plasma concentration ($\mu g\, mL^{-1}$)
0.5	5.36
1.0	9.35
2.0	17.18
4.0	25.78
8.0	29.78
12.0	26.63
18.0	19.40
24.0	13.26
36.0	5.88
48.0	2.56
72.0	0.49

in Figs 6.19 and 6.20, respectively. From these data a number of parameters can be derived.

The elimination half life and the elimination rate constant are obtained from the semiloga-rithmic plot of plasma concentration against time (Fig. 6.20):

the elimination half life $(t_{1/2}) = 10\,h$
the elimination rate constant $K = 0.693/t_{1/2} = 0.693/10\,h = 0.0693\,h^{-1}$
the y-axis intercept $= \frac{K_a F X_0}{V(K_a - K)} = 67\,\mu g\, mL^{-1}$ for a 500 mg dose.

The absorption rate constant and the absorption phase half life are obtained from the residual or feathering method. From the data in Fig. 6.20, the differences between the observed and the extrapolated plasma concentrations are calculated (Table 6.6, column 4) and are then plotted against time (column 1) on semilogarithmic paper.

From Figure 6.21 we can calculate:

- the half life of the absorption phase $(t_{1/2})_{abs} = 2.8\,h$
- the absorption rate constant $(K_a) = 0.693/2.8\,h = 0.247\,h^{-1}$

Please note that absorption rate constant is much greater than the elimination rate constant ($K_a \gg K$).

The apparent volume of distribution is calculated from the amount (mass) of absorbable drug at the site of administration at time $t = 0$, $(X_a)_{t=0}$. This

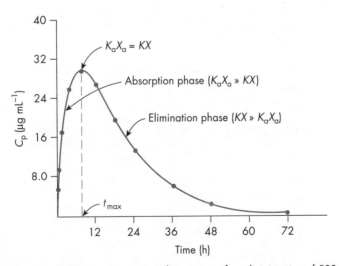

Figure 6.19 Plasma concentration (C_p) versus time on rectilinear paper for administration of 500 mg dose of drug using values in Table 6.5. X_a, amount of absorbable drug at the absorption site at time t; K_a and K, first-order absorption and elimination rate constants, respectively; $K_a X_a$ and KX, first-order rates of absorption and elimination, respectively.

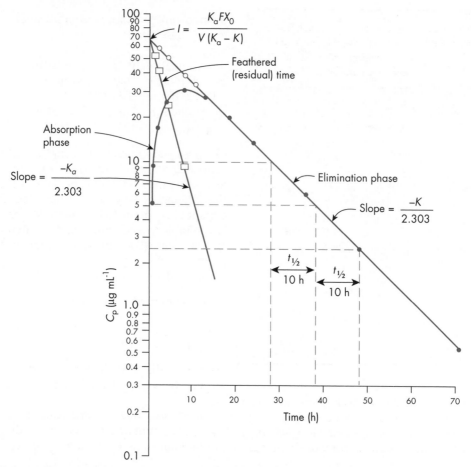

Figure 6.20 Plasma concentration (C_p) versus time on semilogarithmic paper for administration of 500 mg dose of drug using values in Table 6.5. The observed plasma concentrations (●) are extrapolated back (○) and then the feathered (residual) method is used to get the residual concentration (□) plot. Other abbreviations as in Fig. 6.6.

Table 6.6 Method of residuals to calculate the difference between the extrapolated and observed plasma concentrations values using the data in Table 6.5 plotted as in Fig. 6.20

Time (h)	$(C_p)_{extrap}$ ($\mu g\ mL^{-1}$)	$(C_p)_{obs}$ ($\mu g\ mL^{-1}$)	$(C_p)_{diff}$ ($\mu g\ mL^{-1}$)
0.5	65.0	5.36	59.64
1.0	62.0	9.95	52.05
2.0	58.0	17.18	40.82
4.0	50.0	25.78	24.22
8.0	39.0	29.78	9.22

$(C_p)_{extrap}$, extrapolated plasma concentrations; $(C_p)_{obs}$, observed plasma concentrations; $(C_p)_{diff}$, difference between extrapolated and observed values for each time in the absorption phase.

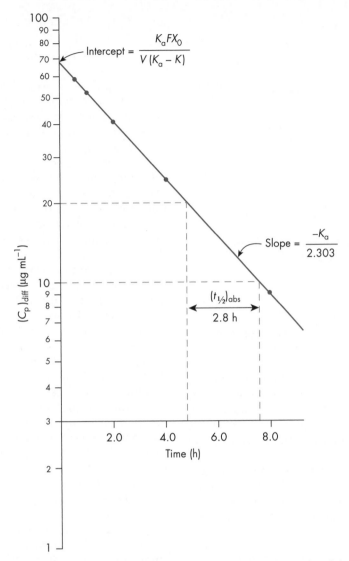

Figure 6.21 Feathered (residual) plot of the differences $[(C_p)_{diff}]$ between the observed and the extrapolated plasma concentrations in Fig. 6.20 (as given in Table 6.6, column 4) plotted against time on semilogarithmic paper. $(t_{1/2})_{abs}$, absorption half life; other abbreviations as in Fig. 6.6.

equals the dose $= X_0 = 500$ mg if it is assumed that the fraction absorbed $(F) = 1.0$. Please note that this assumption is made solely for purpose of demonstrating how to use this equation for the determination of the apparent volume of distribution.

$$\text{Intercept} = \frac{K_a F X_0}{V(K_a - K)}$$

where $\text{intercept} = 67\,\mu\text{g mL}^{-1}$; $K_a = 0.247\,\text{h}^{-1}$; $F = 1.0$; and $FX_0 = 500\,\text{mg} = 500\,000\,\mu\text{g}$.

Hence,

$$V = \frac{K_a F D_0}{\text{Intercept}(K_a - K)}$$

$$V = \frac{0.247\,\text{h}^{-1} \times 500\,000\,\mu g}{67\,\mu g/\text{mL}^{-1}(0.247 - 0.0693)\,\text{h}^{-1}}$$

$$V = \frac{123500\,h^{-1}\,\mu g}{67\,\mu g/mL^{-1}(0.177\,h^{-1})}$$

$$V = \frac{123500}{11.906} = 10372.92\,mL \quad \text{or} \quad 10.37\,L$$

The peak time can be obtained from the graph (Fig. 6.19): $t_{max} = 8.0\,h$. Or it can be calculated using the equation:

$$t_{max} = \frac{\ln(K_a/K)}{K_a - K}$$

Since $K_a = 0.247\,h^{-1}$ and $K = 0.0693\,h^{-1}$,

$$t_{max} = \frac{\ln\,(0.247/0.0693)}{(0.247 - 0.0693)} = \frac{\ln\,(3.562)}{(0.1777)}$$

Since $\ln 3.562 = 1.2703$, then

$$t_{max} = 1.2703/0.1777 = 7.148\,h.$$

Please note that administration of a different dose (250 or 750 mg) of the same drug via same dosage form, same formulation and same route of administration will have absolutely no effect on peak time. However, administration of the same drug (either same or different dose) via a different dosage form, different routes of administration and/or different formulation may result in a different peak time.

If we administer 500 mg of the same drug to the same subject by the intramuscular route and found the absorption rate constant (K_a) to be $0.523\,h^{-1}$, will the peak time be shorter or longer? Please consider this.

The peak plasma concentration can be obtained from Fig. 6.19: $(C_p)_{max} = 29.78\,\mu g\,mL^{-1}$. Or it can be caculated using Eq. 6.16:

$$(C_p)_{max} = \frac{K_a F X_0}{V(K_a - K)}[e^{-Kt_{max}} - e^{-K_a t_{max}}]$$

$$\frac{K_a F X_0}{V(K_a - K)} = \text{Intercept} = 67\,mg\,mL^{-1}.$$

We know that $K_a = 0.247\,h^{-1}$, $K = 0.0693\,h^{-1}$ and $t_{max} = 7.148\,h$. Substituting these values in the equation gives:

$$(C_p)_{max}$$
$$= 67\,\mu g\,mL^{-1}[e^{-0.0693 \times 7.148} - e^{-0.247 \times 7.148}]$$

$$(C_p)_{max} = 67\,\mu g\,mL^{-1}[e^{-0.495} - e^{-1.765}]$$

$$e^{-0.495} = 0.6126, \text{ and } e^{-1.765} = 0.1720.$$

Hence, $(C_p)_{max} = 67\,\mu g\,mL^{-1}\,[0.6126 - 0.1720] = 67\,\mu g\,mL^{-1}\,[0.4406] = 29.52\,\mu g\,mL^{-1}$.

Please note that peak plasma concentration is *always* directly proportional to the administered dose (assuming the first-order process and passive diffusion are operative) of a drug. Therefore, following the administration of 250 mg and 750 mg doses of the same drug via the same formulation, the same dosage form and the same route of administration, plasma concentrations of $14.76\,\mu g\,mL^{-1}$ and $44.28\,\mu g\,mL^{-1}$, respectively, will result.

It is important to recognize that the intercept of plasma concentration versus time data will have concentration units; therefore, the value of the intercept will also be directly proportional to the administered dose of the drug. In this exercise, therefore, the value of the intercept of the plasma concentration versus time data for a 250 mg and 750 mg dose will be $33.5\,\mu g\,mL^{-1}$ and $100.5\,\mu g\,mL^{-1}$, respectively.

Is it true that the larger the difference between the intercept of the plasma concentration–time data and the peak plasma concentration, the slower is the rate of absorption and longer is the peak time?

Is it accurate to state that the larger the difference between the intercept of the plasma concentration time data and the peak plasma concentration, the larger is the difference between the absorption rate constant and the elimination rate constant? Please consider.

6.12 Flip-flop kinetics

Flip-flop kinetics is an exception to the usual case in which the absorption rate constant is greater than the elimination rate constant ($K_a > K$). For a drug absorbed by a slow first-order process, such as certain types of sustained-release formulations, the situation may arise where the elimination rate constant is greater than the absorption rate constant ($K > K_a$). Since the terminal linear slope of plasma drug

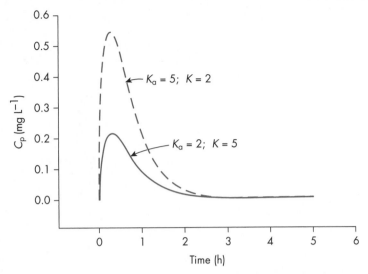

Figure 6.22 Comparison of a regular (−−−) and a flip-flop (—) oral absorption model. In this simulation, the apparent volume of distribution/fraction of administered dose available to reach the general circulation and the dose are the same for both plots; but the values of the elimination rate constant (K) and the absorption rate constant (K_a) are flipped.

concentration versus time plotted on semilogarithmic co-ordinates always represents the slower process, this slope is related to the absorption rate constant; the slope of the feathered line will be related to the elimination rate constant. Figure 6.22 compares a regular and a flip-flop oral absorption model.

In this simulation, the lower graph (solid line) represents the flip-flop situation. Because of a larger value for the elimination rate constant, the flip-flop graph has both a smaller AUC and a smaller $(C_p)_{max}$ than the normal graph. However, both the regular and flip-flop curves have the same shape and the same t_{max} (0.305 h).

When fitting plasma drug concentration data to the one-compartment extravascular model by non-linear regression, estimates for the elimination rate constant and absorption rate constant from regular and flip-flop approaches will have exactly the same correlation coefficient, indicating an equally good fit to the model. Whether the computerized fit gives the regular or the flip-flop result is simply a matter of which initial parameter estimates were input into the computer.

So, is there any way to tell which fit represents reality?

One sure way is to have an unambiguous value of the drug's elimination half life (and therefore of the elimination rate constant) determined from a study in which the drug is administered intravenously. Another strong indication that the regular model is the correct model is the situation where the extravascular administration is of a type that should not have any kind of slow, extended absorption. An example of this is an immediate release tablet or a capsule. This type of dosage form should not have an absorption half life that is slower than its elimination half life.

Problem set 2

Problems for Chapter 6

Question 1

Table P2.1 gives the plasma drug concentrations (C_p) that were obtained following the oral administration of 1 g dose of a drug.

Plot the data and, using the plot, determine the following.

a. The elimination half life ($t_{1/2}$) and the elimination rate constant (K).
b. The absorption half life, $(t_{1/2})_{abs}$.
c. The absorption rate constant (K_a).
d. The observed and calculated peak time (t_{max}).
e. The observed and calculated peak plasma concentrations, $(C_p)_{max}$.

Table P2.1

Time (h)	Plasma concentrations (mg%)
0.25	3.00
0.50	4.60
1.00	5.70
1.50	5.60
2.00	4.80
3.00	3.20
4.00	2.00
5.00	1.20
6.00	0.75
7.00	0.46

f. The y-axis intercept.

Compare:

g. The observed peak time (t_{max}) with the calculated peak time.
h. The observed and the calculated peak plasma concentrations ($C_p)_{max}$.

Question 2

Promethazine (Phenergan) is a widely used antihistaminic, antiemetic and sedative drug. Zamen *et al.* (1986) undertook a study to determine the dose proportionality of promethazine from the tablet dosage form. Following the administration of one tablet containing either 25 or 50 mg of promethazine, plasma concentrations were measured (Table P2.2).

Plot the data and, using the plot, determine the following.

a. The elimination half life ($t_{1/2}$) for each dose.
b. The elimination rate constant (K) for each dose.
c. The absorption half life, $(t_{1/2})_{abs}$, for each dose.
d. The absorption rate constant (K_a) for each dose.
e. The observed and computed peak time (t_{max}) for each dose.
f. The observed and computed peak plasma concentrations, $(C_p)_{max}$, for each dose.
g. The y-axis intercept for each dose.
h. The apparent volume of distribution (V).
i. The fraction of drug absorbed (F).
j. The characteristics of a plot on rectilinear paper of peak time (t_{max}) against the administered dose (then make an important observation).
k. The characteristics of a plot on rectilinear paper of peak plasma concentrations, $(C_p)_{max}$,

Table P2.2

Time (h)	Mean plasma concentrations (ng mL^{-1})[a]	
	25 mg tablet (lot 1821448)[b]	50 mg tablet (lot 1821148)[b]
0.5	0.12 ± 0.45	0.26 ± 0.75
1.0	2.20 ± 1.76	3.62 ± 3.05
1.5	5.38 ± 4.26	6.65 ± 4.15
2.0	6.80 ± 4.42	10.74 ± 3.67
3.0	6.91 ± 3.42	12.54 ± 6.22
4.0	6.32 ± 2.90	11.20 ± 4.42
6.0	4.25 ± 2.00	8.54 ± 3.04
8.0	3.60 ± 1.53	6.48 ± 2.43
10.0	2.72 ± 1.27	4.85 ± 1.66
12.0	2.30 ± 1.35	4.05 ± 2.07
24.0	0.67 ± 0.94	1.70 ± 1.64

[a] Mean $\pm$ SD of 15 determinations.
[b] Products made by Wyeth Laboratory.

against the administered dose (make an important observation).
l. Lag time (t_o), if any.

Problem-solving exercise

Procainamide is used for the treatment of ventricular tachyarrhythmia. It is administered intravenously, orally and intramuscularly, and its therapeutic range is 4 to $8\,\mu g\,mL^{-1}$. When a 750 mg dose is administered intravenously to a normal healthy subject:

- the elimination half life $= 3\,h$
- the apparent volume of distribution $= 140\,L$ or $2\,L\,kg^{-1}$
- % excreted in urine $= 65\%$
- % metabolite (N-acetylprocainamide) $= 35\%$.

Please note that the elimination half ($t_{1/2}$), the elimination rate constant (K), the apparent volume of distribution (V) and the systemic clearance (Cl_s) of a drug are independent of the route of administration.

When a tablet containing 250 mg procainamide is administered orally to a normal healthy subject:

- the absorption rate constant (K_a) $= 2.8\,h^{-1}$
- the intercept of the plasma concentration time profile $= 1.665\,\mu g\,mL^{-1}$
- the fraction of dose absorbed (i.e. reaching the general circulation) $= 85.54\%$.

Determine the following from the available information.

1. Peak time (t_{max}) and peak plasma concentration [$(C_p)_{max}$] following the administration of a 250 mg and 500 mg tablet.
2. Whether the administered oral dose (i.e. 250 mg tablet) will provide the peak plasma concentration high enough to control arrhythmia.
3. If not, how many tablets (250 mg strength) will be required to control arrhythmia?
4. Determine the absorbable amount of drug remaining at the site of administration (X_a) and the amount of drug in the body and/or blood (X) at a time when the rate of absorption is equal to the rate of elimination for extravascularly administered dose of 500 mg via tablet.
5. Determine the rate of absorption and the rate of elimination, at peak time, following the administration of a 250 mg and a 500 mg tablet.
6. Indicating the appropriate graphical coordinates (rectilinear or semilogarithmic), sketch the profiles of rate of absorption against the dose administered and rate of elimination against dose administered. What will be the relationship between the rate of absorption and the rate of elimination at peak time?
7. Is it possible to determine the absorption rate constant (K_a) and the peak time from the knowledge of peak plasma concentration, the apparent volume of drug distribution, the elimination half life and the amount of drug remaining at the site of administration at peak time? Only if the answer is yes, show all the steps involved in the calculation.
8. In a 70 kg patient with renal impairment, the elimination half life ($t_{1/2}$) of procainamide is reported to be 14 h (range, 9–43 h). Following the administration of a 250 mg procainamide tablet to this subject, the absorption rate

constant and the intercept on the y-axis of the plasma concentration–time profile were reported to be $2.8\,h^{-1}$ and $1.556\,\mu g\,mL^{-1}$, respectively. Assume no change in volume of distribution from the $2\,L\,kg^{-1}$ value in normal subjects. Determine the systemic (Cl_s), renal (Cl_r) and metabolic (Cl_m) clearances following the administration of this 250 mg procainamide tablet. Also determine t_{max}, the time of peak plasma level. Will these values change for a 750 mg dose administered intravenously? In a *normal subject*, peak time was observed to be 0.97 h. Determine the percentage difference in peak time in normal and renally impaired subjects, with respect to the normal value of a 750 mg dose intravenously.

9. What will be the peak time in this renally impaired patient following the administration of a 500 mg tablet of an identical formulation.

10. What will be the procainamide peak plasma concentration in this renally impaired subject following the administration of a 500 mg tablet of an identical formulation.

11. Show the relationship between the area under the plasma concentration–time curve $(AUC)_0^\infty$ and the systemic clearance of a drug in a renally impaired patient.

Answers

The problem set provides plasma concentration versus time data following the administration of a drug by an extravascular route (oral). Once again, it is assumed that the administered drug follows the first-order process and exhibits the characteristics of a one-compartment model. The following are our answers to these questions and it is possible that your answers may differ from these for the reasons discussed in Problem set 1.

Question 1 answer

a. $t_{1/2} = 1.4\,h$
   $K = 0.495\,h^{-1}$.

b. Employing the feathering or residual or curve stripping method:

$$(t_{1/2})_{abs} = 0.425\,h.$$

c. $K_a = 1.630\,h^{-1}$.

d. Observed $t_{max} = 1\,h$ (graphical method) calculated $t_{max} = 1.05\,h$ (equation method).

e. $(C_p)_{max} = 5.70\,mg\,\%$ (graphical method)
   $(C_p)_{max} = 5.796\,mg\,\%\,(5.796\,mg\,100\,mL^{-1})$
   (equation method).

f. The y-intercept of the plasma concentration versus time profile is $14\,mg\,\%$.

g. The observed t_{max} is simply the time of the highest recorded plasma drug concentration; therefore, it will be exactly equal to one of the time points at which blood was collected. The calculated t_{max} is not restricted to a time at which blood was collected; moreover, its value will be based on the curve that best fits all the data points. Calculated t_{max} will, therefore, be more accurate.

h. The observed $(C_p)_{max}$ is simply the highest recorded plasma drug concentration and, as for t_{max}, it will occur at one of the time points at which blood was collected. The calculated $(C_p)_{max}$ is not restricted to a time at which blood was collected but is based on the pharmacokinetic fit to all the plasma drug concentration versus time data; it will, therefore, be more accurate.

Note: Peak plasma concentration is always directly proportional to the dose administered, regardless of the route of administration or the health of the subject (healthy or renally impaired) as long as a first-order process is occurring. Therefore, administration of a 500 mg dose of the same drug via identical formulation, dosage form and route of administration will give a y-intercept of $7\,mg\,\%$ and a peak plasma concentration of $2.898\,mg\,\%$ $(2.898\,mg\,100\,mL^{-1})$. The peak plasma concentration in a renally impaired subject will be higher than in a normal subject; nonetheless, it will be directly proportional to the administered dose.

Question 2 answer

This question involves two different doses of an identical drug (promethazine) in an identical dosage form (tablet), via an identical route of administration (oral) of an identical formulation (made by the same manufacturer). Plasma concentration versus time data were plotted on suitable semilogarithmic graph paper. As mentioned above, greater variation can occur in the values in parts a–d because of the technique employed. This variation, in turn, will be reflected in the answers for the peak time, peak plasma concentration and the intercept of the plasma concentration versus time profile.

a. 25 mg tablet, $t_{1/2} = 5.25$ h
   50 mg tablet, $t_{1/2} = 5.50$ h.
   (Do not be concerned about the 0.25 h difference [insignificant] in the elimination half life of the drug; this reflects the graphical method employed.)

b. 25 mg tablet, $K = 0.132\,h^{-1}$
   50 mg tablet, $K = 0.126\,h^{-1}$.
   (Ignore the small difference in the elimination rate constants.)

c. Use the feathering or residual or curve-stripping method to determine from the feathered or residual line of $(C_p)_{diff}$ against time on a semilogarithmic graph paper. As mentioned above, there may be greater variation in these values because of the technique employed. This variation, in turn, will be reflected in the answers for the peak time, peak plasma concentration and the intercept of the plasma concentration versus time profile.

   25 mg tablet, $t_{1/2} = 0.625$ h
   50 mg tablet, $t_{1/2} = 0.700$ h.

d. 25 mg tablet, $K_a = 1.109\,h^{-1}$
   50 mg tablet, $K_a = 0.990\,h^{-1}$.

e. The observed and computed peak time for each dose:
   25 mg tablet, $t_{max} = 3.00$ h (graphical method)
   50 mg tablet, $t_{max} = 3.00$ h (graphical method)
   25 mg tablet, $t_{max} = 2.178$ h (calculated method)
   50 mg dose, $t_{max} = 2.385$ h (calculated method).

   Note that doubling the dose did not alter the peak time.

f. 25 mg tablet, $(C_p)_{max} = 6.91\,ng\,mL^{-1}$ (graphical method)
   50 mg tablet, $(C_p)_{max} = 12.54\,ng\,mL^{-1}$ (graphical method).
   Is the peak plasma concentration for a 50 mg dose approximately twice that of 50 mg dose? Note the units of concentration ($ng\,mL^{-1}$; $1\,mg = 1000\,\mu g$; $1\,\mu g = 1000\,ng$).
   25 mg tablet, $(C_p)_{max} = 6.476\,ng\,mL^{-1}$ ($6.476\mu g\,L$) (calculated method)
   50 mg tablet, $(C_p)_{max} = 11.63\,ng\,mL^{-1}$ (calculated method).
   Once again, note the approximate directly proportional relationship between the peak plasma concentration and the administered dose.
   The intercept values for the plasma concentration versus time profiles are as follows:
   25 mg tablet, intercept $= 9.8\,ng\,mL^{-1}$.
   For 50 mg tablet, intercept $= 18.0\,ng\,mL^{-1}$.

g. 25 mg tablet, intercept $= 9.8\,ng\,mL^{-1}$ (graphical method)
   50 mg tablet, intercept $= 18.0\,ng\,mL^{-1}$ (graphical method).
   These two values are reasonably close for graphical estimates.

h. Notice that V cannot be calculated for an extravascular dose without knowledge of F, the bioavailable fraction. The best that one can do is to calculate the ratio V/F:

   $$V/F = X_0 K_a / (I)(K_a - K)$$

   where I is the y-axis intercept.
   For 25 mg dose, $V/F =$
   $(25)(1.109)/(9.8)(1.109 - 0.132) = 2.90\,L$
   For 50 mg dose, $V/F =$
   $(50)(0.990)/(18.0)(0.990 - 0.126) = 3.18\,L$.
   Again, reasonably close for graphical estimates.

i. For reasons explained above in (h), F cannot be calculated with the information at hand.

j. Your plot should show no significant changes in t_{max} as a function of dose.

k. Within the limits of accuracy of the graphically derived answers, your plot should show direct proportionality between dose and $(C_p)_{max}$.

1. The extrapolated line and the feathered line intersect virtually at the y-axis, indicating the absence of any lag time.

Problem-solving exercise answer

1a. $$t_{max} = \frac{\ln(K_a/K)}{K_a - K} = \frac{\ln(2.8\,h^{-1}/0.231\,h^{-1})}{2.8\,h^{-1} - 0.231\,h^{-1}}$$

$$t_{max} = \frac{2.4949}{2.569\,h^{-1}}$$

$t_{max} = 0.971\,h$ or 58.25 min for a 250 mg dose.

Please note that since peak time is *independent of the dose administered*, for a 500 mg tablet, the peak time will be identical (i.e. 0.971 h or 58.25 min). However, if an identical dose or even a different dose of procainamide is administered through a different extravascular route (e.g intramuscular), different dosage form (e.g. solution, capsule, controlled release tablet) or different formulation (e.g. tablet made by a different manufacturer or the same manufacturer with a different formulation), the peak time may be different. This is because the absorption rate constant may change with route of administration, dosage form and formulation.

b. $(C_p)_{max}$ is given by

$$(C_p)_{max} = I(e^{-Kt_{max}} - e^{-K_a t_{max}})$$

where I is the y-axis intercept of the line extrapolated from the terminal linear segment of the plasma concentration versus time curve on semilogarithmic coordinates. We know from the available information that the absorption rate constant (K_a) and the elimination rate constant (K) are $2.8\,h^{-1}$ and $0.231\,h^{-1}$, respectively, and the calculated peak time is 0.971 h. The intercept of the plasma concentration versus time data for a 250 mg tablet is reported to be $1.665\,\mu g\,mL^{-1}$. Substituting these values in the equation will provide $(C_p)_{max}$:

$(C_p)_{max} = 1.665\,\mu g\,mL^{-1}(e^{-0.231\times0.971} - e^{-2.8\times0.971})$
$(C_p)_{max} = 1.665\,\mu g\,mL^{-1}(e^{-0.2243} - e^{-2.7188})$
$(C_p)_{max} = 1.665\,\mu g\,mL^{-1}(0.7990 - 0.06595)$
$(C_p)_{max} = 1.220\,\mu g\,mL^{-1}$ for a 250 mg dose.

2. The therapeutic range for the drug is 4–$8\,\mu g\,mL^{-1}$. This, therefore, suggests that 250 mg dose is insufficient to produce the pharmacological effect and a larger dose will be needed. Furthermore, the relationship between the peak plasma concentration and the dose administered is directly proportional (linear pharmacokinetics). Therefore, following the administration of a 500 mg dose peak plasma concentration will be $2.440\,\mu g\,mL^{-1}$. This dose will also be *inadequate* to provide a procainamide plasma concentration within therapeutic range.

3. Administration of four to six tablets of 250 mg strength or three tablets of 500 mg strength or two tablets of 750 mg strength, however, will yield procainamide plasma concentration of $4.88\,\mu g\,mL^{-1}$ for the 1000 mg dose and $7.32\,\mu g\,mL^{-1}$ for a 1500 mg dose (linear pharmacokinetics) (within the therapeutic range).

4. When the rate of absorption ($K_a X_a$) is equal to the rate of elimination (KX), $t = t_{max}$; in other words, rate of absorption and rate of elimination become equal *only at peak time*:

$$(X_a)_t = FX_0 e^{-K_a t}$$

The absorbable fraction F is 0.8554, or 85.54%. When $t = 0$; $e^{-Kat} = 1.0$; and $K_a = 2.8\,h^{-1}$. Therefore, for a 250 mg dose, the absorbable amount of drug at the site of administration at $t = 0$ is $(X_a)_{t=0} = 0.8554 \times 250\,mg \times 1 = 213.85$ mg.
When $t = t_{max}$, $F(Xa)_0 = 213.85$ mg.
At t_{max}, $(X_a) = F(X_a)_0 e^{-K_a t_{max}}$, where t_{max} 0.970 h and $K_a = 2.8\,h^{-1}$.
So at t_{max}, $(X_a) = 213.85\,mg \times e^{-2.8 \times 0.970}$
$= 213.85\,mg \times e^{-2.716}$
$= 213.85\,mg \times 0.066138$
At t_{max}, $(X_a) = 14.14\,mg$ (the absorbable amount of drug remaining at the site of administration at peak time).
Therefore, for the 500 mg dose (linear pharmacokinetics), the absorbable amount of drug remaining at the site of administration at peak time is 24.28 mg.
The amount of drug in the blood $(X)_{max}$ at peak time:

$$(X)_{max} = (C_p)_{max} \times V$$

Peak plasma concentration for a 250 mg tablet is $1.22\,\mu g\,mL^{-1}$ and the apparent volume of distribution is $140\,000\,mL$. Therefore, the amount of drug in the blood/body at peak time:

$(X)_{max} = 1.22\,\mu g\,mL^{-1} \times 140\,000\,mL = 170.8\,mg$

For 500 mg dose (applying linear pharmacokinetics), the amount of drug in the blood/body at peak time, $(X)_{max}$, is:

$2.44\,\mu g\,mL^{-1} \times 140\,000\,mL = 341.6\,mg$.

5. These calculations show that, following the administration of a 250 mg tablet and 500 mg tablet, the amount of drug ultimately reaching the general circulation is 213.85 mg and 427.7 mg, respectively (85.54% of dose; note that the fraction reaching the general circulation is *independent* of the dose administered). At peak time for the 250 mg tablet, the amount of drug remaining at the site of administration and the amount of drug in the blood/body are 14.09 mg and 170.80 mg, respectively. At peak time for the 500 mg tablet, the amount of drug remaining at the site of administration and the amount of drug in the blood/body are 28.18 mg and 341.6 mg, respectively.

Therefore, the amount of drug eliminated at peak time for a 250 mg tablet is 213.85 mg $(14.09\,mg + 170.80\,mg) = 28.91\,mg$.

By linear pharmacokinetics, the amount of drug eliminated at peak time is 57.82 mg for the 500 mg tablet.

At peak time, rate of absorption $(K_a X_a)$ = rate of elimination (KX):

$K_a(X_a)_{max} = KX_{max}$.

For the 250 mg tablet:

rate of absorption $= K_a(X_a)_{max} = 2.8\,h^{-1} \times 14.09\,mg = 39.45\,mg\,h^{-1}$

rate of elimination $= K(X_a)_{max} = 0.231\,h^{-1} \times 170.80\,mg = 39.45\,mg\,h^{-1}$.

For the 500 mg tablet:

rate of absorption $= 2.8\,h^{-1} \times 28.18\,mg = 78.90\,mg\,h^{-1}$

rate of elimination $= 0.231\,h^{-1} \times 341.6\,mg = 78.90\,mg\,h^{-1}$.

Calculations provided here support and confirm the theory that *only* at peak time do the rate of absorption and the rate of elimination become equal, regardless of the dose administered, chosen extravascular route, chosen dosage form, chosen formulation of a dosage form and health of the subject (normal or renally impaired). However, the *time* at which rates become equal can be different.

6. A graph on rectilinear coordinates of rate of absorption against dose administered is given in Fig. P2.1. The relationship between the rate of absorption and the rate of elimination at peak time is shown in Fig. P2.2.

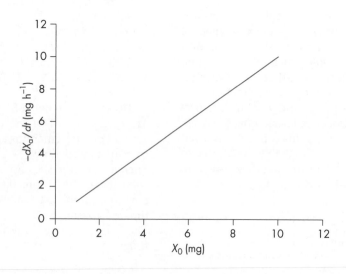

Figure P2.1

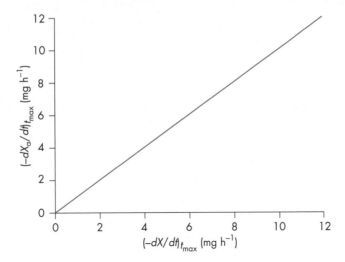

Figure P2.2

7. The following approach will permit determination of the absorption rate constant and peak time. As shown above, only at peak time does the rate of absorption equal the rate of elimination: $K_a(X_a)_{max} = KX_{max}$.

Rearranging this equation gives:

$$K_a = \frac{KX_{max}}{(X_a)_{max}}$$

Once the absorption and elimination rate constants are known, calculation of peak time is possible by using the equations in Answer 4. Since 65% of the dose is excreted in urine as procainamide and 35% as N-acetylprocainamide (metabolite), for a 750 mg intravenous bolus dose, the amount excreted at time infinity is dose × % excreted.

For procainamide, the amount excreted is 750 mg × 0.65 = 487.50 mg.

For N-acetylprocainamide, the amount excreted is 750 mg × 0.35 = 262.5 mg.

8. We know that:

$K = 0.693/t_{1/2} = 0.693/14\,h = 0.0495\,h^{-1}$.

$Cl_s = V \times K$

$Cl_s = 140\,000\,mL \times 0.0495\,h^{-1} = 6930\,mL\,h^{-1}$ (6.930 L h^{-1}).

Normal value is 32.34 L h^{-1}. Note that systemic clearance of procainamide in this renally impaired patient is 21.42% of the normal value. Calculate the percentage change in the elimination half life (3 h in normal subject and 14 h in this renally impaired subject) of this drug in this renally impaired patient and compare the answer with the percentage change in the systemic clearance.

$Cl_s \times$ % excreted $= 6930\,mL\,h^{-1} \times 0.65$
  $= 4504.5\,mL\,h^{-1}$ (4.50 L h^{-1}).

$Cl_m = Cl_s \times$ % metabolite $= 6930\,mL\,h^{-1}$
  $\times 0.35 = 2425.5\,mL\,h^{-1}$ (2.42 L h^{-1}).

These clearance values are dose independent and, therefore, will not change for a 750 mg intravenous dose.

Peak time will be:

$$t_{max} = \frac{\ln(K_a/K)}{K_a - K} = \frac{\ln(2.8\,h^{-1}/0.0495\,h^{-1})}{2.8\,h^{-1} - 0.0495\,h^{-1}}$$

$$t_{max} = \frac{4.0354}{2.7505\,h^{-1}} = 1.467\,h.$$

The value of t_{max} is also dose independent and, therefore, will not change for a 750 mg intravenous dose. In a normal subject, peak time was observed to be 0.97 h. The percentage difference in peak time in renally impaired subjects with respect to the normal value is:

$$(1.467 - 0.97)/0.97 = 0.512 = 51.2\%$$

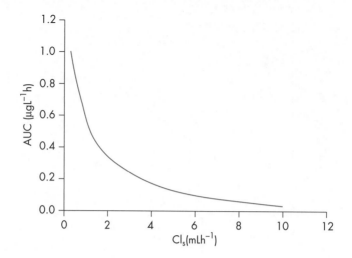

Figure P2.3

This increase in t_{max} indicates slower elimination for the renally impaired patient.

9. Since peak time is independent of the dose administered, peak time for a 500 mg tablet in this renally impaired subject will be identical to that for a 250 mg tablet (1.467 h).

10. $(C_p)_{max}$ is given by:

$$(C_p)_{max} = I(e^{-Kt_{max}} - e^{-K_a t_{max}})$$

The available information is that K_a and K are $2.8\,h^{-1}$ and $0.0495\,h^{-1}$, respectively; peak time has been calculated to be 1.467 h. The intercept of the plasma concentration–time data for a 250 mg tablet was reported to be $1.556\,\mu g$ mL^{-1}. Substituting these values in the equation will provide the following:

$(C_p)_{max} =$
$\quad 1.556\,\mu g\,mL^{-1}(e^{-0.0495 \times 1.467} - e^{-2.8 \times 1.467})$
$(C_p)_{max} = 1.556\,\mu g\,mL^{-1}(e^{-0.0726} - e^{-4.107})$
$(C_p)_{max} = 1.556\,\mu g\,mL^{-1}\,(0.9299 - 0.0164)$
$(C_p)_{max} = 1.421\,\mu g\,mL^{-1}$ for a 250 mg dose.

Note that the relationship between the peak plasma concentration and the dose administered is directly proportional (linear pharmacokinetics). This means that for a 500 mg tablet the peak plasma concentration will be $2.842\,\mu g\,mL^{-1}$.

11. Since

$$(AUC_0^\infty) = \frac{FX_0}{Cl_s}$$

the AUC will be inversely proportional to systemic clearance (Fig. P2.3). If renal clearance represents a significant fraction of systemic clearance, (AUC_0^∞) will increase with decreasing renal function.

Additional reflections. Compare the calculated values of peak time and peak plasma concentration for the 250 and 500 mg doses in normal and renally impaired subjects. Is there a prolongation in peak time (i.e. longer peak time) and elevation in peak plasma concentration in the renally impaired subject following the administration of the same dose? Do these calculations agree with the theory?

7

Bioavailability/bioequivalence

Objectives

Upon completion of this chapter, you will have the ability to:

- define terms bioavailability, absolute bioavailability, comparative bioavailability, bioequivalence, therapeutic equivalence, pharmaceutically equivalent products and pharmaceutical alternatives
- explain the difference between bioequivalence and therapeutic equivalence and describe whether bioequivalence will, in all cases, lead to therapeutic equivalence
- calculate absolute and relative bioavailability
- explain the manner in which parameters reflecting rate and extent of absorption are used to determine bioequivalence between two formulations; use equations to calculate these parameters
- explain the first-pass effect and its influence on bioavailability of a drug
- perform calculations to assess bioequivalency by the method employed by the US Food and Drug Administration (FDA)
- explain the FDA rating system for bioequivalency.

7.1 Introduction

The concept of bioavailability was introduced in 1945 by Oser *et al.* during studies of the relative absorption of vitamins from pharmaceutical products. At that time it was called "physiological availability." Since then, many definitions have been used and proposed by various scientists: some defining it as the availability of active drug at the site of action, others as the likely availability of the active ingredients or drugs to the receptors, etc. All these definitions turned out to be far more euphemistic than accurate.

The bioavailability concept entered the political arena in the late 1960s as a result of:

- the increasing number of prescriptions being written generically
- probability that formulary systems would be established in an increasing number of situations
- the activity in many US states to repeal anti-substitution laws
- the existence of laws limiting or extending the pharmacist's role in drug product selection
- pronouncements by the US Federal Government, and other governments, that they would purchase drugs on the basis of price.

7.2 Important definitions

Bioavailability

"The relative amount of an administered dose that reaches the general circulation and the rate at which this occurs" (American Pharmaceutical Association, 1972).

"The rate and extent to which the active ingredient or therapeutic moiety is absorbed from a product and becomes available at the site of drug action" (US Food and Drug Administration, 1977).

The US Food and Drug Administration (FDA) definition was not well received by many experts and scholars in this field, particularly among the academic community, for the reasons that drug concentrations are seldom monitored at the site of action in bioavailability studies and, very frequently, the site of action may not even be known. Furthermore, current guidelines of the FDA require manufacturers to perform bioavailability and bioequivalence studies by monitoring drug in plasma and/or urine.

Pharmaceutically or chemically equivalent products

Pharmaceutical or chemical equivalence means that two or more drug products contain equal amounts of the same therapeutically active ingredient(s) in identical dosage forms, and that these dosage forms meet the requirements such as purity, content uniformity and disintegration time as established by the *United States Pharmacopeia* and/or *National Formulary*.

Bioequivalence

Bioequivalence means that two or more chemically or pharmaceutically equivalent products produce comparable bioavailability characteristics in any individual when administered in equivalent dosage regimen (parameters compared include the area under the plasma concentration versus time curve (AUC) from time zero to infinity $(AUC)_0^\infty$, maximum plasma concentration and the time of peak concentration).

Pharmaceutical alternatives

Pharmaceutical alternatives are drug products that contain the same therapeutic moiety but differ in salt or ester form, in the dosage form or in the strength. Also, controlled-release dosage forms are pharmaceutical alternatives when compared with conventional formulations of the same active ingredients. For example, Atarax (hydroxyzine HCl) and Vistaril (hydroxyzine palmoate) are examples of different salts; as are Tofranil (imipramine HCl) and Tofranil PM (imipramine palmoate). Keflex Capsules (cephalexin) and Keftab Tablets (cephalexin HCl) are different salts and different dosage forms. Calan SR and Isoptin SR are both controlled release dosage forms of verapamil HCl; while Calan and Isoptin are a conventional tablet dosage forms of the same salt. Wellbutrin XL and Wellbutrin SR both are controlled release dosage forms of bupropion HCl; however, the mechanisms of drug release are different.

Pharmaceutical alternatives are not interchangeable. (Why is this?)

Therapeutic equivalence

Therapeutic equivalence signifies that two or more chemically or pharmaceutically equivalent products essentially produce the same efficacy and/or toxicity in the same individuals when administered in an identical dosage regimen.

Please compare the definition of therapeutic equivalence with the definition of bioequivalence and examine the differences, if any, between these two definitions. Would you consider them to be the same? Would bioequivalent products guarantee or assure therapeutic effectiveness? Please discuss these issues in a study group.

7.3 Types of bioavailability

There are two types of bioavailability;

- absolute
- comparative (or relative).

Absolute bioavailability

Absolute bioavailability is assessed by comparing the values of $(\text{AUC})_0^\infty$ and/or cumulative mass of drug excreted in the urine (X_u), obtained following the administration of a drug in an extravascular dosage form and an equal dose of the same drug intravenously (intravenous bolus) (Fig. 7.1). If doses are not equal, they may be adjusted mathematically.

From area under the plasma concentration–time curve data

Absolute bioavailability (extent) = fraction of drug absorbed (F):

$$\frac{\dfrac{(\text{AUC}_0^\infty)_{\text{extravascular}}}{\text{Dose}_{\text{extravascular}}}}{\dfrac{(\text{AUC}_0^\infty)_{\text{IV}}}{\text{Dose}_{\text{IV}}}}$$

or

$$F = \frac{(\text{AUC}_0^\infty)_{\text{oral}}}{(\text{AUC}_0^\infty)_{\text{IV}}} \times \frac{\text{Dose}_{\text{IV}}}{\text{Dose}_{\text{oral}}} \qquad (7.1)$$

From urinary data

Figure 7.2 shows the cumulative amount of drug in urine following different administration routes.

Again, absolute bioavailability (extent) = fraction of drug absorbed (F):

$$\frac{\dfrac{(X_u)_{t=7t_{1/2}}^{\text{extravascular}}}{\text{Dose}_{\text{extravascular}}}}{\dfrac{(X_u)_{t=7t_{1/2}}^{\text{IV}}}{\text{Dose}_{\text{IV}}}}$$

or

$$F = \frac{(X_u)_{t=7t_{1/2}}^{\text{oral}}}{(X_u)_{t=7t_{1/2}}^{\text{IV}}} \times \frac{\text{Dose}_{\text{IV}}}{\text{Dose}_{\text{oral}}} \qquad (7.2)$$

Please note that the reference standard, while determining the absolute bioavailability of a drug, must always be an intravenous solution since the drug administered intravenously is presumed to be always "completely bioavailable." Furthermore, the value of $(\text{AUC})_0^\infty$ (Eq. 7.1) or the value of $X_u = {}_{7t\frac{1}{2}}$ (Eq. 7.2) for the intravenous solution, (the reference standard) must always be in the denominator of the respective equations. It is important to recognize that the absolute bioavailability or fraction of the administered dose of a drug that reaches the general circulation can equal 1.0 or a number less than 1.0; however, it cannot be greater than 1.0.

Comparative (relative) bioavailability

The ratio comparative (relative) bioavailability is assessed by comparing the bioavailability parameters derived from plasma drug

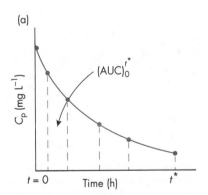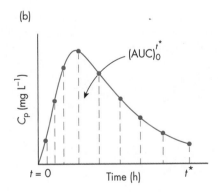

Figure 7.1 Plasma concentration (C_p) versus time data following the administration of a dose of a drug as an intravenous bolus (a) or by an extravascular route (b). $(\text{AUC})_0^{t^*}$, area under the plasma concentration versus time curve from time zero to t^*.

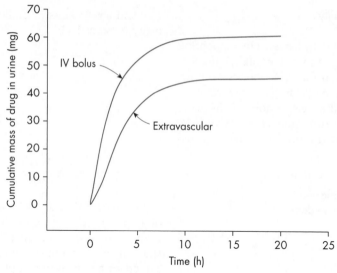

Figure 7.2 A plot of cumulative amount of drug eliminated in urine following the administration of a dose of a drug as an intravenous (IV) bolus and by an extravascular route.

concentration–time plot data and/or urinary excretion data following the administration of a drug in two different dosage forms (i.e. tablet and syrup, capsule and suspension, etc.) and/or two different extravascular routes of administration (i.e. oral and intramuscular). In addition, as we will discuss below under bioequivalence, a special type of relative bioavailability compares a generic formulation with a standard formulation of the same dosage form of the same drug.

When plasma concentration data are utilized in the determination of the comparative (or relative) bioavailability, please note that peak plasma concentrations, $(C_p)_{max}$ and peak times (t_{max}) for the test and the reference products, in addition to the relative fraction of drug absorbed must also be compared.

From plasma concentration versus time data

Figure 7.3 shows plasma drug concentration–time plot data following the administration of a drug by two different routes.

$$F_{rel} = \frac{(AUC_0^\infty)_{tablet}}{(AUC_0^\infty)_{solution}} \times \frac{Dose_{solution}}{Dose_{tablet}}$$

or

$$F_{rel} = \frac{(AUC_0^\infty)_{IM}}{(AUC_0^\infty)_{oral}} \times \frac{Dose_{oral}}{Dose_{IM}} \qquad (7.3)$$

where F_{rel} is the comparative (relative) bioavailability.

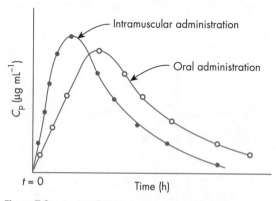

Figure 7.3 A plot of plasma concentration (C_p) versus time data following the administration of the dose of a drug by two different extravascular routes (or this could be via two different dosage forms and the same extravascular route or two different formulations).

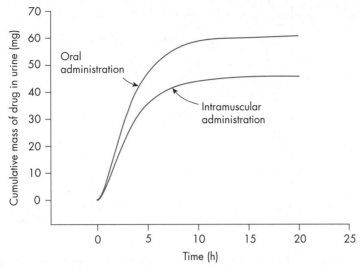

Figure 7.4   A plot of cumulative amount of drug eliminated in urine following the administration of a drug by two different extravascular routes (or this could be via two different dosage forms and same extravascular route, or two different formulations and same dosage form).

From urinary data

Figure 7.4 shows the cumulative amount of drug eliminated in urine following the administration of a drug by two different extravascular routes.

$$F_{rel} = \frac{(X_u)_{t=7t_{1/2}}^{tablet}}{(X_u)_{t=7t_{1/2}}^{solution}} \times \frac{Dose_{solution}}{Dose_{tablet}}$$

or

$$F_{rel} = \frac{(X_u)_{t=7t_{1/2}}^{IM}}{(X_u)_{t=7t_{1/2}}^{oral}} \times \frac{Dose_{oral}}{Dose_{IM}} \qquad (7.4)$$

where F_{rel} is the comparative (relative) bioavailability and X_u is the cumulative mass of drug excreted in urine.

Please note that the reference standard when determining comparative or relative bioavailability of a drug must be chosen by considering which dosage form is being compared with the other dosage form or which route of drug administration is being compared with the other route of drug administration. For example, if we are interested in determining the relative bioavailability of a drug from a tablet dosage form (test product) compared with a solution dosage form (Eq. 7.4), then the solution dosage form becomes the reference standard. Conversely, if we are interested in determining the relative bioavailability of a drug from a solution dosage form (test product) compared with a tablet dosage form, then the tablet dosage form becomes the reference standard. The products being compared can be innovator (brand name) but different dosage forms and/or different routes of drug administration or both generic products in different dosage forms.

Unlike absolute bioavailability, the comparative (relative) bioavailability of a drug can be >1, <1 or 1. The following are some examples of comparative bioavailability studies:

- Valium (diazepam): tablet (oral administration) and intramuscular (innovator products administered via two different extravascular routes)
- Tagamet (cimetidine): tablet and syrup (innovator products administered orally via two different dosage forms)
- cephalexin: capsule dosage form (generic product) marketed by two different manufacturers (different formulations).

7.4 Bioequivalence

Bioequivalence is a type of comparative or relative bioavailability study. However, in a bioequivalence study, $(AUC)_0^\infty$, peak plasma concentration

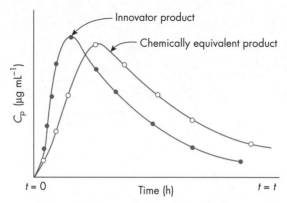

Figure 7.5   A plot of plasma concentration (C_p) versus time data following the administration of a dose of a drug as chemically or pharmaceutically equivalent products (identical dosage forms). One of these (the reference product) must be an innovator product.

and peak time are determined for two or more chemically or pharmaceutically equivalent products (identical dosage forms) where at least one of them is an innovator product (also known as the Brand Name or Reference Standard) (Fig. 7.5).

In this case:

$$F_{rel} = \frac{(AUC)_0^\infty}{(AUC)_0^\infty} \times \frac{Dose_{standard}}{Dose_{generic}}$$

Notice that, for this bioequivalence equation, the AUC for the standard (innovator) product is always in the denominator since it is the standard of comparison for the generic.

The following are some examples of bioequivalence studies

- propranolol: Inderal Tablet (innovator product by Wyeth Laboratories) and propranolol HCl tablet (generic brand)
- perphenazine: Trilafon tablet (innovator product by Schering, Inc.) and perphenazine tablet (generic brand)
- cephalexin: Keflex capsule (innovator product) and cephalexin capsule (generic product)
- sertraline: Zoloft tablet (innovator product by Pfizer) and sertraline HCl tablet (generic product).

Please note that the difference between a bioequivalence study and a comparative bioavailability study is that a bioequivalency study compares a drug formulation with a reference standard that is the innovator product. Moreover both formulations must be identical dosage forms.

The parameters evaluated in a bioequivalency study are $(AUC)_0^\infty$, peak plasma concentrations and peak time.

7.5 Factors affecting bioavailability

Factors affecting bioavailability may be classified into two general categories:

- formulation factors
- physiological factors.

Formulation factors will include, but are not limited to:

- excipients (type and concentration) used in the formulation of a dosage form
- particle size of an active ingredient
- crystalline or amorphous nature of the drug
- hydrous or anhydrous form of the drug
- polymorphic nature of a drug.

Physiological factors will include, among others:

- gastric emptying
- intestinal motility
- changes in gastrointestinal pH
- changes in nature of intestinal wall.

7.6 The first-pass effect (presystemic clearance)

The fraction, *f*, of orally administered drug that successfully passes through gut lumen and gut wall is then taken via the hepatic portal vein to the liver, where metabolism of the drug by enzymes may take place. This extraction by the liver of orally administered drug is called the first-pass effect. The fraction of drug entering the liver that manages to survive the first-pass effect is designated by the notation F^*. We can see that F^* must equal $1 - E$, where E is the hepatic extraction ratio. Compared with an intravenous dose of drug, an oral dose has an extra pass through the liver because it appears first in the portal, not the systemic, circulation. This additional pass through the liver and opportunity for metabolism leads to the first-pass effect. The passage of drug molecules from the gastrointestinal tract to the general circulation and some factors that will play a role, following oral administration, are shown in Figs 6.1 and 6.2 (pp. 98 and 99).

Equation 7.5 shows that the overall extent of bioavailability is the product of two factors reflecting the two steps involved in an orally administered drug reaching the systemic circulation: first, traversing the gastrointestinal membrane and, second, surviving the first-pass effect in the liver.

$$F = f \cdot F^* \qquad (7.5)$$

where F is the fraction of administered drug that eventually reaches the general (systemic) circulation (this is the fraction that would be obtained in an absolute bioavailability calculation); f is the fraction of dose absorbed from gut into the portal circulation (not the systemic circulation); F^* is the fraction of absorbed dose that survives the first-pass effect.

For, example, let us assume that the orally administered dose of a drug is 100 mg; the fraction absorbed into the portal circulation is 0.9 and the fraction that survives the first-pass effect is 0.9. Therefore, $F = f \cdot F^* = 0.9 \times 0.9 = 0.81$ (or 81%). In this example, therefore, 81 mg out of 100 mg of the administered dose will reach the general circulation and will be reflected in the $(AUC)_0^\infty$ and in the amount of drug excreted in urine $(X_u)_\infty$.

Let us assume that the fraction drug reaching the portal circulation is the same (0.9); however, the fraction that survives the first-pass effect is 0.5. Then, $F = f \cdot F^* = 0.9 \times 0.5 = 0.45$ (or 45%). In

this example, therefore, 45 mg out of 100 mg of the administered dose will reach the general circulation and will be reflected in $(AUC)_0^\infty$ and in the amount of drug excreted in urine.

In these examples, although the fraction transferred into the portal circulation is identical, the fraction that survives the first-pass effect is different, resulting in a different amount of drug eventually reaching the general circulation. This difference will be reflected in the values of extent of drug absorption $(AUC)_0^\infty$ and the amount eliminated in urine.

Following this reasoning, is it accurate to state that amount of the administered dose that eventually reaches the general circulation and that is eventually eliminated is influenced by both the fraction of drug reaching the portal circulation and the fraction that survives the first-pass effect (true or false?) Are these fractions additive?

If the amount of the administered dose that eventually reaches the general circulation is smaller, will it be reflected in the $(AUC)_0^\infty$ and peak plasma concentration values?

7.7 Determination of the area under the plasma concentration–time curve and the cumulative amount of drug eliminated in urine

It is clear from discussions so far that knowledge of $(AUC)_0^\infty$ and/or cumulative amount of drug eliminated in urine is absolutely essential to assess any type of bioavailability. Both provide an indication of the extent to which the administered dose of a drug has reached the general circulation. The greater the amount of the administered dose of a drug that reaches the general circulation the greater will be the value of $(AUC)_0^\infty$ and the amount excreted in urine. Is it accurate to state that there is a directly proportional relationship between these two parameters?

The AUC can be determined from plasma concentration versus time data by employing the trapezoidal rule or an appropriate equation (depending on the route of drug administration and the compartmental model chosen). In any case, the use of an equation requires the knowledge of pharmacokinetic parameters such as the apparent volume of distribution, the absorption rate constant, the elimination rate constant, the amount of drug excreted and/or eliminated in urine at time infinity or the amount of metabolite in urine at time infinity, systemic clearance, renal clearnance and metabolic clearance. (Please review these concepts in Chapters 3 and 4.)

The amount of drug excreted in urine can be determined from urinary data, requiring collection of urine samples up to at least $7t_{1/2}$ (elimination half lives) of the drug. At this point, 99% of the administered dose of a drug is eliminated and, therefore this procedure provides a fairly accurate estimate of bioavailability.

Determination of the area under the plasma concentration–time curve from intravenous bolus administration

From our earlier discussion of intravenous bolus administration (Ch. 3, for the one-compartment model) we know that, for intravenously administered drug,

$$C_p = \frac{X_0}{V}e^{-Kt} \tag{7.6}$$

where C_p is plasma concentration at time t; X_0 is the administered dose; V is the apparent volume of distribution; and K is the first-order elimination rate constant. We also know:

$$(AUC)_0^\infty = \int_0^\infty C_p dt \tag{7.7}$$

Hence,

$$\int_0^\infty C_p dt = \frac{X_0}{V}\int_0^\infty e^{-Kt} dt$$

$$\int_0^\infty C_p dt = \frac{-X_0}{VK}[e^{-Kt}]_0^\infty = \frac{-X_0}{VK}[e^{-Kt_\infty} - e^{-Kt_0}]$$

When $t = \infty$, $e^{-Kt} = 0$, and when $t = 0$, $e^{-Kt} = 1.0$. Therefore,

$$\int_0^\infty C_p dt = \frac{X_0}{VK} \tag{7.8}$$

where C_p is the plasma concentration at time t; X_0 is the dose; V is the apparent volume of distribution; and K is the elimination rate constant.

Recognizing that X_0 is the administered dose and VK is the systemic clearance $(Cl)_s$,

$$\int_0^\infty C_p dt = (AUC)_0^\infty = \frac{Dose}{Cl_s} \tag{7.9}$$

This is another way to obtain $(AUC)_0^\infty$, which shows that AUC is directly proportional to the administered dose (i.e. that it exhibits linear pharmacokinetics) (Fig. 7.6).

Determination of the area under the plasma concentration–time curve from extravascular route of drug administration

From Ch. 6 we know that, for a drug administered by an extravascular route:

$$(C_p)_t = \frac{K_a FX_0}{V(K_a - K)}[e^{-Kt} - e^{-K_a t}] \tag{7.10}$$

From Eq. 7.7, we know that:

$$(AUC)_0^\infty = \int_0^\infty C_p dt$$

Hence, integration of Eq. 7.10 yields the following:

$$\int_0^\infty C_p dt = \frac{K_a FX_0}{V(K_a - K)}\int_0^\infty [e^{-Kt} - e^{-K_a t}] dt$$

$$(AUC)_0^\infty = \frac{K_a FX_0}{V(K_a - K)}\left[\frac{-e^{-Kt}}{K} + \frac{e^{-K_a t}}{K_a}\right]_0^\infty$$

$$(AUC)_0^\infty = \frac{K_a FX_0}{V(K_a - K)}\left[\frac{1}{K} - \frac{1}{K_a}\right] \tag{7.11}$$

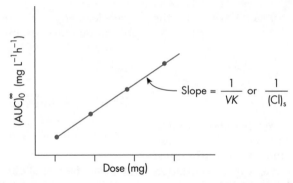

Figure 7.6 The area under the plasma concentration (C_p) versus time curve $(AUC)_0^\infty$ against dose of a drug administered by the intravascular route. Please note that slope of the graph permits the determination of the systemic clearance $(Cl)_s$ of the drug. (Review how to calculate the slope.) K, elimination rate constant; V, apparent volume of distribution.

$$(AUC)_0^\infty = \frac{K_a F X_0}{V(K_a - K)}\left[\frac{K_a - K}{KK_a}\right]$$

$$(AUC)_0^\infty = \frac{FX_0}{VK} = \frac{(X_a)_{t=0}}{Cl_s} \qquad (7.12)$$

where FX_0 is the fraction drug absorbed into the systemic circulation multiplied by the administered dose (this is the amount of drug available to reach the general circulation); VK is the systemic clearance $(mL\,h^{-1}\,kg^{-1})$ of the drug. Please recall that the systemic clearance of the drug is generally independent of the route of drug administration.

If the drug under consideration undergoes metabolism or the first-pass effect, then $F = f \cdot F^*$ and

$$(AUC)_0^\infty = \frac{FX_0}{VK} = \frac{f \times F^* X_0}{VK} = \frac{f \times F^* X_0}{Cl_s} \qquad (7.13)$$

where F is the fraction of the dose of drug that is absorbed into the systemic circulation; f is the fraction of drug traversing the gastrointestinal tract membrane and reaching the portal circulation; F^* is the fraction that survives the first-pass effect in the liver; FX_0 is the effective dose, or the amount of the administered dose of a drug that ultimately reaches the general (systemic) circulation; and $(Cl)_s$ is the systemic clearance.

We know from earlier discussion that for an intravenous solution:

$$(AUC)_0^\infty = \frac{X_0}{VK} \qquad (7.14)$$

For an extravascular route, Eq. 7.12:

$$(AUC)_0^\infty = \frac{FX_0}{VK}$$

If we take the ratio of $(AUC)_0^\infty$ for an extravascular route to that for an intravenous solution,

$$\frac{(AUC_0^\infty)_{oral}}{(AUC_0^\infty)_{IV}} = \frac{\frac{FX_0}{VK}}{\frac{X_0}{VK}} = F = \text{absolute bioavailability}$$

where VK is the systemic clearance of a drug, which is assumed to be independent of the route of administration.

Determination of the extent of absorption

One can also determine the extent of absorption [i.e. $(AUC)_0^\infty$] for an extravascularly administered dose of a drug by following the trapezoidal rule as shown in Eq. 7.7. (In case you have forgotten the trapezoidal rule (very often memory has a very short half life), please review the section regarding use of trapezoidal rule in Ch. 4.)

$$(AUC)_0^\infty = \int_0^\infty C_p dt$$

$$(AUC)_0^\infty = \int_0^\infty C_p dt = \int_0^{t^*} C_p dt + \int_{t^*}^\infty C_p dt$$

However, since we do not have blood samples after $t = t^*$, we cannot actually measure $(AUC)_{t^*}^\infty$.

Mathematically one can obtain $(AUC)_{t^*}^{\infty}$ by the following equation:

$$\int_{t^*}^{\infty} C_p dt = \frac{(C_p)^*}{K} \tag{7.15}$$

where $(C_p)^*$ is the last observed plasma concentration $(t = t^*)$ and K is the elimination rate constant (h^{-1}). In order for this formula to work, $(C_p)^*$ must be in a region of the plasma drug concentration versus time curve that is linear when plotted on semilogarithmic co-ordinates. Then,

$$(AUC)_0^{\infty} = \int_0^{t^*} C_p dt + \frac{(C_p)^*}{K}$$

or

$$(AUC)_0^{\infty} = (AUC)_0^{t^*} + (AUC)_{t^*}^{\infty} \tag{7.16}$$

This is shown in Figure 7.7.

The value of $(AUC)_0^{t^*}$ can be computed by using the trapezoidal rule (Ch. 4) (Fig. 4.6). It is also important to note that Eq. 7.15 is applicable only for a one-compartment model following oral or intravenous bolus administration.

Alternatively, one may use Eq. 7.11 to compute $(AUC)_0^{\infty}$ following the administration of drug by an extravascular route:

$$(AUC)_0^{\infty} = \frac{K_a F X_0}{V(K_a - K)} \left[\frac{1}{K} - \frac{1}{K_a} \right]$$

where K and K_a are the first-order elimination and absorption rate constants, respectively.

Since $\frac{K_a F X_0}{V(K_a - K)} =$ intercept (e.g. $ng\,mL^{-1}$), we have:

$$(AUC)_0^{\infty} = (Intercept) \left[\frac{1}{K} - \frac{1}{K_a} \right] \tag{7.17}$$

This is demonstrated in Fig. 7.8.

Assessing the rate of absorption

The rate of absorption is assessed by comparing the following two parameters:

- peak time (t_{max})
- peak plasma concentration $(C_p)_{max}$.

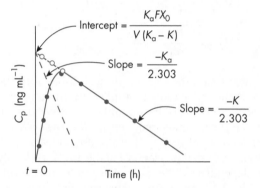

Figure 7.8 A semilogarithmic plot of plasma concentration (C_p) versus time for a drug administered by an extravascular route. X_0, dose; K_a and K, first-order absorption and elimination rate constants, respectively; F, fraction absorbed for the extravascular dosage form; V, apparent volume of distribution.

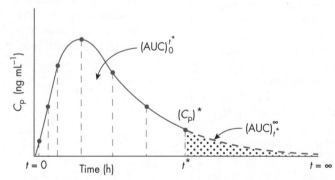

Figure 7.7 A typical plot of plasma concentration (C_p) versus time data following administration of a drug by an extravascular route, showing components of total area under the plasma concentration–time curve (AUC).

(However, keep in mind that the parameter peak plasma concentration can also be affected by the extent of absorption.)

For significance and methods used for computation of these two parameters, please refer to the section Extravascular routes of administration (Ch. 6).

7.8 Methods and criteria for bioavailability testing

1. The general procedure involves administering a drug to healthy human subjects, collecting blood and/or urine samples, analyzing the samples for drug content and tabulating and graphing results.

2. For comparative bioavailability studies, a crossover design must be conducted to minimize individual subject variation. A crossover study means that each subject receives each of the dosage forms to be tested. Tables 7.1 through 7.3 show the design of crossover studies.

3. A minimum of 12 subjects is recommended; however, 18 to 24 subjects are normally used to increase the database for statistical analysis.

4. In addition to informed written consent from each subject, physical examination and

Table 7.1 Example of a two-way crossover design to determine bioequivalency

Sequence group	No. subjects/group	Period[a]	
		I	II
A	6	Brand name (standard) drug	Generic
B	6	Generic	Brand name (standard) drug

[a] Gray shading indicates a washout period when no drug is given.

Table 7.2 Example of a balanced three-way crossover design for a bioequivalency study

Sequence group	No. subjects/group	Period[a]		
		I	II	III
A	4	Brand name (standard) drug	Generic 1	Generic 2
B	4	Generic 1	Generic 2	Brand name (standard) drug
C	4	Generic 2	Brand name (standard) drug	Generic 1
D	4	Brand name (standard) drug	Generic 2	Generic 1
E	4	Generic 1	Brand name (standard) drug	Generic 2
F	4	Generic 2	Generic 1	Brand name (standard) drug

[a] Gray shading indicates a washout period when no drug is given.

Table 7.3   Example of a balanced four-way crossover design for a bioequivalency study

Sequence group	No. subjects/ group	Period[a]			
		I	II	III	IV
A	6	Brand name (standard) drug	Generic 3	Generic 1	Generic 2
B	6	Generic 1	Brand name (standard) drug	Generic 2	Generic 3
C	6	Generic 2	Generic 1	Generic 3	Brand name (standard) drug
D	6	Generic 3	Generic 2	Brand name (standard) drug	Generic 1

[a] Gray shading indicates a washout period when no drug is given.

laboratory testing are also required to establish them as healthy volunteers.

5. Usually the volunteers fast overnight and drug is taken in the morning with a prescribed amount of water.

Figures 7.9 and 7.10 are examples of plasma concentration versus time data obtained following the administration of an identical dose of a drug via different formulations. In Fig. 7.9, although the rate of absorption is higher from formulation A and is similar in extent to B, it is not the preferred formulation because the peak plasma concentration is much higher than the minimum toxic concentration (i.e. outside the therapeutic range). In Fig. 7.10, by comparison, it is quite obvious that the rate and extent of absorption are similar for two out of three formulations (formulations A and B); however, formulation C exhibits much slower and lesser absorption compared with A and B.

When plasma concentration versus time data are not as obviously and clearly different, as they are in Figs 7.9 and 7.10, the following procedure is recommended for the assessment of bioavailability of two drugs in order to make a decision as to which formulation is better.

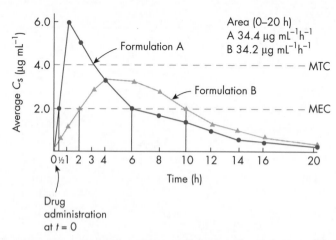

Figure 7.9   Assessment of the rate and extent of the drug absorption from two different formulations (A and B) of the same drug. C_s, serum concentration; MTC, minimum toxic concentration; MEC, minimum effective concentration.

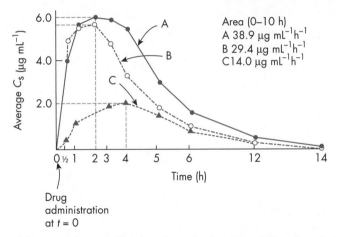

Figure 7.10 Assessment of the rate and extent of the drug absorption from three different formulations (A–C) of a drug. C_s, serum concentration.

Bioavailability testing

Drug product selection

1. Check the criteria for bioavailability testing.
2. Compare bioavailability parameters for products being tested: $(AUC)_0^\infty$, peak plasma concentration, peak time and/or amount of drug excreted in urine $(D_u)_\infty$.
3. Examine the information provided for statistical analysis.
4. Determine the percentage differences for each parameter between products being tested.
5. Apply the 20% rule as a rough indicator in the absence of statistical analysis.
6. Know the use of the drug being tested: is onset of action more important or duration? What is the therapeutic range? Is it narrow or broad?

Statistical terms used in bioavailability testing

Average. The number obtained by adding a group of numbers and dividing by the number of numbers in this group.

Analysis of variance (ANOVA). A procedure, found in any statistical computer package that statistically analyzes data. Among other things, it gives a statistic called the standard error.

Bar over a letter (e.g. $\overline{X}$). This indicates average.

Bioequivalence. This is the statistical equivalence between the generic and the standard (brand name) formulation of drug for the "big three" parameters: peak plasma drug concentration $[(C_p)_{max}]$, time of peak plasma drug concentration (t_{max}), and area under the plasma drug versus time concentration curve (AUC). The FDA looks at the data of the study and decides whether these have proved bioequivalence or not.

Confidence interval (CI). This is the probability (chance), expressed as a percentage, that the next bit of data will fall within a given range of values. The 90% CI is narrower (tighter) than the 95% CI.

Control. This is the point of reference in an experimental study. In the case of a bioequivalency study, the control data are the data for the brand name drug.

Crossover. A study design where the same subjects receive both formulations (with a washout period in between). This design minimizes error owing to differences between subjects, since a given subject is used as his/her control. Therefore, differences between formulations will not be confounded by intersubject variability.

Distribution (frequency distribution). This is the plot of the number of times a response occurs versus the value of the response. For example, if the number of times an AUC ratio (generic/standard) falls within

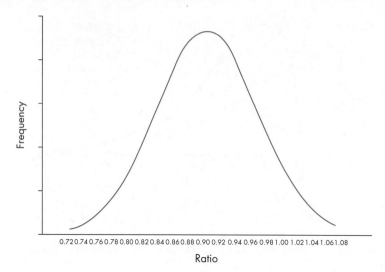

Figure 7.11 A frequency distribution.

each of the small ranges in Fig. 7.11 is plotted, the greatest frequency occurs between 0.90 and 0.92. The frequencies decline for ranges on each side of this range. For purposes of making statistically based conclusions, the most useful distributions are in the shape of bell-shaped curves (normal distributions).

Formulation. This is the same drug in the same dosage form produced by two different pharmaceutical companies. In the example study below, formulation 1 is the generic and formulation 2 is the standard (brand name) product.

Frequency distribution. *See* distribution.

Group. *See* sequence group.

Logarithmic transformation (LT). This is taking the log to base *e* (ln) of the raw data.

Mean. *See* average.

Median. This is the value at which 50% of the values are smaller and 50% of the values are larger; the median is sometimes used instead of the mean.

Period. Period I is the first part of the study. This is followed by washout of drug and then crossover of subjects for the second part of the study, Period II.

Sequence group. Group A receives the generic first and, after a washout period, then receives the brand name formulation. Vice versa for Sequence group B.

Standard error (SE). This is a statistic that tells the variability in the data.

t. This is a number derived from a statistical table called "Values of the *t* statistic." The value of *t* is affected by the number of subjects in the study and by the percentage confidence interval.

Washout. This is the time for drug to be eliminated from the body, after which the second period of the study may proceed. Seven drug elimination half lives are usually sufficient.

Bioequivalency testing: an example

Twelve subjects (normal healthy volunteers) were assigned at random to one of two groups, A or B. The six subjects in group A received a single oral dose (250 mg) of a generic formulation (formulation 1) of a calcium channel blocker. Based on 10 plasma drug concentrations determined from each subject, $(AUC)_0^\infty$ values were calculated. After waiting a suitable number of days (≥ 7 elimination drug half lives) to allow washout of virtually all drug, these same six subjects were given the same dose of the standard (brand name) drug (formulation 2). Blood concentrations were again taken and a new set of $(AUC)_0^\infty$ values were calculated. The sequence of receiving the generic drug in the first time period and the standard in the second time period was labeled sequence A. Subjects in group A underwent sequence A.

Table 7.4

Subject	Sequence group	Period I			Period II		
		Formulation	AUC	ln AUC	Formulation	AUC	ln AUC
1	A	1	12.11	2.49	2	24.06	3.18
2	B	2	15.84	2.76	1	31.94	3.46
3	A	1	27.09	3.30	2	25.80	3.25
4	B	2	37.17	3.62	1	33.53	3.51
5	B	2	46.89	3.85	1	39.63	3.68
6	A	1	33.18	3.50	2	28.98	3.37
7	A	1	37.13	3.61	2	39.84	3.68
8	B	2	55.59	4.02	1	52.47	3.96
9	A	1	25.11	3.22	2	40.08	3.69
10	B	2	40.13	3.69	1	25.73	3.25
11	B	2	24.33	3.19	1	29.63	3.39
12	A	1	31.67	3.46	2	38.78	3.66

AUC, area under the plasma concentration–time curve.

The six subjects in sequence group B received the standard (formulation 2) in period I and the generic (formulation 1) in period II. AUC values and their natural logarithm transformations are shown in Table 7.4.

The mean (average) of all the AUCs resulting from taking the generic $\overline{X}_1$ was 31.60 (in AUC units). The mean for the standard $\overline{X}_2$ was 34.79. The ratio $\overline{X}_1/\overline{X}_2$ was 0.9083. That is, the generic was within 10% of the standard mean. Is that good enough for bioequivalence?

Use of the confidence interval

The current bioequivalence rule is not to use the ratio of means, as above, but instead to use the 90% confidence interval around the ratio of medians (another statistical measure of central tendency). When this confidence interval is calculated, it must fall within 80–125% of the standard or the products are considered to lack bioequivalence (that is, bioequivalence has not been proven).

So, what is a confidence interval and how do you calculate it? If an AUC is chosen at random from a subject who received the generic drug formulation, then another AUC is chosen at random from a subject who received the standard drug formulation, and if the ratio $AUC_{generic}/AUC_{standard}$ was then calculated, it would be highly unusual to exactly hit the mean or median value determined by using all the $AUC_{generic}/AUC_{standard}$ ratios. However, there must be a range of ratios within which the calculated ratio has a 90% chance of fitting, and an even wider range of ratios that the ratio has a 95% chance of being within. There is only a small (5%) chance that our ratio would be outside this latter range. (The extreme case is that our ratio would have a 100% chance of being within the infinitely wide range of all possible ratios.) The "90% chance" range is the 90% confidence interval; while the wider "95% chance" range is the 95% confidence interval (Fig. 7.12).

The 90% confidence interval for the ratio of medians is

$$\exp\left(\overline{X}_{LT_1} - \overline{X}_{LT_2} \pm (t)(\text{SE})\right)$$

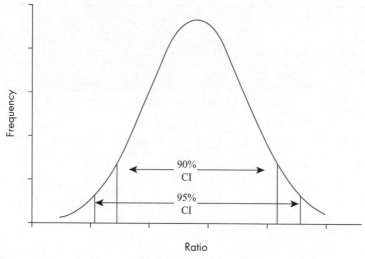

Figure 7.12 The 90% and 95% confidence intervals (CI).

where $\overline{X}_{LT_1}$ is the average of the ln AUC values of the generic; $\overline{X}_{LT_2}$ is the average of the ln AUC values of the standard; t is obtained from a statistical table (it equals 1.812 for a 90% confidence interval for this 12 subject crossover experiment); and SE is the standard error from an analysis of variance of the ln transformed data.

For these data, the analysis of variance produced SE = 0.0633, $\overline{X}_{LT_1} = 3.4025$, and $\overline{X}_{LT_2} = 3.4967$. Therefore, $\exp(\overline{X}_{LT_1} - \overline{X}_{LT_2} - (t)(SE)) = e^{-0.20887} = 0.8115$, and $\exp(\overline{X}_{LT_1} - \overline{X}_{LT_2} + (t)(SE)) = e^{+0.02053} = 1.0207$.

Does this confidence interval fall within the FDA limits of 0.80–1.25 (80–125%)? The answer is "Yes" (at the low end, the answer is: "Yes, by a whisker.") So, the generic has passed its bioequivalence test with respect to AUC values.

However, the procedure must be repeated for maximum plasma concentration (ln C_{pmax}) data and, for some drugs, for peak time data (t_{max} or ln t_{max}) also! If the generic clears all these hurdles, it is declared bioequivalent to the standard.

Interpretation of the Food and Drug Administration's 90% confidence interval formula

The following formula was used above for the 90% confidence interval for the ratio of geometric means (which is the best estimate we can get of the 90% interval for the ratio of medians):

$$\exp(\overline{X}_{LT_1} - \overline{X}_{LT_2} \pm (t)(SE))$$

which is just another way of saying:

$$e^{(\overline{X}_{LT_1} - \overline{X}_{LT_2} \pm (t)(SE))}$$

This is a great calculating formula, but it is a little less than intuitive for seeing what is really going on. So the rules of logs can be used to get the equivalent expression:

$$\frac{\exp(\overline{X}_{LT_1})}{\exp(\overline{X}_{LT_2})} \pm (\exp(t)(SE))$$

The first part of the above expression:

$$\frac{\exp(\overline{X}_{LT_1})}{\exp(\overline{X}_{LT_2})}$$

represents the ratio of the geometric means of the generic AUC values to the standard AUC values. Numerically, it equals (30.039/33.006) = 0.9101. The entire expression may be re-expressed as the range 0.9101/(exp(t)(SE)) to (0.9101)(exp(t)(SE)), which equals 0.9101/1.1215 to (0.9101)(1.1215), or 0.8115 to 1.0207. This latter range is the 90% confidence interval around 0.9101.

The last step is to see whether this range can fit through the FDA's criterion, which is the fixed size 0.80 to 1.25. (In this case, it does.)

Of course, the process would have to be repeated for peak plasma concentration also. A generic drug would have to pass on at least these two bioequivalence parameters in order to be allowed by the FDA.

Presentation of bioavailability data

Figure 7.13 is an example of relevant information typically presented for bioavailability data by a good manufacturer.

Tables 7.5 and 7.6 show bioavailability parameter values and pharmacokinetic parameter values for theophylline following the oral administration

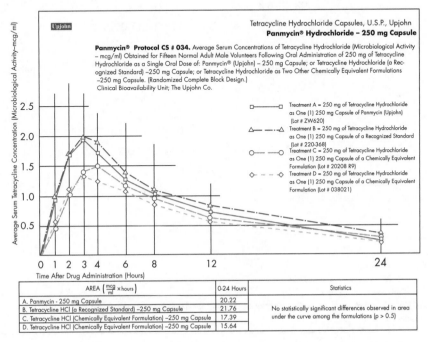

Figure 7.13   An example of comparative bioavailability data.

Table 7.5 Bioavailability parameters for theophylline after oral administration of 300 mg dose through liquid or capsule dosage forms to 14 subjects

Parameter (mean ± SE)	Formulation		Statistical significance
	Liquid	Capsule	
AUC^a (μg mL^{-1}h)			
Observed[b]	98.0 ± 6.4	104.0 ± 8.3	NS ($p > 0.05$)
Calculated[c]	95.0 ± 6.4	118.0 ± 11.0	
C_{max} (μg mL^{-1})			
Observed[b]	11.5 ± 0.7	15.1 ± 1.2	Significant ($p < 0.05$)
Calculated[c]	10.3 ± 0.6	11.5 ± 0.7	
t_{max} (h)			
Observed[b]	1.24 ± 0.3	0.98 ± 0.30	NS ($p > 0.05$)
Calculated[c]	1.20 ± 0.2	0.92 ± 0.20	
F_{rel}[d]			
Observed[b]	–	1.01 ± 0.06	NS ($p > 0.05$)
Calculated[c]	–	1.09 ± 0.04	

See text for abbreviations.
[a] From zero to infinity.
[b] Based on actual assay values in serum.
[c] Based on computer fit of data to a one-compartment model.
[d] Corrected for interindividual variation in elimination.

From Lesko *et al.* (1979). Pharmacokinetics and relative bioavailability of oral theophylline capsules. *J Pharm Sci* 68: 1392–1394. Copyright 1979. Reprinted with permission of John Wiley & Sons, Inc.

Table 7.6 Pharmacokinetic parameters for theophylline after oral administration of 300 mg dose through liquid or capsule dosage forms to 14 subjects

Parameter (mean ±SE)	Formulation		Statistical significance
	Liquid	Capsule	
K_a (per h)	5.22 ± 1.18	13.98 ± 3.10	Significant ($p < 0.05$)
$(t_{1/2})_{abs}$ (h)	0.27 ± 0.07	0.18 ± 0.16	NS ($p > 0.05$)
t_0 (h)[a]	0.047 ± 0.017	0.143 ± 0.038	Significant ($p < 0.05$)
K_E (per h)	0.12 ± 0.01	0.11 ± 0.01	NS ($p > 0.05$)
$(t_{1/2})_{elim}$ (h)	6.19 ± 0.31	6.98 ± 0.61	NS ($p > 0.05$)
V (L kg^{-1})	0.42 ± 0.02	0.38 ± 0.01	NS ($p > 0.05$)
Cl_B (ml min^{-1} kg^{-1})	0.84 ± 0.06	0.70 ± 0.07	NS ($p > 0.05$)

abs, absorption; elim, elimination.
[a] Where t_0 is equal to the absorption lag time.

From Lesko *et al.* (1979). Details as above. Reprinted with permission of John Wiley & Sons, Inc.

of a 300 mg dose via liquid and capsule dosing forms to 14 subjects (Lesko *et al.* 1979).

From the data presented in Tables 7.5 and 7.6 please attempt to answer the following questions:

1. Were the data in these tables for a comparative bioavailability study or a bioequivalence study?
2. Will these data permit you to assess the absolute bioavailability of theophylline?
3. Which parameters, reported in the two tables, show statistically significant difference in two dosage forms?
4. Do you see significant differences in fundamental pharmacokinetic parameters such as the elimination half life, the elimination rate constant, the apparent volume of distribution and systemic clearance for this drug (Table 7.6) when it is administered via different dosage forms? Would you expect this?
5. Do you agree with the reported values of the absorption rate constant (Table 7.6) for theophylline from liquid and capsule dosage forms?
6. If there is a significant difference in the absorption rate constant, as reported in Table 7.6, should the difference in peak time be statistically significant? Please mull over this question. Or is there a typographical and/or calculation error in the reported value of the absorption rate constant? Please ponder? Will this change the conclusion?

7.9 Characterizing drug absorption from plasma concentration versus time and urinary data following the administration of a drug via different extravascular routes and/or dosage forms

This requires either

- monitoring drug in the blood (plasma or serum concentration data)
- monitoring drug in urine.

Monitoring drug in blood

Figure 7.14 represents plasma concentration versus time data following the administration of an

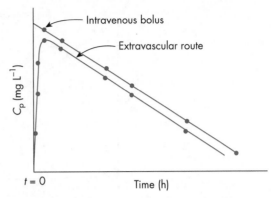

Figure 7.14 Plasma concentration (C_p) versus time following the administration of an identical dose of a drug by intravascular and extravascular routes (fast oral absorption).

identical dose of a drug by an intravascular or extravascular route. The absorption of drug from the extravascular route can be described as rapid and complete in this case since peak time is very short and peak plasma concentration is almost identical to initial plasma concentration for an intravenous bolus. Since the plasma concentration values are very close to each other for the intravascular and extravascular routes, the $(AUC)_0^\infty$ values are likely to be almost identical.

Figure 7.15 represents plasma concentration versus time data following the administration of an identical dose of a drug by intravascular or extravascular routes. The absorption of drug from the extravascular route can be described as slow but virtually complete. Since peak time is long and peak plasma concentration is much lower than the initial plasma concentration for an intravenous bolus, this can be attributed to slower absorption. The $(AUC)_0^\infty$ for the intravascular and extravascular routes may be identical. If this assumption is applicable, then the extent of drug absorption is identical.

Figure 7.16 represents plasma concentration versus time data following the administration of three different doses of a drug via identical formulation and identical dosage form. Since the only difference here is the dose administered, it is reflected in peak plasma concentration and in $(AUC)_0^\infty$. Please note that these differences result only from differences in the administered dose (linear kinetics). Also, please note that peak time remains unaffected.

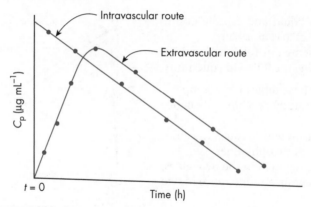

Figure 7.15   Plasma concentration (C_p) versus time following the administration of an identical dose of a drug by intravascular and extravascular routes (slow oral absorption).

Monitoring drug in the urine

Figure 7.17 represents data for the cumulative amount of drug in urine against time following the administration of an identical dose of a drug by an intravascular and extravascular route. The absorption of the drug from the extravascular route can be described as slow but complete (fraction of oral drug absorbed, 1). The cumulative amount of drug in urine, at most times, differs (lower for the extravascular route than for the intravascular route); however, by a time equal to

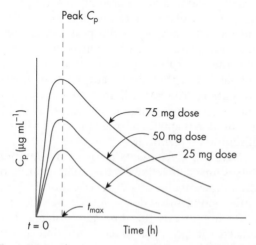

Figure 7.16   Plasma concentrations (C_p) versus time following the administration of different doses of a drug via identical formulation of an identical dosage form. Peak concentration occurs at t_{max}.

seven half lives of the drug, the cumulative amount in urine is identical from each route.

Rate of excretion method

Figure 7.18 represents cumulative amount of drug in urine against time following the administration of different absorbed doses of a drug by an intravascular or extravascular route. The absorption of the drug from the extravascular route can be described as slow and incomplete (fraction of oral drug absorbed, <1). The cumulative amount of drug in urine is lower for the orally administered drug at all times, even at $t = \infty$.

Figure 7.19 represents the rate of excretion against average time profile following the administration of an identical dose of a drug via an intravascular or extravascular route. The absorption of drug from the extravascular route can be described as rapid and complete. This profile is the same as that presented in Fig. 7.14. The time at which maximum rate of elimination occurs is very short and the maximum elimination rate for the oral dose is almost identical to that for an intravenously administered dose.

Figure 7.20 represents the rate of elimination versus average time profile following the administration of an identical dose of a drug by an intravascular and extravascular route. The absorption of drug from the extravascular route can be described as slow but virtually complete. This profile is the same as that presented in Fig. 7.15. The time of peak rate elimination for the oral dose is

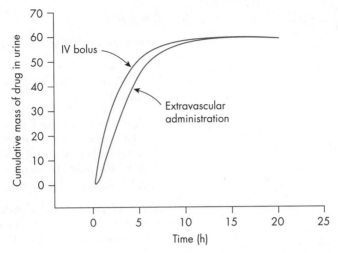

Figure 7.17 Cumulative amount of drug in urine versus time following the administration of an identical dose of a drug by intravascular (IV) and extravascular routes. Fraction of oral drug absorbed = 1.

longer than for the intravenously administered dose and the maximum rate of elimination is smaller. The cumulative amount in urine at seven half lives can be identical from each route.

7.10 Equivalency terms

Figure 7.21 is a flowchart showing how various types of equivalence are determined for two drug products.

7.11 Food and Drug Administration codes

Codes are published by the FDA for every multi-source product listed in the Orange Book (listing of the approved drug products). The two basic classifications into which multi-source drugs have been placed are indicated by the first letter of the code:

A: drug products that the FDA considers to be therapeutically equivalent to other pharma-ceutically equivalent products

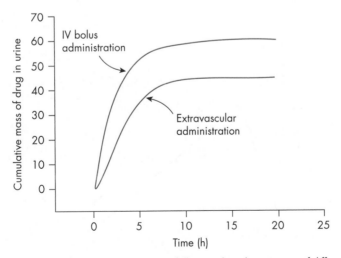

Figure 7.18 Cumulative amount of drug in urine versus time following the administration of different absorbed doses of a drug (fraction of oral drug absorbed <1) by intravascular (IV) and extravascular routes.

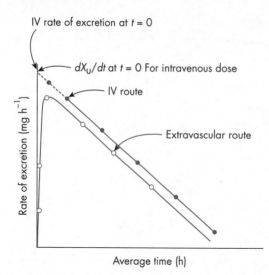

Figure 7.19 Rate of excretion of drug (dX_u/dt) versus average time following the administration of an identical dose of a drug by intravascular (IV) and extravascular routes where there is fast oral absorption.

B: drug products that the FDA does not consider, at this time, to be therapeutically equivalent to other pharmaceutically equivalent products (i.e. drug products for which actual or potential bioequivalence problems have not been resolved by adequate evidence of bioequivalence).

Group A

Within group A there are two subgroups.

1. No known or suspected bioequivalence problems: These are designated as AA, AN, AO, AP or AT

   AA: for conventional dosage forms
   AN: for aerosol products
   AO for injectable oil solutions
   AP for injectable aqueous solutions
   AT for topical products.

2. Actual or potential bioequivalence problems have been resolved with adequate *in vivo* or *in vitro* evidence supporting bioequivalence. These are designated as AB.

Group B

This group has also been divided into subgroups:
BC: for controlled-release tablets
BD: for dosage forms and active ingredients with documented bioequivalence problems
BE: for enteric coated tablets
BP: for active ingredient and dosage forms with potential bioequivalence problems
BR: for suppository and enema for systemic use
BS: for products having drug standard deficiency
BT: for topical products
BX: for insufficient data.

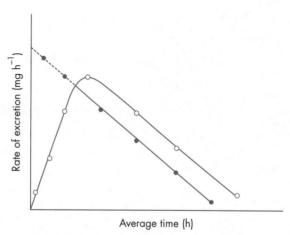

Figure 7.20 Rate of excretion of drug (dX_u/dt) versus average time following the administration of an identical dose of a drug by intravascular (IV) and extravascular routes where there is slow oral absorption.

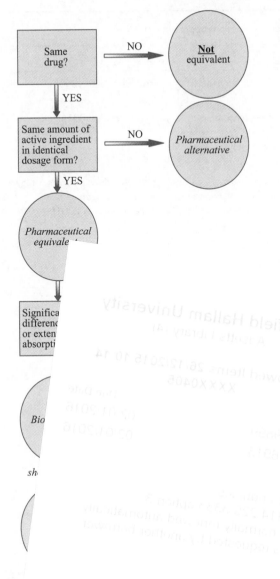

```
┌──────────────┐        NO        ╭──────────╮
│    Same      │ ──────────────▶  │   Not    │
│    drug?     │                  │equivalent│
└──────────────┘                  ╰──────────╯
        │ YES
        ▼
┌──────────────┐        NO        ╭──────────────╮
│Same amount of│ ──────────────▶  │Pharmaceutical│
│active ingred.│                  │ alternative  │
│in identical  │                  ╰──────────────╯
│dosage form?  │
└──────────────┘
        │ YES
        ▼
   Pharmaceutical
     equivale...

   Significa...
   differenc...
   or exten...
   absorpti...

      Bio...

      sh...
```

Figu...
len...
len...

7.12 Fallacies on bioequivalence

Many "experts" have stated certain opinions concerning bioavailability problems as if they were facts in order to promote entirely different political goals. As a result many fallacies have arisen.

Fallacy 1 *If a drug product passes official* (United States Pharmacopeia *or* British National Formulary) *standards then this assures bioavailability in humans.* Perhaps there are few studies which demonstrate significant therapeutic differences among drug products containing the same active ingredient(s), which have also met compendial standards, but there have been no studies which show that these standards are suitable for assuring bioavailability or therapeutic equivalence. Also the confusing of therapeutic differences with differences in bioavailability is inexcusable – these are not interchangeable terms.

Fallacy 2 *If drug products containing the same ac-*
...dient(s) do have different bioavailabilities
...rent therapeutic differences, then this
...gnized in clinical use of the drug and
... the scientific literature. There are two
...that illustrate this fallacious argu-
...st, thiazide KCl tablets were used
...r 5 years before a serious problem
...tified: hundreds of users developed
...g ulcers of the small bowel, many
...g surgery and some resulting in death.
...digoxin tablets were used clinically
...ly years without reports that there were
...nces in bioavailability and in therapeu-
...ponses from one manufacturer's tablet
...next. When, finally, such reports were
...shed, and it was conclusively shown that
...ablets of digoxin, both of which passed
...mpendial standards in FDA laboratories,
...markedly different bioavailability.

...y 3** In vitro *rate of dissolution tests can*
...lose differences in bioavailability and/or
...rapeutic effects without parallel data on
...same drug products in human. It has been
...ssible with some drug products to correlate
...sults of *in vitro* rate of dissolution tests with
...sults attained in human. However, *in vitro* rate of dissolution tests alone, without data in humans, will tell us nothing with respect to what may happen in humans.

Fallacy 4 *Bioavailability must always be related to pharmacological effects or clinical response.* The definition of bioavailability, provided by the American Pharmaceutical Association says

Table 7.7 Evidence of generic bioinequivalence for certain formulations approved by FDA

Trade name	Generic	Class	Problem	Reference
Clozaril	Clozapine	Atypical antipsychotic	Lower C_p max for generic	Ereshefsky *et al.* (2001)
			Greater incidence of psychological decompensation and lower metabolite levels with generic	Kluznik *et al.* (2001)
			FDA required new bioequivalence study; generic currently on market	http: www.fda.gov/cder/drug/infopage/clozapine.htm accessed March 2001)
Dilantin	Phenytoin	Antiepileptic	31% lower total phenytoin levels for generic	Rosenbaum *et al.* (1994)
			30% lower total and free phenytoin levels for generic	Leppik *et al.* (2004)
Depakene	Valproic acid	Antiepileptic	Breakthrough seizure on substitution of generic	MacDonald *et al.* (1987)
Tegretol	Carbamazepine	Antiepileptic	Complications, when switching to generic	Pedersen *et al.* (1985)
			Complications, when switching to generic	Welty *et al.* (1992)
			Differences in bioavailability	Meyer *et al.* (1992)
			Three generics were compared with Tegretol: two failed for AUC and $(C_p)_{max}$; the other failed for $(C_p)_{max}$	Olling *et al.* (1999)
Combined study	Phenytoin, valproic acid, and carbamazepine	Antiepileptic	10.8% of 1333 patients reported problems, including reappearance of convulsions, when switching to generic form	Crawford *et al.* (1996)

AUC, area under the plasma concentration–time curve; $(C_p)_{max}$, maximum plasma concentration.

nothing about the relationship of bioavailability to either pharmacological activity or clinical response.

Fallacy 5 *Differences in bioavailability from one manufacturer's product to the next are less important than differences between the labeled dose and average potency as determined by chemical assay* in vitro *or in vivo* in an animal system.

7.13 Evidence of generic bioinequivalence or of therapeutic inequivalence for certain formulations approved by the Food and Drug Administration

Table 7.7 shows certain pharmaceutical products showing evidence of clinical bio**in**equivalence despite having passed the FDA requirements for bioequivalence.

Problem set 3

Problems for Chapter 7

Question 1

Tse and Szeto (1982) reported on the bioavailability of theophylline following single intravenous bolus and oral doses in beagle dogs (Table P3.1). Plasma theophylline concentrations after intravenous and oral administration were described by a one-compartment open model. The doses administered were as follows:

- intravenous bolus: 50 mg aminophylline (85% theophylline)
- oral administration (A): Elixophylline (theophylline, 100 mg capsules); administered one capsule
- oral administration (C): Aminophylline (aminophylline, 200 mg tablets); administered one tablet.

Plot the data and, using the plot, determine the following.

Table P3.1

Time (h)	Plasma theophylline concentrations ($\mu g\,mL^{-1}$)		
	Intravenous bolus	Oral administration A	Oral administration C
0.25	4.70	0.40	1.65
0.50	4.40	2.40	12.65
0.75	4.10	6.95	14.30
1.00	3.95	11.15	15.70
1.50	3.75	11.15	13.90
2.00	3.60	9.50	14.60
3.00	2.95	8.45	13.75
4.00	2.75	8.15	11.15
6.00	2.05	6.65	10.00
8.00	1.45	4.60	7.30
12.00	0.80	2.90	3.60
24.00	0.25	1.00	0.85

a. The elimination half life ($t_{1/2}$) of theophylline following the administration of intravenous solution, oral capsule and oral tablet doses.

b. The elimination rate constant (K) of theophylline following the administration of intravenous solution, oral capsule and oral tablet doses.

c. The apparent volume of distribution (V) of theophylline from the intravenous bolus data.

d. The absorption half life, $(t_{1/2})_{abs}$, and the absorption rate constant (K_a) for each orally administered theophylline dose.

e. The area under the plasma concentration–time curve, $(AUC)_0^{24}$, by trapezoidal rule for each dose.

f. Using the trapezoidal data for $(AUC)_0^{24}$ determined in (e), calculate the total area under the plasma concentration–time curve $(AUC)_0^\infty$ for each dose.

g. Employing equations determine $(AUC)_0^\infty$ for both the intravenous and the extravascular routes.

h. Using the values of $(AUC)_0^\infty$ calculated in (g), determine the absolute bioavailability (i.e. fraction F) of the administered dose reaching the general circulation for the two orally administered (i.e. capsule and tablet) theophylline doses.

i. Find the relative extent of bioavailability (F_{rel}) of theophylline from the 200 mg tablet dosage form compared with the capsule dosage form. Is this the same as bioequivalency?

Question 2

Prednisolone (11,17,21-trihydroxypregna-1,4-dien-3,20-dione) is a potent corticosteroid that is offered for the palliative treatment of rheumatoid arthritis and various other diseases. Partly because of its low solubility, prednisolone is on a list of drugs susceptible to bioavailability problems. Tembo *et al.* (1977) reported on the bioavailability of seven different commercially available prednisolone tablets. Table P3.2 gives the average prednisolone plasma concentrations for two commercial products: Delta-Cortef 5 mg (Upjohn lot 945CB) and prednisolone 5 mg (McKesson, lot 3J215). Each subject ingested 10 mg prednisolone with 180 mL water.

Plot the data and, using the plot, determine the following for each.

a. The elimination half life ($t_{1/2}$) of prednisolone from each product.

b. The elimination rate constant (K) of prednisolone from each product.

Table P3.2

Time (h)	Mean plasma concentrations (ng mL^{-1})	
	Delta-Cortef (Upjohn)	Prednisolone (McKesson)
0.25	71.7	31.2
0.50	157.0	136.0
1.00	240.0	211.0
2.00	205.0	200.0
3.00	179.0	163.0
4.00	153.0	144.0
6.00	90.6	89.5
8.00	53.2	49.1
12.00	17.3	17.1
24.00	2.3	2.0

c. The absorption rate constant (K_a) of prednisolone from each product.

d. The observed and calculated peak time (t_{max}) and peak plasma concentration, $(C_p)_{max}$, for prednisolone from each product.

e. The area under the plasma concentration time curve, $(AUC)_0^\infty$, by the trapezoidal method and by calculation using the equation for prednisolone from each product.

f. An assessment of the rate and extent of absorption of prednisolone from each product.

g. If these two chemically and/or pharmaceutically equivalent products are bioequivalent. The assessment should be based on the results presented in this study.

h. An assessment of whether these two products are therapeutically equivalent.

Question 3

Nash *et al.* (1979) administered fenoprofen (Nalfan) in capsule form to 12 healthy male volunteers, who were allocated to three equal groups. In a random three-way cross-over study, all the subjects in each group received a single capsule containing 60, 165 or 300 mg of fenoprofen equivalent. Blood samples were collected over 12 h and the plasma concentrations (C_p) of fenoprofen measured. The mean fenoprofen plasma concentrations are provided in Table P3.3.

a. Does this study permit an assessment of the absolute bioavailability of fenoprofen? Explain your answer.

b. Determine the elimination half life ($t_{1/2}$) of fenoprofen for each administered dose.

c. Determine the elimination rate constant (K) of fenoprofen for each administered dose.

d. Determine the absorption rate constant (K_a) of fenoprofen for each administered dose.

e. Determine the peak time (t_{max}) and peak plasma concentration $(C_p)_{max}$ for each administered dose (observe the relationship between peak time and dose administered and peak plasma concentration and dose administered).

f. Calculate the area under the plasma concentration versus time curve, $(AUC)_0^\infty$, for each administered dose. Observe the relationship between this and the administered dose.

Table P3.3

Time (h)	Mean plasma concentrations (mg L^{-1})		
	60 mg dose	165 mg dose	300 mg dose
0.0	0.0	0.0	0.0
0.25	1.6	2.9	4.4
0.50	4.0	10.4	15.8
0.75	4.7	13.8	21.1
1.0	4.8	13.8	22.2
1.5	4.3	13.6	21.9
2.0	4.8	11.2	22.1
2.5	3.9	9.7	18.1
3.0	2.9	7.9	15.4
4.0	2.2	5.7	10.8
6.0	1.0	3.1	7.0
8.0	0.5	1.5	3.7
12.0	0.2	0.5	1.5

g. Show graphically, or by calculation, whether the pharmacokinetics of fenoprofen is dose independent (linear). *Hint*: plot a concentration versus time curve for each administered dose.

Problem-solving exercise

1. Procainamide is used for the treatment of ventricular tachyarrhythmia. It is administered intravenously, orally and intramuscularly, and its therapeutic range is 4–8 µg mL^{-1}. When a 750 mg dose is administered intravenously,

- elimination half life ($t_{1/2}$) = 3 h
- apparent volume of distribution (V) = 2 L kg^{-1} (or 140 L in a 70 kg person)
- % excreted in urine = 65%
- % metabolite (N-acetylprocainamide) = 35%.

When a tablet containing 250 mg procainamide is administered orally to a normal subject:

- absorption rate constant (K_a) = 2.8 h^{-1}
- intercept (I) of the plasma concentration time profile = 1.665 µg mL^{-1}.

Determine the following from the available information.

1. The systemic clearance (Cl_s), renal clearance (Cl_r), and metabolic clearance (Cl_m) in normal subjects.
2. The absolute bioavailability (F) of procainamide from tablet dosage form in a normal subject by employing two different methods.
3. Is the absolute bioavailability of the drug influenced by the dose administered? Is the absolute bioavailability influenced by renal impairment?

   In patients with renal impairment, the elimination half life of procainamide is reported to be 14 h (range, 9–43 h). When a 250 mg procainamide tablet is administered to a renally impaired subject, the absorption rate constant and the elimination rate constant are reported to be $2.8\,h^{-1}$ and $0.0495\,h^{-1}$, respectively. However, the intercept of the plasma concentration–time profile is observed to be $1.556\,\mu g\,mL^{-1}$.
4. Determine the absolute bioavailability of procainamide from tablet dosage form in patients with renal impairment by employing two different methods and observe the influence of renal impairment or systemic clearance of drug on the absolute bioavailability.

Answers

The problem set includes three questions. Question 1 provides the plasma concentration versus time data following the administration of a drug by intravenous as well as extravascular routes. Such data are necessary to assess the absolute bioavailability of a drug.

Question 2 provides the plasma concentration–time data following the oral administration a drug by a tablet dosage form. Note that one of the products is a brand name (innovator) product and other is a chemically equivalent product. Such a study type allows the determination of whether the chemically equivalent product is, indeed, bioequivalent.

Question 3 also provides plasma concentration–time data following the administration of the three different doses of a drug via identical dosage form, identical formulation and identical route of administration. Here, the only difference is the administered dose.

Question 1 answer

a. Intravenous bolus dose, $t_{1/2} = 5.75\,h$
   100 mg theophylline capsule, $t_{1/2} = 5.75\,h$
   200 mg aminophylline tablet, $t_{1/2} = 5.75\,h$.
   Note that the elimination half life of a drug remains unaffected by the dose administered, the route of drug administration and the chosen dosage form.
b. Since the elimination half life of a drug is unchanged, the elimination rate constant should also be unchanged. Therefore, $K = 0.1205\,h^{-1}$. The answer may differ if you observe small differences in the elimination half life of the drug. Note that the elimination rate constant of a drug remains unaffected by the dose administered, the route of drug administration and the chosen dosage form.
c. The apparent volume of distribution of theophylline can be calculated from the plasma concentration–time data for an intravenous bolus dose and employing the equation $V = Dose/(C_p)_0$.

   $V = 8854.16\,mL\ (8.854\,L)$.

   The 50 mg aminophylline (salt value, 0.85) represents 42.50 mg theophylline. Therefore, dose of theophylline is 42.5 mg and initial theophylline plasma concentration (from the intercept on the y-axis of the concentration–time plot) is $4.8\,\mu g\,mL^{-1}$. Like other fundamental pharmacokinetics parameters of a drug, the apparent volume of distribution is also independent of the dose administered, route of administration and the chosen dosage form of a drug.
d. The feathering or residual or curve stripping method was used. The $(C_p)_{diff}$ versus time values for both 100 mg theophylline capsule and 200 mg aminophylline (i.e. 170 mg theophylline) were plotted on semilogarithmic coordinates.

   100 mg theophylline capsule:
   $(t_{1/2})_{abs} = 0.1875\,h$

$K_a = 3.696 \, h^{-1}$.

200 mg aminophylline tablet:

$(t_{1/2})_{abs} = 0.200 \, h$

$K_a = 3.465 \, h^{-1}$.

Please note that the difference between the absorption rate constant (K_a) and the elimination rate constant (K), or the ratio of absorption rate constant over the elimination rate constant, is quite large for each orally administered dosage form. Consequently, the peak time value is likely to be quite small (short peak time), suggesting a rapid drug absorption and quick onset of action for both dosage forms.

e,f. The AUC from $t = 0$ to the last observed plasma concentration was calculated by employing a trapezoidal rule. Then the AUC from the last observed plasma concentration (24 h) until $t = \infty$ was calculated by employing the equation $(AUC)_{24}^{\infty} = (C_p)_{24}/K$. These values were then added to yield $(AUC)_0^{\infty}$.

Intravenous bolus dose 50 mg aminophylline (i.e. 42.5 mg theophylline):

$(AUC)_0^{24} = 33.380 \, \mu g \, mL^{-1} \, h$

$(AUC)_{24}^{\infty} = 2.0746 \, \mu g \, mL^{-1} \, h$

$(AUC)_0^{\infty} = 35.454 \, \mu g \, mL^{-1} \, h$.

100 mg theophylline capsule:

$(AUC)_0^{24} = 96.293 \, \mu g \, mL^{-1} \, h$

$(AUC)_{24}^{\infty} = 8.298 \, \mu g \, mL^{-1} \, h$

$(AUC)_0^{\infty} = 104.591 \, \mu g \, mL^{-1} \, h$.

200 mg aminophylline tablet (i.e. 170 mg theophylline):

$(AUC)_0^{24} = 137.2124 \, \mu g \, mL^{-1} \, h$

$(AUC)_{24}^{\infty} = 7.0539 \, \mu g \, mL^{-1} \, h$

$(AUC)_0^{\infty} = 144.266 \, \mu g \, mL^{-1} \, h$.

g. $(AUC)_0^{\infty} = X_0/VK$

Intravenous bolus dose, 50 mg aminophylline (i.e. 42.5 mg theophylline):

$X_0 = 42\,500 \, \mu g$

$V = 8854.16 \, mL$

$K = 0.1205 \, h^{-1}$

$Cl_s = 1066.926 \, mL \, h^{-1}$

$(AUC)_0^{\infty} = 39.834 \, \mu g \, mL^{-1} \, h$.

Notice that this answer is slightly different from that obtained by the trapezoidal method:

$$(AUC)_0^{\infty} = \left(\frac{K_a F X_0}{(V)(K_a - K)} \right) \left(\frac{1}{K} - \frac{1}{K_a} \right)$$

100 mg theophylline capsule:

$(AUC)_0^{\infty} = 104.366 \, \mu g \, mL^{-1} \, h$.

200 mg aminophylline tablet (i.e. 170 mg theophylline):

$(AUC)_0^{\infty} = 160.202 \, \mu g \, mL^{-1} \, h$.

Therefore, for 100 mg of theophylline, $(AUC)_0^{\infty}$ 94.236 $\mu g \, mL^{-1} \, h$.

h. $F = [(AUC_0^{\infty})_{capsule}/X_{capsule}]/[(AUC_0^{\infty})_{i.v.\ bolus}/X_{i.v.\ bolus}]$

100 mg theophylline capsule:

[104.366/100 mg theophylline]/[39.834/42.5 mg theophylline]

[104.366/100 mg theophylline]/[93.73/100 mg theophylline]

[104.366]/[93.73] = 1.11

Absolute bioavailability of theophylline from the capsule dosage form was determined to be 1.11. Please note that the absolute bioavailability cannot be greater than 1; the results obtained here may be attributed to the methods employed in the determination of AUC values as well as other graphical methods employed in determination of pharmacokinetics parameters.

The authors of this article reported the F value to be slightly greater than 1.0. It may be postulated that the type of animals used in this study, the computation methods employed as well as other unknown sources of variability in the data may also have contributed to the atypical results.

For a 200 mg aminophylline tablet (equivalent to 170 mg theophylline), the same equation is employed and the absolute bioavailability of theophylline from the tablet dosage form was determined to be 0.905: 90.50% of the administered dose reached the general circulation.

Please note that the absolute bioavailability of a drug may vary if the formulation or the dosage form or route of administration differs. For example, if a 100 mg aminophylline tablet of an identical formulation was administered to the same subjects, the absolute bioavailability would be exactly half that for the 200 mg dose because of linear pharmacokinetics.

i. Using the $(AUC)_0^\infty$ of the theophylline capsule as a reference standard (in the denominator of the equation) and that of the aminophylline tablet as a test product (in the numerator), F_{rel} is determined by:

$$F_{rel} = [(AUC_0^\infty)_{tablet}/X_{tablet}]/[(AUC_0^\infty)_{capsule}/X_{capsule}]$$

$$[160.202/170 \text{ mg theophylline}]/[104.366/100 \text{ mg theophylline}]$$

$$= [0.94236]/[1.04366] = 0.903.$$

In assessing bioequivalency, in addition to $(AUC)_0^\infty$, the peak time and peak plasma concentration of each dosage form under consideration would need to be compared. Moreover, in a bioequivalency study, these comparisons are not done by calculating simple ratios. Instead they are performed by rather sophisticated statistical techniques, as described in Chapter 7. The calculation below of peak time (t_{max}) and peak plasma concentration (C_p)$_{max}$ for the tablet and capsule dosage forms performs a very simple comparison of the values.

100 mg theophylline capsule:
observed $t_{max} = 1$ or 1.5 h
calculated $t_{max} = 0.957$ h.

200 mg aminophylline tablet:
observed $t_{max} = 1$ h
calculated $t_{max} = 1.00$ h.

Note that the peak time is not affected by the dose administered. Also note that the calculated peak times of the two dosage forms are quite similar.

100 mg theophylline capsule:
observed $(C_p)_{max} = 11.15 \, \mu g \, mL^{-1}$
calculated $(C_p)_{max} = 11.20 \, \mu g \, mL^{-1}$.

200 mg aminophylline tablet:
observed $(C_p)_{max} = 15.70 \, \mu g \, mL^{-1}$
calculated $(C_p)_{max} = 17.104 \, \mu g \, mL^{-1}$.

As 200 mg aminophylline is equivalent to 170 mg theophylline, the dose of theophylline is 1.7 times greater than the dose of theophylline administered via capsule dosage form.

200 mg aminophylline tablet adjusted for the dose difference:
observed $(C_p)_{max} = 9.235 \, \mu g \, mL^{-1}$
calculated $(C_p)_{max} = 10.06 \, \mu g \, mL^{-1}$.

This peak plasma concentration is not too far away from the value of 11.20 obtained above for the capsule. A formal bioequivalence calculation would prove if this were close enough to say that there was equivalency in peak plasma concentration for the two dosage forms.

Question 2 answer

This question constitutes a *bioequivalence study* (a type of comparative bioavailability).

a. Delta-Cortef tablet $t_{1/2} = 3.25$ h
   prednisolone tablet $t_{1/2} = 3.25$ h.
b. Since the elimination half life for prednisolone from each product is identical, the elimination rate constants (K) should be identical: $K = 0.213 \, h^{-1}$.
c. The feathering or residual or curve stripping method is used to determine the absorption half life, $(t_{1/2})_{abs}$, and K_a for the two products and semilogarithmic plots of $(C_p)_{diff}$ versus time were obtained.
   Delta-Cortef tablet: $(t_{1/2})_{abs} = 0.260$ h and $K_a = 2.665 \, h^{-1}$
   prednisolone tablet: $(t_{1/2})_{abs} = 0.300$ h and $K_a = 2.31 \, h^{-1}$.
d. The peak values can be observed (graphical method, reading from the plot of plasma concentration against time) or derived by calculation from equations:

Delta-Cortef tablet:
observed $t_{max} = 1.0$ h
calculated $t_{max} = 1.030$ h.

Prednisolone tablet:
observed $t_{max} = 1.0$ h
calculated $t_{max} = 1.136$ h.

Delta-Cortef tablet:
observed $(C_p)_{max} = 240 \, ng \, mL^{-1}$
calculated $(C_p)_{max} = 236.41 \, ng \, mL^{-1}$.

Prednisolone tablet:
observed $(C_p)_{max} = 211 \, \text{ng mL}^{-1}$
calculated $(C_p)_{max} = 224.47 \, \text{ng mL}^{-1}$.

e. Delta-Cortef tablet:
trapezoidal rule,
$(\text{AUC})_0^\infty = 1374.098 \, \text{ng mL}^{-1} \text{h}$
employing equation,
$(\text{AUC})_0^\infty = 1382.27 \, \text{ng mL}^{-1} \text{h}$.

Prednisolone tablet:
trapezoidal rule, $(\text{AUC})_0^\infty = 1280.54 \, \text{ng mL}^{-1} \text{h}$
employing equation,
$(\text{AUC})_0^\infty = 1342.51 \, \text{ng mL}^{-1} \text{h}$.

f. This is asking for a comparison of the rate and extent of absorption of prednisolone from a generic product (in this case a pharmaceutically equivalent product) and an innovator product (Brand name product). The rates of absorption are close for both products. The extent of absorption is assessed by comparing the $(\text{AUC})_0^\infty$ values. These are also close for both products, indicating similar extent of absorption.

g. If the confidence interval for the ratio of median value for AUC_{test} to median value for $\text{AUC}_{standard}$ is between 80 and 125% (within ±20–25%), the test product is judged to be bioequivalent to the reference product. In actual practice, the drug company seeking to show bioequivalence is required to provide a statistical analysis of the data. Since we do not have this analysis, we do not have enough information to decide whether the products are bioequivalent or not.

h. The presumption is that two bioequivalent products will also be therapeutically equivalent. However, since we have not proven bioequivalence, we can make no assertion about possible therapeutic equivalence for these two products.

Question 3 answer

This question provides plasma concentration versus time data following the administration of different doses of fenoprofen administered as a capsule dosage form. Since the same drug is administered through the same dosage form and, presumably, same formulation, to the same healthy subjects, there should not be significant differences in the elimination half life, elimination rate constant, peak time, the absorption rate constant and a few other pharmacokinetics parameters. Note that the peak plasma concentration, the intercept of the plasma concentration versus time plot on the *y*-axis and the area under the plasma concentration–time curve, however, will be different for each dose. In fact, these will all be directly proportional to dose since we are dealing with a drug eliminated by a linear (first order) process.

We plotted plasma concentration versus time data on semilogarithmic paper and obtained the following results.

a. Since the intravenous data are not provided and/or available, one *cannot* determine the absolute bioavailability of this drug from the available data.

b. The elimination half life is 2.3 h for the 60 mg dose, 2.2 h for the 165 mg dose and 2.6 h for the 300 mg dose.

c. The elimination rate constant (K) is $0.301 \, \text{h}^{-1}$ for the 60 mg dose, $0.315 \, \text{h}^{-1}$ for the 165 mg dose and $0.266 \, \text{h}^{-1}$ for the 300 mg dose.

   The results obtained are within the margin of error in the graphical process and, therefore, clearly suggest that the elimination half life and the elimination rate constant are independent of the dose administered.

d. Employing the feathering or residual or curve stripping method, the absorption half life, $(t_{1/2})_{abs}$ and the absorption rate constant (K_a) were determined for each dose of fenoprofen capsule. Then semilogarithmic plots of $(C_p)_{diff}$ versus time were made.

60 mg capsule:
$(t_{1/2})_{abs} = 0.175 \, \text{h}$
$K_a = 3.96 \, \text{h}^{-1}$.

165 mg capsule:
$(t_{1/2})_{abs} = 0.237 \, \text{h}$
$K_a = 2.924 \, \text{h}^{-1}$.

300 mg capsule:
$(t_{1/2})_{abs} = 0.2625 \, \text{h}$
$K_a = 2.64 \, \text{h}^{-1}$.

e. *60 mg capsule:*
calculated $t_{max} = 0.704 \, \text{h}$
calculated $(C_p)_{max} = 5.083 \, \text{mg L}^{-1}$.

165 mg capsule:
calculated $t_{max} = 0.854$ h
calculated $(C_p)_{max} = 14.99$ mg L^{-1}.

300 mg capsule:
calculated $t_{max} = 0.966$ h.
calculated $(C_p)_{max} = 23.64$ mg L^{-1}

Please note the relationship between the value for the intercept on the y-axis of the plasma concentration versus time profiles and the administered dose, as well as peak plasma concentration and the administered dose. These should be observed to be directly proportional to dose.

f. *60 mg capsule*:
trapezoidal rule, $(AUC)_0^\infty = 20.914$ mg L^{-1} h
employing equation,
$(AUC)_0^\infty = 20.873$ mg L^{-1} h.

165 mg capsule:
trapezoidal rule, $(AUC)_0^\infty = 56.962$ mg L^{-1} h
employing equation,
$(AUC)_0^\infty = 62.317$ mg L^{-1} h.

300 mg capsule:
trapezoidal rule, $(AUC)_0^\infty = 111.189$ mg L^{-1} h
employing equation,
$(AUC)_0^\infty = 114.94$ mg L^{-1} h.

g. Once again, please note the relationship between the value of the intercept on the y-axis of the plasma concentration versus time profiles and the administered dose, as well as the area under the plasma concentration versus time curve. These should be observed to be directly proportional to dose, indicating linear kinetics.

Problem-solving exercise answer

1. Please note that the elimination half life, the elimination rate constant, the apparent volume of distribution and the systemic clearance of a drug are independent of the route of administration.

Systemic clearance:
$Cl_s = VK$
$K = 0.693/t_{1/2} = 0.693/3$ h $= 0.231$ h^{-1}
$Cl_s = V \times K = 140\,000$ mL $\times 0.231$ h^{-1},
or 2000 mL kg^{-1} $\times 0.231$ h^{-1}
$Cl_s = 32\,340$ mL h^{-1} (32.34 L h^{-1}) or 462 mL kg^{-1} h^{-1}.

Renal clearance:
$Cl_r = K_u V$
$K_u = K \times \%$ excreted $= 0.231$ h^{-1} $\times 0.65 = 0.150$ h^{-1}
$Cl_r = 0.150$ h^{-1} $\times 140.0$ L
$Cl_r = 21.021$ L h^{-1} (21021 mL h^{-1})

or

$Cl_r = 0.150$ h^{-1} $\times 2.0$ L kg^{-1} $= 0.3$ L kg^{-1} h^{-1}

or

$Cl_r = Cl_s \times \%$ excreted
$Cl_r = 32.34$ L h^{-1} $\times 0.65 = 21.021$ L h^{-1}
(21021 mL h^{-1}).

Metabolic clearance:

$Cl_m = K_m V$
$K_m = K \times \%$ metabolite $= 0.231$ h^{-1} $\times 0.35 = 0.0808$ h^{-1}
$Cl_m = 0.0808$ h^{-1} $\times 140.0$ L
$Cl_m = 11.319$ L h^{-1} (11319 mL h^{-1})

or

$Cl_m = 0.0808$ h^{-1} $\times 2.0$ L kg^{-1} $= 0.1616$ L kg^{-1} h^{-1}

or

$Cl_m = Cl_s \times \%$ metabolite
$Cl_m = 32.34$ L h^{-1} $\times 0.35 = 11.319$ L h^{-1}
or 11319 mL h^{-1}.

The above calculations can be checked by employing the following procedures:
$K = K_u + K_m$
$Cl_s = Cl_r + Cl_m$

2. *Method A*. The area under the plasma concentration–time curve $(AUC)_0^\infty$ and/or the amount of drug eliminated in urine (X_u) for at least up to seven half lives of the drug must be known to assess any type of bioavailability. To determine absolute bioavailability, these parameters must be known for a drug dose administered by intravenous solution (reference standard) and by the extravascular route.

Intravenous dose:

$$(AUC)_0^\infty = \frac{X_0}{VK} \text{ or } \frac{X_0}{Cl_s}$$

$$(AUC)_0^\infty = \frac{750\,000\,\mu g}{32\,340\,mL\,h^{-1}}$$

$$(AUC)_0^\infty = 23.1911\,\mu g\,L^{-1}\,h.$$

Alternatively,

$$(AUC)_0^\infty = \frac{X_0}{VK}$$

and since

$$\frac{X_0}{V} = (C_p)_0$$

Therefore, $(AUC)_0^\infty = (C_p)_0/K$
$(C_p)_0 = Dose/V = 750\,000\,\mu g/140\,000\,mL =$
$5.3571\,\mu g\,mL^{-1}$ and $K = 0.231\,h^{-1}$
$(AUC)_0^\infty = 5.3571\,\mu g\,mL^{-1}/0.231\,h =$
$23.1911\,\mu g\,mL^{-1}\,h.$

Extravascular route:

$$(AUC)_0^\infty = I\left(\frac{1}{K} - \frac{1}{K_a}\right)$$

$$I = \frac{K_a F X_0}{V(K_a - K)}$$

$I = 1.665\,\mu g\,mL^{-1}; K_a = 2.8\,h^{-1}$ and
$K = 0.231\,h^{-1}$.
$(AUC)_0^\infty = 1.665\,\mu g\,mL^{-1}[1/0.231\,h^{-1} -$
$1/2.8\,h^{-1}]$
$(AUC)_0^\infty = 1.665\,\mu g\,mL^{-1}[4.3290 - 0.3571\,h]$
$(AUC)_0^\infty = 1.665\,\mu g\,mL^{-1}[3.9718\,h] =$
$6.6131\,\mu g\,mL^{-1}\,h$ for a 250 mg dose

$$F = \left[\frac{(AUC_{tablet})_0^\infty}{(AUC_{i.v})_0^\infty}\right]\left[\frac{(X_{i.v.})_0}{(X_{tablet})_0}\right]$$

$$= \left(\frac{6.6131\,\mu g\,mL^{-1}\,h}{23.1911\,\mu g\,mL^{-1}\,h}\right)\left(\frac{750\,mg}{250\,mg}\right)$$

$F = 0.8554$ or 85.54%

Please note that, since the $(AUC)_0^\infty$ is directly proportional to the dose administered (linear pharmacokinetics), the absolute bioavailability or fraction of the administered dose reaching the general circulation is independent of the dose administered. What will the rectilinear plot of absolute bioavailability against dose look like? It is also important to recognize that if the same drug is administered via another dosage form, via different formulations of the same dosage

form or via a different extravascular route, it is conceivable that the absolute bioavailability may be different. Analogously, peak time and peak plasma concentration may also be different. Therefore, the same drug, when administered via different routes, different dosage forms or different formulations may manifest different rates and extents of absorption and, therefore, differ in their bioavailability (review definition of bioavailability).

Method B. The following equation can also be used to determine *F*:

$$(AUC)_0^\infty = \frac{FX_0}{VK}\ \text{or}\ \frac{FX_0}{Cl_s}$$

where, $VK = Cl_s$
Rearrangement of this equation yields

$$F = \frac{(AUC)_0^\infty(V)(K)}{X_0}$$

For the 250 mg tablet $(AUC)_0^\infty = 6.6131\,\mu g\,mL^{-1}\,h$ and $VK = 32340\,mL\,h^{-1}$ (obtained from intravenous bolus data and assumed to be independent of the route of drug administration).

$$F = \frac{(6.6131\,\mu g\,mL^{-1}\,h) \times (32340\,mL\,h^{-1})}{25000\,\mu g}$$

$$F = 0.8554\ \text{or}\ 85.54\%.$$

3. Doubling the dose will double the $(AUC)_0^\infty$ and, therefore, absolute bioavailability will remain uninfluenced by the administered dose.

4. *Method A.* Determination of *F* in renal impairment from AUC.
Intravenous bolus dose of 750 mg in a renally impaired patient:

$$(AUC)_0^\infty = \frac{X_0}{VK}\ \text{or}\ \frac{X_0}{Cl_s}$$

$K = 0.693/t_{1/2} = 0.693/14\,h = 0.0495\,h^{-1}$
$Cl_s = VK = 140\,000\,mL \times 0.0495\,h^{-1} =$
$6930\,mL\,h^{-1}$ $(6.930\,L\,h^{-1};$
normal value $32.34\,L\,h^{-1})$.

So,

$$(AUC)_0^\infty = \frac{750\,000\,\mu g}{6930\,mL\,h^{-1}}$$

$$= 108.225\,\mu g\,mL^{-1}\,h.$$

Alternatively,

$$(AUC)_0^\infty = \frac{X_0}{VK}$$

and since

$$\frac{X_0}{V} = (C_p)_0$$

$$(AUC)_0^\infty = \frac{(C_p)_0}{K}$$

$(C_p)_0 = Dose/V = 750\,000\,\mu g /140\,000\,mL$
$= 5.3571\,\mu g\,mL^{-1}$
$K = 0.0495\,h^{-1}$.

Therefore,
$(AUC)_0^\infty = 5.3571\,\mu g\,mL^{-1}/0.0495\,h^{-1}$
$(AUC)_0^\infty = 108.224\,\mu g\,mL^{-1}\,h$.

Please note that in a normal subject, for a 750 mg dose, $(AUC)_0^\infty = 23.1911\,\mu g\,mL^{-1}\,h$.

Oral dose of 250 mg procainamide in a renally impaired subject:

$$(AUC)_0^\infty = I\left(\frac{1}{K} - \frac{1}{K_a}\right)$$

$$I = \frac{K_a F(X_a)_0}{V(K_a - K)} = \frac{K_a F X_0}{V(K_a - K)}$$

$K_a = 2.8\,h^{-1}$
$K = 0.0495\,h^{-1}$
$I = 1.556\,\mu g\,mL^{-1}$.
Therefore,

$(AUC)_0^\infty = 1.556\,\mu g\,mL^{-1}[1/0.0495\,h^{-1} - 1/2.8\,h^{-1}]$
$(AUC)_0^\infty = 1.556\,\mu g\,mL^{-1}[20.2020 - 0.3571\,h]$
$(AUC)_0^\infty = 1.556\,\mu g\,mL^{-1}[19.8449\,h]$
$= 30.878\,\mu g\,mL^{-1}\,h$. (In a normal subject, for a 250 mg tablet, the $(AUC)_0^\infty$ is $6.6131\,\mu g\,mL^{-1}\,h$.)

Then,

$$F = \left[\frac{(AUC_{tablet})_0^\infty}{(AUC_{i.v.})_0^\infty}\right]\left[\frac{(X_{i.v.})_0}{(X_{tablet})_0}\right]$$

$$F = \left(\frac{30.878\,\mu g\,mL^{-1}\,h}{108.224\,\mu g\,mL^{-1}\,h}\right)\left(\frac{750\,mg}{250\,mg}\right)$$

$F = 0.8554$ or 85.54%

Method B. Absolute bioavailability may also be computed by using the following approach:

$$(AUC)_0^\infty = \frac{FX_0}{VK} \text{ or } \frac{FX_0}{Cl_s}$$

where $VK = Cl_s$. Rearrangement of the equation yields:

$$F = \frac{(AUC)_0^\infty (V)(K)}{X_0}$$

For a 250 mg tablet in a renally impaired subject, $(AUC)_0^\infty = 30.878\,\mu g\,mL^{-1}\,h$.
$VK = 6930\,mL\,h^{-1}$ (normal value 32 340 mL h^{-1}). (Again this value is from intravenous bolus data and assumed to be independent of the route of drug administration.)

$$F = \frac{(30.878\,\mu g\,mL^{-1}\,h)\times(6930\,mL\,h^{-1})}{25000\,\mu g}$$

$F = 0.8554$ or 85.54%.

From the results obtained, draw your own conclusion with regard to the influence of renal impairment on the absolute bioavailability of a drug.

8

Factors affecting drug absorption: physicochemical factors

Objectives

Upon completion of this chapter, you will have the ability to:

- explain why dissolution is usually the rate-limiting step in the oral absorption of a drug
- explain the significance of drug dissolution on drug absorption and bioavailability
- explain factors that can affect dissolution rate (Noyes–Whitney equation), which, in turn, may affect bioavailability
- describe means of optimizing dissolution rate.

8.1 Dissolution rate

In order for absorption to occur, a drug or a therapeutic agent must be present in solution form. This means that drugs administered orally in solid dosage forms (tablet, capsule, etc.) or as a suspension (in which disintegration but not dissolution has occurred) must dissolve in the gastrointestinal (GI) fluids before absorption can occur (Fig. 8.1).

8.2 Dissolution process

When solid particles are in the GI tract, a saturated layer of drug solution builds up very quickly on the surfaces of the particles in the liquid immediately surrounding them (called the diffusion layer) (Fig. 8.2). The drug molecules then diffuse through GI content to the lipoidal membrane where diffusion across the gastrointestinal membrane and absorption into the circulation takes place.

There are two possible scenarios for drug dissolution:

1. Absorption from solution takes place following the *rapid dissolution of solid particles*. In this case, the absorption rate is controlled by the rate of diffusion of drug molecules in GI fluids and/or through the membrane barrier.
2. Absorption from solution takes place following *slow dissolution of solid particles*. In this process, the appearance of drug in the blood (absorption) is controlled by the availability of drug from solid particles into the GI fluid (i.e. *dissolution is the rate-limiting step*). Hence, the rate of absorption and bioavailability are dependent upon how fast the drug dissolves in the GI fluid. Generally, for hydrophobic drugs, the rate of absorption and bioavailability may be improved by increasing the rate of dissolution.

159

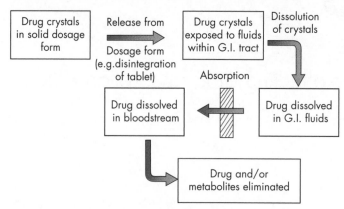

Figure 8.1 Some of the steps involved in the absorption of drugs administered orally from solid dosage forms. GI, gastrointestinal.

8.3 Noyes–Whitney equation and drug dissolution

The Noyes–Whitney equation was developed from careful observation of the dissolution behavior of solids in a solvent system (Fig. 8.3). The equation, in many aspects, is similar to Fick's law of diffusion (Ch. 5).

The specific dissolution rate constant (K_1) is a constant for a specific set of conditions, although it is dependent on temperature, viscosity, agitation or stirring (which alters the thickness of diffusion layer) and volume of the solvent.

The Noyes–Whitney equation tells us that the dissolution rate (dC/dt) of a drug in the GI tract

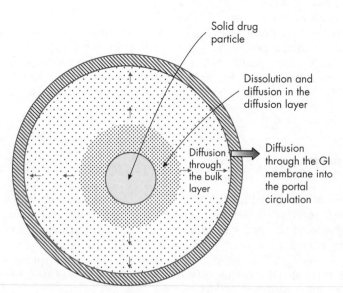

Figure 8.2 The dissolution process. GI, gastrointestinal.

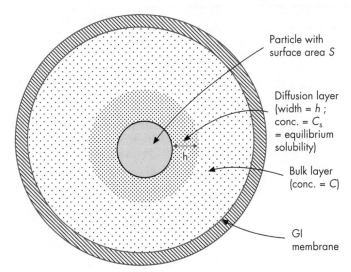

Particle with
surface area S

Diffusion layer
(width = h ;
conc. = C_s
= equilibrium
solubility)

Bulk layer
(conc. = C)

GI
membrane

Figure 8.3 Noyes–Whitney dissolution rate law. dC/dt, dissolution rate of a drug; K, dissolution rate constant; D, diffusion coefficient; h, thickness of the diffusion layer; S, surface area of the undissolved solid drug; C_s, solubility of drug in solvent; C, concentration of drug in gastrointestinal (GI) fluid; $C_s - C$, concentration gradient; K_1, specific dissolution rate constant.

depends on:

- diffusion coefficient (D) of a drug
- surface area (S) of the undissolved solid drug
- saturation, or equilibrium, solubility (C_s) of the drug in the GI fluid
- thickness of the diffusion layer (h).

$$dC/dt = KDS/h(C_s - C)$$

The concentration of drug in GI fluid (C) is generally not a significant factor because the continuous removal of drug, through the absorption process, prevents a significant build up of drug in the GI fluid. Furthermore, the Noyes–Whitney equation suggests that there are two main variables that govern the dissolution of a drug in the GI tract:

- surface area of a solid drug
- saturation or equilibrium solubility of a drug in the GI fluid.

The surface area of the powder (drug) can be controlled by controlling the drug's particle size. The equilibrium solubility of a drug can be controlled

by a proper selection of soluble salts (rather than use of the less-soluble free acid or base form), the selection of different crystal forms or hydrated forms, or perhaps modifications in chemical structure.

8.4 Factors affecting the dissolution rate

Some of the more important factors that affect the dissolution rate, especially, of slowly dissolving or poorly soluble substances, are:

- surface area and particle size
- solubility of drug in the diffusion layer
- the crystal form of a drug
- the state of hydration
- complexation
- chemical modification.

Surface area and particle size

Of all possible manipulations of the physico-chemical properties of drugs to yield better dissolution, the reduction of the particle size of the drug has been the most thoroughly investigated. A drug dissolves more rapidly when its surface area is increased. This increase in surface area is accomplished by reducing the particle size of the drug. This is the reason why many poorly soluble and slowly dissolving drugs are marketed in micronized or microcrystalline form (i.e. particle size of 2–10 μm).

The reduction in particle size and, therefore, surface area is accomplished by various means (e.g. milling, grinding and solid dispersions).

The use of solid dispersions provides an innovative means of particle size reduction and has received considerable attention recently. Solid dispersions are prepared by dissolving the drug and carrier in a suitable solvent and solidifying the mixture by cooling or evaporation (Box 8.1).

Among listed drugs in the box, griseofulvin and digoxin have been most comprehensively studied since the dissolution is the rate-limiting step in the absorption of these drugs. Jounela *et al.* (1975) showed that decreasing the particle size of digoxin from 102 μm to approximately 10 μm resulted in 100% increase in bioavailability (Figs 8.4 to 8.6 are examples).

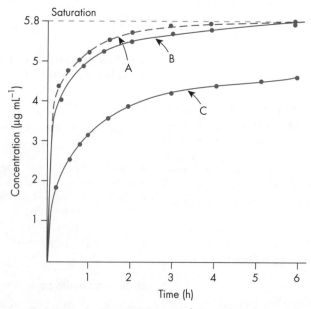

Figure 8.4 Rate of dissolution of norethisterone acetate in 0.1 mol L^{-1} HCL at 37 °C. A, micronized powder; B, micronized powder in coated tablet form; C, non-micronized material in coated tablet form. (With permission from Gibian *et al.* 1968.)

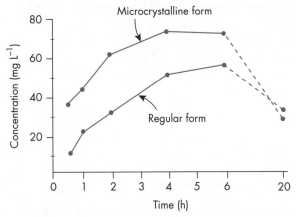

Figure 8.5 Blood sulfadiazine concentration in human following the administration of a 3 g dose. (Reinhold JG *et al.*(1945). A comparison of the behavior of microcrystalline sulfadiazine with that of regular sulfadiazine in man. *Am J Med Sci* 210:141. Reprinted with permission: Wolters Kluwer Health, Baltimore, MD.)

The smaller the particle size the larger the specific surface and the faster the dissolution. Reduction in the particle size alone, however, is not enough to improve the dissolution rate of drug particles, especially, for hydrophobic drugs. For these, the effective surface area is more important. The effective surface area can be increased by the addition of a wetting agent into the formulation of tablets, capsules, suspensions, and so on. The more commonly used wetting agents include tweens, spans, sodium and lauryl sulfate. These agents lower the contact angle between an aqueous liquid and a hydrophobic particle. For example, Ceclor (cefaclor) suspension contains:

cefaclor monohydrate
cellulose
FDC Red 40
flavor
xanthum gum
sucrose
sodium lauryl sulfate (wetting agent).

The importance of incorporating a surface-active agent lies in the fact that physiological

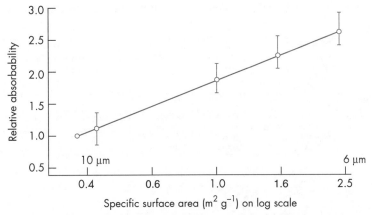

Figure 8.6 Effect of specific surface on bioavailability of griseofulvin. Relative absorbabilty was based on the area under the curve of blood concentration versus time. Specific surface is the surface area/unit weight of powder. It was derived as $6/(\rho d_v)$, where ρ is density (g mL^{-1}) of powder and d_v is volume diameter of powder particles. (Wagner 1964, *Am J Med Sci*, 210:141. Reprinted with permission, Wolters Kluwer Health, Baltimore, MD.)

Table 8.1 Influence of surface active agent on the absorption of Phenacetin

Character of suspension	$(C_p)_{max}$ (μg mL^{-1})	Urinary recovery (% of dose)
Fine, with polysorbate 80	13.5	75
Fine	9.6	51
Medium	3.3	57
Coarse	1.4	48

$(C_p)_{max}$, maximum plasma concentration.

From Prescott et al. (1970). The effects of particle size on the absorption of phenacetin in man. *Clin Pharmacol Ther* 11: 496. Reprinted with permission from Macmillon Publishers Ltd.

surface-active agents such as bile salts and lysolecithin facilitate the dissolution and absorption in the small intestine of drugs that are poorly water soluble.

Table 8.1 illustrates the influence of a surface-active agent on the absorption of phenacetin.

Reduction in particle size, however, is not always desirable. For example, Slow K tablets incorporate a matrix that slowly releases potassium in order to minimize GI tract irritation. Simulatly, Macrodantin is a formulation of large crystals of nitrofurantoin, which will dissolve slowly and thereby minimize irritation.

Solubility of a drug in the diffusion layer

If the solubility of a drug can be appreciably increased in the diffusion layer, the drug molecules can rapidly escape from the main particle and travel to the absorption site. This principle is used to increase the solubility of weak acids in the stomach. The solubility of weak acids increases with an increase in pH because the acid is transformed into an ionized form, which is soluble in aqueous GI content (Figure 8.7).

The pH of a solution in the diffusion layer can be increased by;

- using a highly water-soluble salt of a weak acid;
- mixing or combining a basic substance into a formulation (e.g. NaHCO$_3$ [sodium bicarbonate], calcium carbonate, magnesium oxide, and magnesium carbonate] [MgCO$_3$]); examples include Bufferin (aspirin), which contains aluminum dihydroxyamino acetate and

Area	Diffusion layer surround-ing particles		Bulk liquid of GI tract	Bulk liquid of GI tract	GI membrane (separates gastrointestinal tract from portal circulation)
pH	5		2	2	
Event	Dissolu-tion: salt of weak acid drug	Diffu-sion	Precipita-tion (small particles)	Redissolu-tion and diffusion of acidic drug	Traversal across GI membrane and absorption into portal circulation

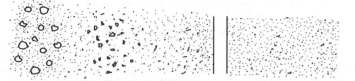

Figure 8.7 Dissolution process in the stomach from the surface of a highly water soluble salt. GI, gastrointestinal.

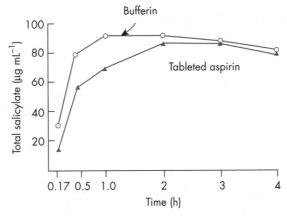

Figure 8.8   Comparison of two preparations of aspirin in regard to serum concentration of total salicylate over a 4 h period. (Hollister *et al.* 1972, *Clin Pharmacol Ther* 13:1).

MgCO$_3$ (Fig. 8.8), and Alka-Seltzer, which contains NaHCO$_3$ and aspirin;

- increasing the pH of the GI content by the use of antacids (however, the fact that antacids strongly adsorb many drugs, limits the use of this method).

Crystalline versus amorphous form

Some drugs exist as either crystalline or amorphous form. As the amorphous form is always more soluble than the crystalline form, there is

the possibility that there will be significant differences in their bioavailability. The amorphous form of the antibiotic novobiocin (Albamycin) is 10 times more soluble than the crystalline form and has similar differences in dissolution rate (Table 8.2). The data in the table demonstrate the difference in the plasma concentration between crystalline and amorphous forms.

Crystalline forms

Many drugs exist in more than one crystalline form, a property known as polymorphism. Drug

Table 8.2   Differences in Novobiocin plasma levels as a function of salt form, crystalline form, and amorphous form

Time after dose (h)	Plasma concentration (μg mL^{-1})			
	Amorphous (acid)	Calcium salt	Sodium salt	Crystalline (acid)
0.5	5.0	9.0	0.5	ND
1	40.0	16.4	0.5	ND
2	29.5	26.8	14.6	ND
3	22.3	19.0	22.2	ND
4	23.7	15.7	16.9	ND
5	20.2	13.8	10.4	ND
6	17.5	10.0	6.4	ND

After Mullins and Macek (1960). ND = not detectable.

molecules exhibit different space–lattice arrangement in crystal form in each polymorph. Though chemically the same, polymorphs differ substantially with regards to physicochemical properties. These properties include solubility, dissolution rate, density and melting point, among others. Solubility and dissolution rate, in turn, will likely influence the rate of absorption.

At any one temperature and pressure, only one crystal (polymorph) form will be stable. Any other polymorph found under these condition is metastable and will eventually convert to the stable form, but the conversion may be very slow (sometime can take years). The metastable form is a higher energy form and usually has a lower melting point, greater solubility, and faster dissolution rate. Examples are chloramphenicol palmitate (Aguir *et al.* 1967) and sulfameter (Khalil *et al.* 1972). This sulfanilamide is reported to have six polymorphs. Crystalline form II is about twice as soluble as crystalline form III. Studies in normal subjects showed that the rate and extent of absorption is approximately 40% greater from form II. Table 8.3 provides a few examples of drugs that exhibit polymorphism.

State of hydration

The state of hydration of a drug molecule can affect some of the physicochemical properties of a drug. One such property that is significantly influenced by the state of hydration is the aqueous solubility of the drug. Often the anhydrous form of an organic compound is more soluble than the hydrate (with some exceptions). This difference in solubility is reflected in differences in the dissolution rate. An excellent study was performed by Poole *et al.* (1968) on ampicillin, a penicillin derivative that is available as the anhydrous form (Omnipen) and the trihydrate form (Polycillin). The results are shown in Figs. 8.9 through 8.14).

Complexation

Formation of a complex of drugs in the GI fluid may alter the rate and, in some cases, the extent of absorption. The complexing agent may be a substance normal to the GI tract, a dietary component or a component (excipient) of a dosage form.

Table 8.3 Some drugs which exhibit polymorphism

Name of drug	Number of polymorphs	Number of amorphs	Number of pseudo-polymorphs
Ampicillin	1		1
Betamethasone	1	1	
Caffeine	1		1
Chloramphenicol palmitate	3	1	
Chlordiazepoxide HCl	2		1
Cortisone acetate	8		
Erythromycin	2		
Indometacin	3		
Prednisone	1		1
Progesterone	2		
Testosterone	4		

From "Polymorphism and pseudopolymorphism of drugs." Table 2.3 in Florence AT and Atwood D (1981). *Physicochemical Principles of Pharmacy*, 1st ed., page 21. With kind permission of Springer Science and Business Media.

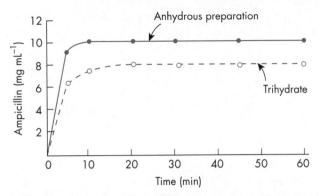

Figure 8.9   Solubility of ampicillin in distilled water at 37 °C. (Poole, J (1968). Physicochemical factors influencing the absorption of the anhydrous and trihydrate forms of ampicillin. *Curr Ther Res*, 10: 292–303. With permission Excerpta Medica, Inc.)

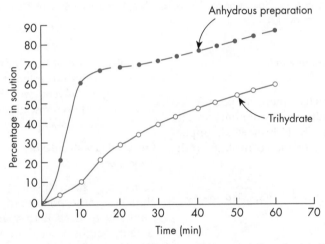

Figure 8.10   Dissolution of ampicillin in distilled water at 37 °C from trade capsule formulations. (Poole, J., Physicochemical factors influencing the absorption of the anhydrous and trihydrate forms of ampicillin. *Curr Ther Res*, 10, 292–303, 1968 Details as above.)

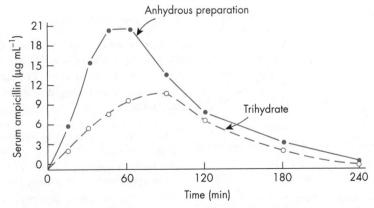

Figure 8.11   Mean serum concentrations of ampicillin in dogs after oral administration of 250 mg doses of trade oral suspensions. (Poole, J., 1968. Details as above.)

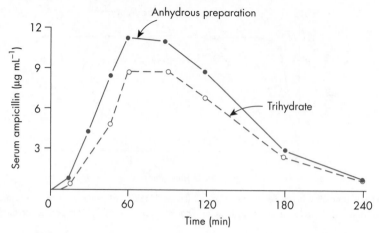

Figure 8.12   Mean serum concentrations of ampicillin in dogs after oral administration of 250 mg doses of trade capsules. (Poole, J., 1968. Details as above.)

Complexing with a substance in the gastrointestinal tract

Intestinal mucus, which contains the polysaccharide mucin, can avidly bind streptomycin and dihydrostreptomycin (E. Nelson *et al*, unpublished data). This binding may contribute to the poor absorption of these antibiotics. Bile salts in the small intestine interact with certain drugs, including neomycin and kanamycin, to form insoluble and non-absorbable complexes.

Complexing with a dietary component

Tetracycline forms insoluble complexes with calcium ions. Absorption of these antibiotics is substantially reduced if they are taken with milk, certain food or other sources of calcium such as some antacids. In the past, the incorporation of dicalcium phosphate as a filler in tetracycline dosage forms also reduced its bioavailability.

Complexing with excipients

The most frequently observed complex formation is between various drugs and macromolecules such as gums, cellulose derivatives, high- molecular-weight polyols and non-ionic surfactants. Mostly, however, these complexes are reversible with little effect on the bioavailability of drugs. There are, however, some exceptions. Phenobarbital, for example, forms an insoluble complex with polyethylene glycol 4000 (PEG 4000). The dissolution and absorption rates of phenobarbital containing this polyol are reported to be markedly reduced (Singh *et al*. 1966).

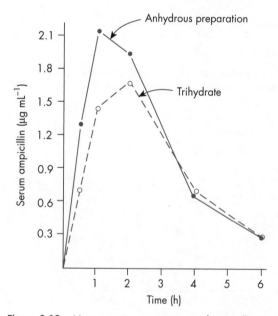

Figure 8.13   Mean serum concentrations of ampicillin in human subjects after oral administration of 250 mg doses of oral suspensions. (Poole, J., 1968. Details as above.)

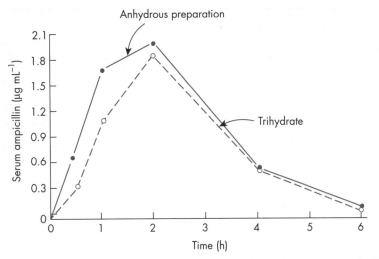

Figure 8.14   Mean serum concentrations of ampicillin in human subjects after oral administration of 250 mg doses of oral trade capsules. (Poole, J., 1968. Details as above.)

Perhaps a more rewarding application of complex formation is the administration of a water-soluble complex of a drug that would be, otherwise, incompletely absorbed because of poor water solubility. Hydroquinone, for example, forms a water-soluble and rapidly dissolving complex with digoxin (Higuchi *et al.* 1974). An oral formulation containing the hydroquinone–digoxin complex resulted in faster absorption compared with the standard tablet of digoxin.

Cyclodextrins (α, β, γ) are some newer complexing agents generating considerable interest and showing promise for the future.

Chemical modification

Alteration of chemical form requires a modification in the actual chemical structure of a drug.

Ideally, a drug molecule should have sufficient aqueous solubility for dissolution, an optimum partition coefficient, high diffusion through lipid layers and stable chemical groups. Such an ideal molecule usually does not exist. Hence, chemical modifications are generally directed toward that part of a molecule which is responsible for hindrance of the overall absorption process.

An example is the increase in lipid solubility achieved by chemical modification by tetracycline to give the derivative doxycycline. Doxycycline (Vibramycin) is more efficiently absorbed from the intestine than is tetracycline, partly because of better lipid solubility and partly because of a decreased tendency to form poorly soluble complexes with calcium.

Absorption of erythromycin is much more efficient when the estolate form is used instead of the ethyl succinate ester form (Grifith *et al.* 1969).

Chemical changes related to lipid solubility and its effect on GI absorption are best exemplified by barbiturates, as seen in Table 8.4, in which an increase in lipid solubility is directly related to absorption from the colon.

Another clear example in this category of two different chemical forms is tolbutamide (Orinase) and its sodium salt. The dissolution rate of disodium tolbutamide is approximately 5000 times greater than tolbutamide at pH 1.2, and approximately 275 times at pH 7.4. Administration of the sodium salt results in a rapid and pronounced reduction in blood glucose (not desired) to approximately 67–70% of control levels. The more slowly dissolving tolbutamide (free acid) produces a more gradual decrease in blood sugar (Fig. 8.15).

Table 8.4   Comparison of barbiturate absorption in rat colon and lipophilicity

Barbiturate	Partition coefficient[a]	Log (partition coefficient)	Percentage absorbed
Barbital	0.7	−0.15	12
Aprobarbital	4.9	0.69	17
Phenobarbital	4.8	0.68	20
Allylbarbituric acid	10.5	1.02	23
Butethal	11.7	1.07	24
Cyclobarbital	13.9	1.14	24
Pentobarbital	28.0	1.45	30
Secobarbital	50.7	1.71	40
Hexethal	>100	>2.0	44

[a] Chloroform/water partition coefficient of undissociated drug.

Reprinted with permission from Shanker LS (1960). On the mechanism of absorption from the gastrointestinal trat. *J. Med. Pharm. Chem.* 2:343. Copyright 1960 American Chemical Society.

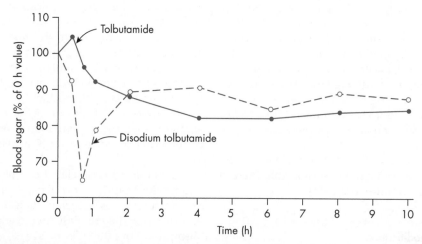

Figure 8.15   Effect of dissolution rate on the absorption and biological response of tolbutamide (1.0 g) and sodium tolbutamide (1.0 g equivalent) when formulated in compressed tablets. From Wagner JG (1961). Biopharmaceutics: absorption aspects. *J. Pharm. Sci.* 50:359. Reprinted with permission John Wiley & Sons, Inc.

9

Gastrointestinal absorption: role of the dosage form

Objectives

Upon completion of this chapter, you will have the ability to:

- predict the effect of the dosage form (solution, suspension, capsule, tablet) on gastrointestinal absorption
- predict the effect of formulation and processing factors (diluents, disintegrants, lubricants, etc.) on gastrointestinal absorption
- explain and describe the utility of the correlation of *in vivo* and *in vitro* studies.

9.1 Introduction

The main purpose of incorporating a drug in a delivery system is to develop a dosage form that possesses the following attributes:

- contains the labeled amount of drug in a stable form until its expiration date
- consistently delivers the drug to the general circulation at an optimum rate and to an optimum extent
- is suitable for administration through an appropriate route
- is acceptable to patients.

All the physicochemical properties of drugs (i.e. particle size, pH, pK_a, salt form, etc.) will contribute to the dosage form design. Additionally, additives incorporated into the dosage form (e.g. diluents, binders, lubricants, suspending agents) often may alter the absorption of a therapeutic agent from a dosage form.

Published studies have demonstrated that, with virtually any drug, a two- to five-fold difference in the rate and/or extent of absorption can routinely be produced by using a specific dosage form or formulation.

For example, a difference of more than 60-fold has been found in the absorption rate of spironolactone (Aldactone) from the worst formulation to the best formulation. The peak plasma concentration following the administration of the same dose ranged from 0.06 to $3.75\,\mu g\,L^{-1}$.

Recognizing the fact that drug must dissolve in the gastrointestinal (GI) fluid before it can be absorbed, the bioavailability of a drug would be expected to decrease in the following order:

solution > suspension > capsule > tablet > coated tablets.

Although this ranking is not universal, it does provide a useful guideline.

Some of the effects are shown in Fig. 9.1.

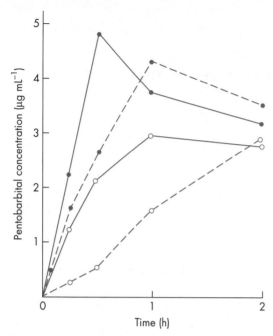

Figure 9.1   Pentobarbital concentrations in plasma after a single 200 mg dose in various dosage forms. Aqueous solution (●–●); aqueous suspension (●--●); tablet, sodium salt (○–○); tablet, acid (○--○). (With permission from Sjorgen *et al* (1965.)

9.2 Solution (elixir, syrup and solution) as a dosage form

A solution dosage form is widely used for cough and cold preparations and other drugs, particularly for pediatric patients. Drugs are generally absorbed more rapidly from solution. The rate-limiting step is likely to be gastric emptying, particularly when the drug is administered after meals.

When a salt of an acidic drug is used to formulate a solution, there is the possibility of precipitation in the gastric fluid. Experience, however, suggests that these precipitates are usually finely divided (have a large surface area) and, therefore, are easily redissolved.

Many drugs, unless converted to water-soluble salts, are poorly soluble. Solutions of these drugs can be prepared by adding co-solvents such as alcohol or polyethylene glycol or surfactants.

Certain materials such as sorbitol or hydrophilic polymers are added to solution dosage forms to improve pourability and palatability by increasing viscosity. This higher viscosity may slow gastric emptying and absorption.

The major problem of the solution dosage form is the physicochemical stability of the dissolved drug(s).

9.3 Suspension as a dosage form

A well-formulated suspension is second to a solution in efficiency of absorption. Dissolution is the rate-limited factor in absorption of a drug from a suspension. However, drug dissolution from a suspension can be rapid if very fine or micronized powders are used. (These have a larger surface area or specific surface.)

Drugs formulated in tablet and capsule dosage forms may not achieve the state of dispersion in the GI tract that is attainable with a finely subdivided, well-formulated suspension (Fig. 9.2).

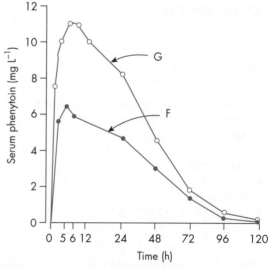

Figure 9.2   Phenytoin concentrations in serum after a 600 mg oral dose in aqueous suspensions containing either micronized (G) or conventional (F) drug. The area under the serum level versus time curve is 40 and 66 mg L^{-1} h^{-1} for F and G, respectively. (With permission from Neuvonen *et al.* (1977).)

Several studies have demonstrated the superior bioavailability characteristics for drugs from suspension compared with those of solid dosage forms. For example, blood concentrations of the antibacterial combination trimethoprim plus sufamethoxazole (Bactrim) were compared in 24 healthy subjects following oral administration of three dosage forms (tablet, capsule and suspension). The absorption rate of each drug was significantly greater from suspension than from tablet or capsule (Langlois *et al.* 1972). However, there were no significant differences in the extent of absorption. Similar findings have been reported for penicillin V and other drugs.

Some important factors to consider in formulating a suspension for better bioavailability are (1) particle size, (2) inclusion of a wetting agent, (3) crystal form and (4) viscosity.

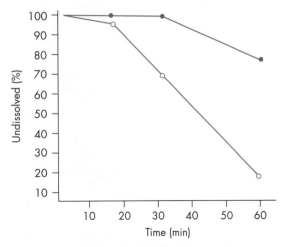

Figure 9.3   Dissolution from hard gelatin capsules containing drug alone (●) or drug and diluent (○).

9.4 Capsule as a dosage form

The capsule has the potential to be an efficient drug delivery system. The hard gelatin shell encapsulating the formulation should disrupt quickly, and expose the contents to the GI fluid, provided that excipients in the formulation and/or the method of manufacture do not impart a hydrophobic nature to the dosage form.

Unlike the tablet dosage form, drug particles in a capsule are not subjected to high compression forces, which tend to compact the powder or granules and reduce the effective surface area. Hence, upon disruption of the shell, the encapsulated powder mass should disperse rapidly to expose a large surface area to the GI fluid. This rate of dispersion, in turn, influences the rate of dissolution and, therefore, bioavailability. It is, therefore, important to have suitable diluents and/or other excipients in a capsule dosage form, particularly when the drug is hydrophobic (Fig. 9.3).

9.5 Tablet as a dosage form

Whereas solutions represent a state of maximum dispersion, compressed tablets have the closest proximity to particles. Since problems in dissolution and bioavailability are generally inversely proportional to the degree of dispersion, compressed tablets are more prone to bioavailability problems. This is primarily because of the small surface area exposed for dissolution until the tablets have broken down into smaller particles (Fig. 9.4).

Factors responsible for the primary breakdown of tablets into granules and their subsequent breakdown into finer particles include:

- type and concentration of a binder
- disintegrating agent
- diluents
- lubricants
- hydrophobicity of the drug
- method of manufacture (wet granulation, dry granulation and direct compression)
- coloring and coating agents used.

From the scheme in Fig. 9.4, it is clear that tablet disintegration and granule deaggregation are important steps in the dissolution and absorption processes. A tablet that fails to disintegrate or which disintegrates slowly may result in incomplete and/or slow absorption; this, in turn, may delay the onset of action.

The importance of disintegration in drug absorption is evident from a study of dipyridamole (Persantine), a coronary vasodilator. In Fig. 9.5,

Sequence of Events in the Absorption Process

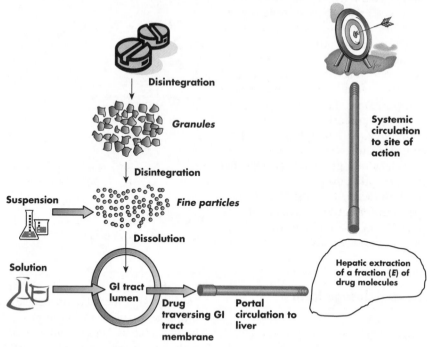

Figure 9.4   Sequence of events in the absorption process GI, Gastrointestinal

it can be seen that the serum appearance of dipyridamole was delayed and variable when the tablets were taken intact but when tablets were chewed before swallowing, the drug appeared in the blood within 5–6 min and the peak serum concentration was higher in every subject.

Similar results have also been reported by Mellinger (1965) for thioridazine (Mellaril) tablets.

It should be noted that routine crushing of tablets should not be recommended. The bioavailability of marketed tablets should be satisfactory. Moreover, crushing of some tablets (e.g. Dulcolax [bisacodyl]) can cause severe side effects, while crushing of tablets intended for controlled or sustained release can cause dose dumping and dangerously high blood concentrations of drug.

Tablet disintegration, though important, is unlikely to be the rate-limiting (slowest) step in the absorption of drugs administered as conventional tablets. In most instances, granule deaggregation and drug dissolution occur at a slower rate than disintegration and are responsible for problems in absorption.

For many years, the accepted laboratory standard for the determination of the release of active ingredient from a compressed tablet has been the disintegration time. However, since the early 1990s, it has become apparent that the disintegration test, in itself, is not an adequate criterion. A tablet may rapidly crumble into fine particles, but the active ingredients may be slowly or incompletely available. Also, a tablet can disintegrate rapidly into granules, but that does not mean that granules will deaggregate into fine particles and that drug particles will dissolve and be absorbed adequately.

The lack of correlation between tablet disintegration time and GI absorption of the active ingredient is shown in Table 9.1.

This study dramatically demonstrates that dissolution rate, rather than disintegration time, is indicative of the rate of absorption from

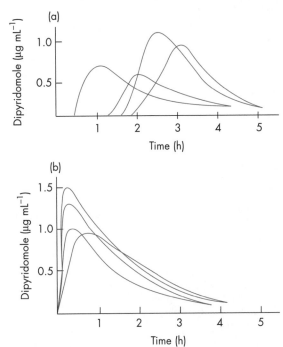

Figure 9.5 Dipyridamole concentrations in the serum of individual subjects after administration of 25 mg oral dose as intact tablets (a) or crushed tablets (b). When tablets are chewed before swallowing, the peak concentration tends to be higher and the peak time tends to be earlier. (Mellinger and Bohorfoush (1966). Blood levels of Persantine in humans. *Arch Int Pharmacodyn* 163: 471–480. Used with permission.)

compressed tablets. Products 1 and 2 were the slowest disintegrating tablets but had the fastest dissolution rate and produced the highest urine drug concentrations.

9.6 Dissolution methods

From the discussion above, it is clear that a dissolution test is much more discriminatory than disintegration is assessing potential *in vivo* performance of various solid dosage forms.

A number of academic, government and industrial scientists have developed dissolution rate tests that have been used to evaluate the *in vitro* dissolution rate of a drug from a dosage form and, hopefully, to correlate it with *in vivo* drug availability. All these methods measure the rate of appearance of dissolved drug in an aqueous fluid (similar to GI fluid) under carefully controlled conditions: temperature, agitation, and pH.

Two official methods given in the *United States Pharmacopeia* and recognized by US Food and Drug Administration (FDA) and, hence, used by the pharmaceutical industry are:

- the rotary basket method
- the paddle method.

These are depicted in Figures 9.6 to 9.8; while a third compendial method is shown in Figure 9.9.

9.7 Formulation and processing factors

There are numerous reports describing the effects of formulation and processing variables on dissolution and bioavailability. All excipients used in the formulation of dosage forms and processes used

Table 9.1 Lack of correlation between disintegration time and gastrointestinal absorption of drug from tablet formulation

Aspirin product	Disintegration time (s)[a]	Mass drug dissolved in 10 min (mg)	Mass drug excreted in urine (mg)
1	256	242	24.3
2	35	205	18.5
3	13	158	13.6
4	<10	165	18.1
5 (average of 2 trials)	<10	127	14.0

[a] *United States Pharmacopeia.*
After Levy (1961).

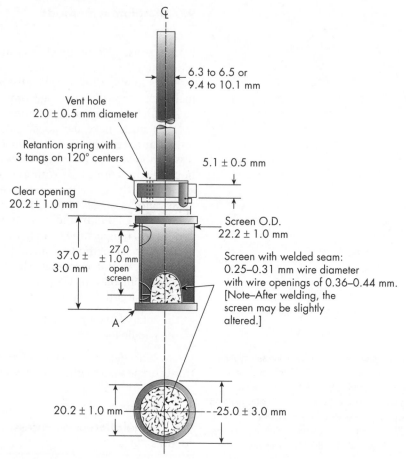

6.3 to 6.5 or
9.4 to 10.1 mm

Vent hole
2.0 ± 0.5 mm diameter

Retantion spring with
3 tangs on 120° centers

5.1 ± 0.5 mm

Clear opening
20.2 ± 1.0 mm

Screen O.D.
22.2 ± 1.0 mm

37.0 ±
3.0 mm

27.0
± 1.0 mm
open
screen

Screen with welded seam:
0.25–0.31 mm wire diameter
with wire openings of 0.36–0.44 mm.
[Note–After welding, the
screen may be slightly
altered.]

A

20.2 ± 1.0 mm   25.0 ± 3.0 mm

Figure 9.6   Basket stirring element. Note: Maximum allowable runout at "A" is ± 1.0 mm when the part is rotated on center line axis with basket mounted.

in the manufacture of these dosage forms can influence the dissolution rate and drug availability.

Diluents

Adsorption of some drugs, especially vitamins, on diluents such as kaolin, Fuller's earth or bentonite can occur in capsule and tablet dosage forms. The physical adsorption can retard dissolution and, hence, bioavailability. Some calcium salts (e.g. dicalcium phosphate) are extensively used as diluents in tablet and capsule dosage forms. The original use of dicalcium phosphate in a tetracycline capsule formation resulted in poor bioavailability. Lactose tends to react with amine compounds causing discoloration.

Natural and synthetic gums (acacia, tragacanth, polyvinyl pyrrolidone [PVP] and cellulose derivatives) are commonly used as tablet binders or suspending agents in suspension dosage forms. When used in excessive amounts, they usually form a viscous solution in gastric fluid and may slow down dissolution by delaying disintegration.

Disintegrants

The concentration and the type of disintegrating agent used in a tablet dosage form can greatly influence the dissolution and bioavailability of a therapeutic agent. The dissolution rate is usually increased when the concentration of starch is increased in a tablet formulation. The effect of

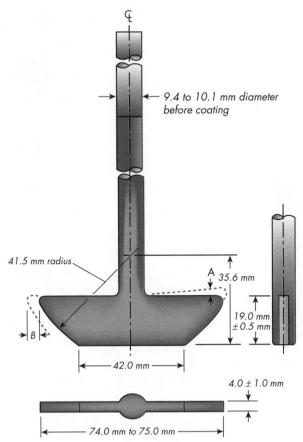

9.4 to 10.1 mm diameter
before coating

41.5 mm radius

A 35.6 mm

19.0 mm
± 0.5 mm

B

42.0 mm

4.0 ± 1.0 mm

74.0 mm to 75.0 mm

Figure 9.7 Paddle stirring element. Notes: (1) A and B dimensions are not to vary more than 0.5 mm when part is rolated on center line axis. (2) Tolerances are ± 1.0 mm unless otherwise stated.

starch concentration on the dissolution of salicylic acid is shown in Fig. 9.10.

Figures 9.11 and 9.12 illustrate how changing the concentration of disintegrant (Veegum) in a tolbutamide tablet formulation can greatly alter bioavailability. A comparison of the commercial product (Orinase) with an experimental formulation that was identical in composition and manufacturing method but contained only 50% of the disintegrant (Veegum) showed that the commercial product displayed higher blood concentrations and greater ability to lower blood glucose than the experimental product.

Types of starch

The dissolution of drugs from tablets can be affected by the type of starch used as a disintegrant

in the tablet formulation. Figure 9.13 clearly suggests that the dissolution of drug was much faster from tablets formulated with specially treated, directly compressible starch.

Tablet lubricants

Magnesium stearate, talc, Compritol and sodium lauryl sulfate are some of the commonly used lubricants. Magnesium stearate and talc are water insoluble and water repellent. Their hydrophobic nature can lower the contact between the dosage form and GI fluids and thereby cause a slower dissolution.

Figure 9.14 shows how magnesium stearate retards the dissolution of salicylic acid from tablets whereas tablets prepared using sodium lauryl sulfate (a soluble hydrophilic wetting agent) as a lubricant had rapid dissolution.

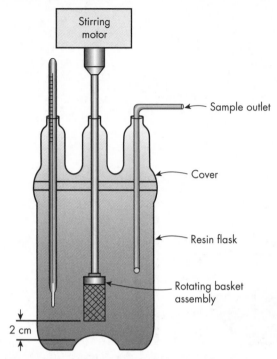

Figure 9.8 Apparatus for dissolution testing by the rotary basket method. This method was retained in the *National Formulary* XIV edition and adopted in *United States Pharmacopeia* XIX edition and retained in both the *National Formulary* XV edition and the *United States Pharmacopeia* XX edition.

Coloring agents

Coloring agents used in the formulation of tablets or other dosage form can sometimes have an adverse effect on dissolution. Figure 9.15 shows the blood concentration of sulfathiazole following administration of tablets containing FDC blue 1 and tablets without dye.

9.8 Correlation of *in vivo* data with *in vitro* dissolution data

Correlation of *in vitro* rate of dissolution with *in vivo* absorption is a topic of significant interest to the pharmaceutical industry because it is a means of assuring the bioavailability of active ingredient(s) from a dosage form. Once such a correlation has been established, quantitative predictions regarding the absorption of drug

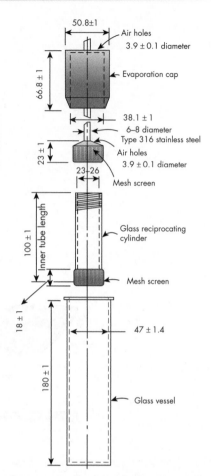

Figure 9.9 USP dissolution testing method 3. © The United States Pharmacopeial Convention, 2009. All rights reserved. Printed with permission.

from new formulations may be made without *in vivo* bioavailability studies.

Many studies have been carried out since the late 1980s in attempts to correlate *in vitro* dissolution with *in vivo* performance. Some studies have found a significant correlation whereas others have been unsuccessful. This limited success in establishing a quantitative correlation is attributed to the fact that absorption is a complicated process. Physiological factors such as gastric emptying time, metabolism of drug by gut wall enzymes or intestinal microflora, and the hepatic first-pass effect can affect the absorption process.

Whether such a correlation is established or not, the greatest value of *in vitro* dissolution lies in the following areas: (1) helping to identify

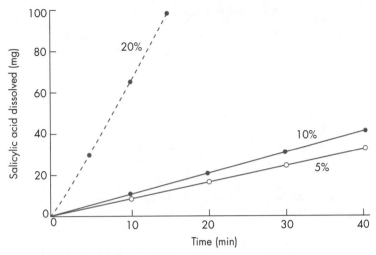

Figure 9.10 Effect of starch (5, 10 and 20%) on the dissolution of salicylic acid. Levy *et al* (1963). *J Pharm Sci* 52: 1047. Reprinted with permission of John Wiley & Sons, Inc.

formulations that may present potential bioequivalence problems and (2) ensuring batch-to-batch bioequivalence once a formulation has been shown to be bioavailable.

Types of correlation

There are two basic types of correlations:

- rank-order correlation
- quantitative correlation.

Rank order correlation

A rank-order correlation is one in which:

- the y variable increases as x increases (implying that the y variable decreases as x decreases)
- the y variable increases as x decreases (implying that the y variable decreases as x increases).

Variables that are definable by an interval scale or ratio scale may be transformed to rank-order forms, which are then treated statistically.

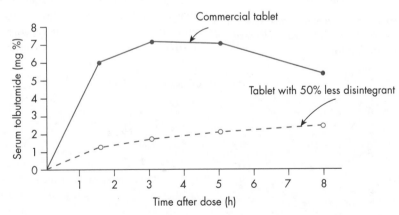

Figure 9.11 Effect of disintegrant (Veegum®) on bioavailability of tolbutamide indicated by serum tolbutamide concentration. Two formulations were administered to healthy, non-diabetic subjects. One was a commercial product (Orinase) and the second was identical in composition and manufacturing method but contained 50% of the amount of disintegrant (Veegum). Varley AB (1968). The generic inequivalence of drugs. *J Am Med Assoc* 206: 1745. Reprinted with permission of the American Medical Association.

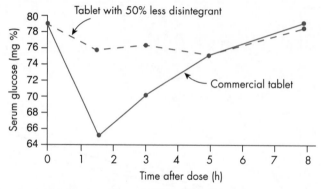

Figure 9.12   Effect of disintegrant (Veegum) on bioavailability of tolbutamide indicated by blood sugar level. Details are given in Fig. 9.11. Varley *et al.* (1968).

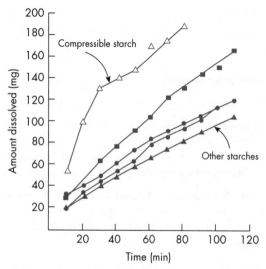

Figure 9.13   Effect of type of starch on drug dissolution. Underwood *et al* (1972). *J Phorm Sc* 61: 239. Reprinted with permission of John wiley & Sons, Inc.

Table 9.2 is an example of "perfect rank-order" and "imperfect rank-order" correlations.

Quantitative correlation

A quantitative correlation is one where the *in vivo* variable y is related to the *in vitro* variable x by one of the following equations:

$$y = a + bx \tag{9.1}$$

$$\ln y = \ln y^0 + bx \tag{9.2}$$

(b can be negative).

These correlations are of a more informative type. However, such a relationship should probably be derived only when there is a theoretical reason for relating variables as indicated by the equation derived. In such correlations, the terms r (often called the correlation coefficient)

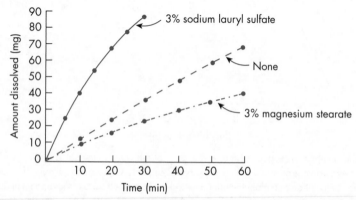

Figure 9.14   Effect of lubricant on dissolution rate of salicylic acid contained in compressed tablets. Levy and Gumtow (1963). *J Pharm Sci* 52: 1139. Reprinted with permission of John Wiley & Sons, Inc.

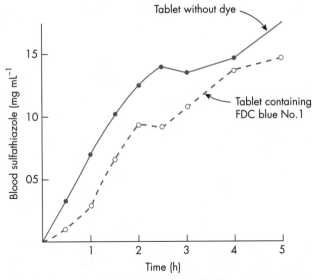

Figure 9.15   Blood concentration of free sulfathiazole following the oral administration of 1 g sulfathiazole crystals with and without the dye FDC blue No.1 to adult human subjects. Tawashi and Piccolo (1972). *J Pharm Sci* 61: 1857. Reprinted with permission of John Wiley & Sons, Inc.

or r^2 (the coefficient of determination) are obtained as evidence of the degree of correlation between the variables.

Correlated variables

Variables derived from *in vivo* data that have been correlated with variables from *in vitro* data

1. Peak plasma concentration, $(C_p)_{max}$
2. Area under the plasma concentration from $t = 0$ to $t = t$ or to $t = \infty$
3. Amount of drug excreted in the urine X_u at time t or at $t = 7t_{1/2}$

4. Urinary excretion rate at a given time t
5. Percentage absorbed plot (Wagner–Nelson method) from plasma or urinary data
6. Pharmacological response, e.g. blood sugar lowering or blood pressure.

Variables derived from *in vitro* data that have been correlated with variables from *in vivo* data

1. Disintegration time
2. Time for a certain percentage of drug to dissolve (i.e. $t_{20\%}$, $t_{50\%}$, etc.)
3. Concentration of drug in dissolution fluid at a given time

Table 9.2   Examples of perfect and imperfect rank order correlations

Perfect rank order correlations						Imperfect rank order correlations			
x	*y*	*x*	*y*	*x*	*y*	*x*	*y*	*x*	*y*
1	1	1	2	1	1	1	2	1	1
2	2	2	4	2	3	2	1	2	2
3	3	3	6	3	8	3	3	3	4
4	4	4	8	4	50	4	4	4	3
5	5	5	10	5	100	5	5	5	5

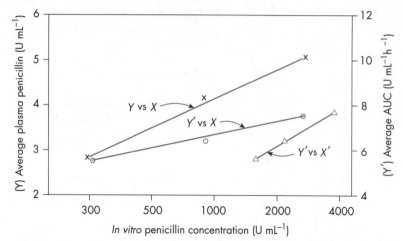

Figure 9.16 The correlation of blood penicillin concentrations at 0.5 h in fasting subjects following the oral administration of three different penicillin V salts (potassium penicillin V, calcium penicillin V and penicillin V) with the *in vitro* rates of dissolution. Line Y vs X is a plot of average plasma penicillin concentration at 0.5 h versus penicillin V in solution after 10 min at pH 2.0. Line Y′ vs X is average (AUC) versus penicillin V in solution after 10 min at pH 2.0. Line Y′ vs X′ is average (AUC) versus penicillin V in solution after 10 min at pH 8.0. In each case, the points from left to right refer to penicillin V, calcium penicillin V and potassium penicillin V. (Juncher *et al.*, 1957).

4. Rate of dissolution
5. Percentage remaining to be dissolved
6. Intrinsic rates of dissolution.

Which variables should be correlated?

The time for 50% of the drug to dissolve *in vitro* ($t_{50\%}$) is a noncompartmental value, indicating the central tendency of the *in vitro* dissolution; however, it suffers from being a single point method. Multiple point methods comparing *in vitro* dissolution rate with *in vivo* input rate are rated most highly by the FDA. (Emami J (2006). In vitro – in vivo correlation: from theory to applications. *J Pharm Pharmaceut Sci* 9(2): 169–189.)

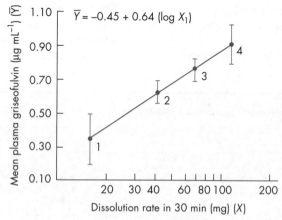

Figure 9.17 *In vivo/in vitro* correlation for griseofulvin. Correlation of average plasma concentration of griseofulvin after a single oral dose of 500 mg in 10 healthy subjects with the amount of griseofulvin dissolved in 30 min in simulated intestinal fluids for four preparations. (Katchen *et al.* (1967). Correlation of dissolution rate and griseofulvin absorption in man. *J Pharm Sci* 56: 1108–1110. Reprinted with permission of John Wiley & Sons, Inc.)

Examples of quantitative correlation

Two examples of quantitative correlation will be discussed: penicillin V and griseofulvin.

Penicillin V

Figure 9.16 shows the correlation of blood concentrations in fasting subjects following the oral administration of three different penicillin V salts: potassium penicillin V, calcium penicillin V and penicillin V.

Griseofulvin

Figure 9.17 compares the mean plasma concentration of griseofulvin at 30 min with the dissolution rate *in vitro* at 30 min in simulated intestinal fluid for four griseofulvin products.

10

Continuous intravenous infusion
(one-compartment model)

Objectives

Upon completion of this chapter, you will have the ability to:

- calculate plasma drug concentration at any time t after an intravenous infusion is initiated
- explain the difference between true steady state and practical steady state
- calculate the infusion rate that will achieve a desired steady-state plasma drug concentration in a particular patient
- describe various methods employed to attain and then maintain a desired steady-state concentration in a patient
- determine the time required to attain practical steady-state conditions when various methods are employed
- calculate an "ideal" bolus/infusion combination for a drug exhibiting one-compartment model characteristics
- employ the salt value (S) to calculate loading and maintenance doses of a drug
- predict plasma drug concentrations at a given time after the cessation of an intravenous infusion
- calculate pharmacokinetic parameters from plasma drug concentration versus time data for an intravenous infusion.

10.1 Introduction

While a single intravenous bolus dose of a drug may produce the desired therapeutic concentration and, therefore, the desired pharmacological effect immediately, this mode of administration is unsuitable when it is necessary to maintain plasma or tissue concentrations at a concentration that will prolong the duration of this effect. We are interested in reaching the therapeutic range and then maintaining drug concentration within the therapeutic range for a longer duration, as shown in Fig. 10.1.

It is common practice, in the hospital setting to infuse a drug at a constant rate (constant rate input or zero-order input). This method (Fig. 10.2) permits precise and readily controlled drug administration.

The infusion rate of a drug is controlled by:

- flow rate (e.g. $mL\,h^{-1}$)

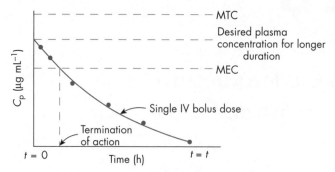

Figure 10.1   A representation of the plasma concentration (C_p) versus time profile following the administration of a single intravenous (IV) bolus dose. MTC, minimum toxic concentration; MEC, minimum effective concentration.

• concentration ($\mu g\,mL^{-1}$, % w/v, etc.) of the drug in solution.

Flow rate is controlled by adjusting the height of an infusion bottle or by regulating the aperture size of the tube that connects the bottle to the needle. When greater precision and control of drug administration is desired, an infusion pump is used.

Theory of intravenous infusion

The drug is administered at a selected or calculated constant rate (Q) (i.e. dX/dt), the units of this input rate will be those of mass per unit time (e.g. $mg\,h^{-1}$). (If necessary, please review Ch. 1,

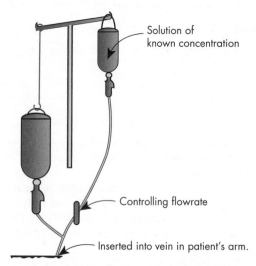

Figure 10.2   Administration of drug at a constant rate (zero-order process) by an intravenous infusion.

Solution of known concentration

Controlling flowrate

Inserted into vein in patient's arm.

where a zero-order (constant rate) output process is discussed.)

The constant rate can be calculated from the concentration of drug solution and the flow rate of this solution, For example, the concentration of drug solution is 1% (w/v) and this solution is being infused at the constant rate of $10\,mL\,h^{-1}$ (solution flow rate). So 10 mL of solution will contain 0.1 g (100 mg) drug. Hence, the units of the infusion rate, (constant rate) = solution flow rate ($mL\,h^{-1}$) × concentration ($\mu g\,mL^{-1}$), will be mass per unit time ($\mu g\,h^{-1}$). In this example, the constant infusion rate will be $10\,mL\,h^{-1}$ multiplied by 100 mg/10 mL, or $0.1\,g\,h^{-1}$ ($100\,mg\,h^{-1}$).

The elimination of drug from the body follows a first-order process. (i.e. $-dX/dt = KX$).

Initially, the rate at which drug enters the body, though constant, is greater than the rate at which drug is eliminated; this allows the drug to reach a certain amount and concentration in the body. Figure 10.3 illustrates the concept of a constant rate (zero order) at which the drug enters the general circulation and the changing rate (first-order rate) of drug elimination.

As time increases following the commencement of a constant rate (Fig. 10.3), the difference between the two rates (i.e. the difference between the rate at which drug enters blood and the rate at which drug leaves blood) becomes smaller and this difference becomes zero at time infinity when rate of elimination equals the rate at which the drug is being administered. Hence, there is no change in mass (amount) of drug or plasma concentration of drug with time as long as the chosen constant rate (zero-order) input is maintained (Fig. 10.4).

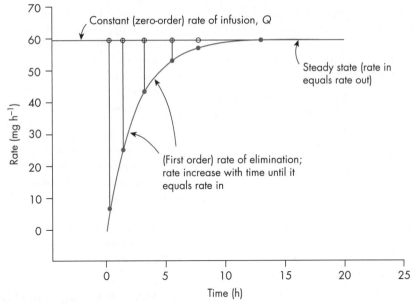

Figure 10.3   A graphical representation of drug administration at a constant rate and drug elimination at a changing (increasing until steady state) rate when a drug is administered as an infusion.

The pharmacokinetic parameters, and the equations required for their computation, following the administration of a drug as an intravenous infusion will be discussed in this chapter. It may be prudent to mention that this topic, owing to its practical application, is of considerable importance and significance for a career as a hospital, clinical or retail

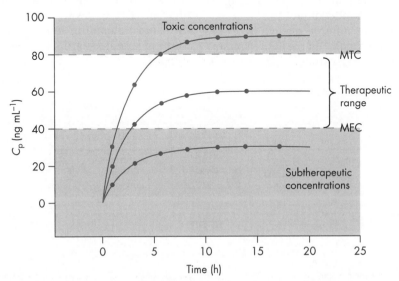

Figure 10.4   A graphical representation of the plasma concentration (C_p) against time profile following the administration of a drug at a constant rate. MTC, minimum toxic concentration; MEC, minimum effective concentration.

pharmacist, and the importance of topic is generally reflected in the pharmacy licencing examinations.

In the following discussion, the following simplifying assumptions are made:

1. The drug we are considering undergoes no metabolism (i.e. monitoring for unchanged parent drug in the blood)
2. The drug exhibits the characteristics of a one-compartment model (rapid distribution).
3. The elimination of the drug follows a first-order process and passive diffusion.

Useful equations and pharmacokinetic parameters

1. Equations for predicting the mass (amount) of drug and plasma concentration at time, t.
2. The steady-state condition and the equation for obtaining the true steady-state plasma concentration. What does steady-state condition mean?
3. The "practical" steady-state condition, the "practical" steady-state plasma concentration, and the time required for attaining this condition.
4. Methods employed to attain the desired plasma concentration instantaneously, or very rapidly, and then maintain it as long as desired, including indefinitely.
5. Calculation of the infusion rate (Q) necessary to attain and then maintain the desired plasma concentration at steady state.
6. Calculation of the loading dose (D_L) necessary to attain the desired plasma concentration instantaneously and the infusion rate (Q) necessary to maintain the plasma concentration at that concentration.
7. Salt form correction value (S) and its utility in pharmacokinetics.
8. Calculation of the two infusion rates (Q_1 and Q_2) required for rapidly attaining and then maintaining the desired plasma concentration.
9. Determination of the elimination half life ($t_{1/2}$), the elimination rate constant (K or K_{el}) and the apparent volume of distribution (V) from post-infusion (i.e. following the cessation of infusion) concentration versus time data and from concentration versus time data obtained during infusion.

10.2 Monitoring drug in the body or blood (plasma/serum)

Drug is monitored in blood under two conditions:

- during infusion (while the drug is being infused)
- in the post-infusion period (following the cessation of infusion).

Figure 10.5 shows the scheme and set up for drug changes in the body or blood under constant infusion. The following text will consider first the issues of sampling during infusions and then those of monitoring drugs after an infusion is stopped.

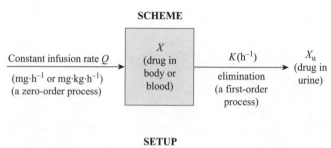

SCHEME

Constant infusion rate Q | X (drug in body or blood) | $K(h^{-1})$ | X_u (drug in urine)

$(mg \cdot h^{-1}$ or $mg \cdot kg \cdot h^{-1})$ (a zero-order process) | | elimination (a first-order process)

SETUP

$$Q(mg\ h^{-1}) \rightarrow X(mg) \xrightarrow{K\ (h^{-1})} X_u(mg)$$

Figure 10.5 Scheme for constant input rate, continuous intravenous infusion. Q, constant input or infusion rate; X, mass (amount) of drug in the blood or body at time t; X_u, mass of unchanged drug in urine at time t; K, first-order elimination rate constant.

10.3 Sampling drug in body or blood during infusion

Since drug is being monitored in the blood, the change in the amount of drug in the blood/body (dX/dt) for the set up described in Fig. 10.5 will be:

$$\frac{dX}{dt} = Q - KX \qquad (10.1)$$

where: dX/dt is the rate of change in the mass or amount of drug in the body (e.g. $mg\,h^{-1}$); Q is the zero-order input or constant infusion rate (e.g. $mg\,h^{-1}$); and KX is the first-order elimination rate (e.g. $mg\,h^{-1}$).

Before proceeding further, and in order to clearly understand the typical plasma concentration versus time profile obtained following the administration of a drug by this approach, it may be imperative and wise to analyze Eq. 10.1 critically.

As stated above in the discussion of the theory of infusion, the rate at which drug enters the body, though constant, is initially greater than the rate at which the drug is being eliminated. Please note that the rate of drug elimination (KX) from body, being a first-order process, increases with time since there is a greater amount of drug in the body (X) as time increases; consequently, the difference between the infusion rate and the elimination rate (i.e. $Q - KX$ in Eq. 10.1) becomes smaller as time increases, eventually reaching zero (Fig. 10.3). When the rate of elimination becomes equal to the rate of infusion (not the other way around) and the difference between two rates becomes zero, there will be no further change in the amount of drug in the blood or body with time. Further, since the apparent of volume of distribution of a drug is constant, the ratio of the amount divided by volume (i.e. concentration) will also be constant. This condition will be attained, theoretically, only at time infinity.

It is highly recommended at this stage that Eq. 10.1 is compared with Eq. 6.4 (p. 100) for differences and similarities, if any. It may become apparent, following careful comparison of the two equations, why plasma concentration versus time profiles look different for a drug administered extravascularly and one administered as an intravenous infusion. It is strongly recommended that you attempt to elicit answers, for the following questions:

Is there any difference between the two equations (Eqs 6.4 and 10.1)?
Is there any difference between the two rates involved in the two equations (Eqs 6.4 and 10.1)?
Is there any difference between the two equations with regards to the rate constants?
Is there any difference in the time at which the maximum plasma concentration is attained following the administration of a drug by an extravascular route and as an intravenous infusion (Eqs 6.4 and 10.1)?
Is there any difference between two equations (Eqs 6.4 and 10.1) with respect to the time at which the difference between the two rates involved in the two equations becomes zero?

Upon integration, Eq. 10.1 yields

$$X = \frac{Q}{K}(1 - e^{-Kt}) \qquad (10.2)$$

Equation 10.2 and Fig. 10.6 indicate that the mass of drug in the body rises asymptotically with time.

In addition to noting that the amount of drug in blood increases asymptotically with time, it should also become apparent from Eq. 10.2 and Fig. 10.6 that the amount of drug in blood is influenced by the chosen infusion rate, the elimination rate constant of the drug and the duration of infusion. However, since the elimination rate constant for a drug is constant, the amount of drug in blood will be influenced by the chosen infusion rate and the duration of infusion; the amount of drug in blood at a given time will be directly proportional to the chosen infusion rate. For two different drugs, however, the amount of each drug in blood at a time will be influenced by the chosen infusion rate, the elimination rate constant of each drug and the duration of the infusion.

Since drug concentration is measured, not the amount of drug, and using Eq. 3.6, which stated

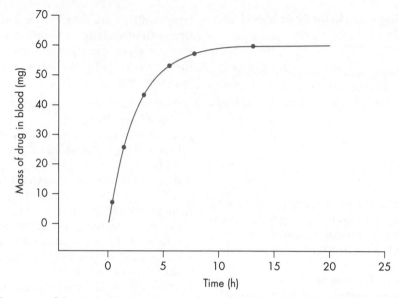

Figure 10.6 The amount of drug in the blood against time during the administration of a drug by intravenous infusion.

that $C_p = X/V$ (or $X = VC_p$), then Eq. 10.2 takes the following form:

$$C_p = \frac{Q}{VK}(1 - e^{-Kt})$$ (10.3)

where C_p is the plasma (or serum) drug concentration at time t; V is the apparent volume of distribution; Q is the constant infusion rate; K is the elimination rate constant; and VK is the systemic clearance (Fig. 10.7).

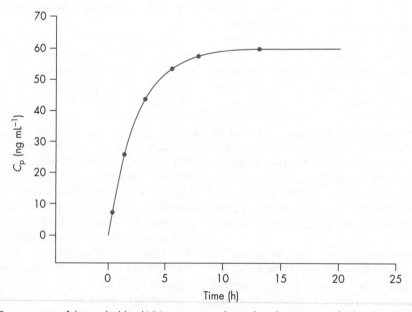

Figure 10.7 Concentration of drug in the blood (C_p) against time during the administration of a drug by intravenous infusion.

Note that Eq. 10.3 is simply a modification of Eq. 10.2 made by introducing the apparent volume of distribution term to convert amount to concentration.

Equation 10.3 clearly indicates that the plasma or serum concentration of a drug increases with time, eventually reaching an asymptotic condition. It should be apparent from Eq. 10.3 and Fig. 10.7 that the plasma concentration of a drug is influenced by the calculated infusion rate, the elimination rate constant, the apparent volume of distribution, the systemic clearance of a drug and the duration of the infusion.

Since the elimination rate constant, the apparent volume of distribution and the systemic clearance for a drug are constant for a given patient receiving a particular drug, the plasma concentration of a drug will be influenced by the chosen infusion rate and the duration of infusion, and the plasma concentration of a drug at a specific time will always be directly proportional (linear pharmacokinetics) to the chosen infusion rate. Should the patient exhibit renal impairment, as indicated by lowered creatinine clearance, this will be reflected in lower systemic clearance of a drug undergoing elimination via the kidneys. Therefore, the same infusion rate will yield a higher, and perhaps toxic, plasma concentration of the drug. It is, therefore, crucial and imperative that the infusion rate of a drug is reduced in a renally impaired patient if the drug in question is eliminated by the kidneys. The magnitude of the adjustment in the infusion rate required in a renally impaired patient will, in turn, depend on the degree of renal impairment.

If two different drugs are administered at an identical infusion rate to a subject, the plasma concentration of each drug at a given time will be influenced by the ratio of the infusion rate to the systemic clearance of each drug (i.e. Q/VK).

True steady state and steady-state plasma concentration ($C_p)_{ss}$

True steady-state condition refers to the condition when the rate of elimination and the rate of infusion become equal, and it occurs, theoretically, only when time is equal to infinity.

Prior to the attainment of a true steady-state condition, the rate of infusion is always greater than the rate of elimination (i.e. $Q \gg KX$); and only at true steady state does $Q = KX$.

The plasma concentration that corresponds to true steady state is referred to as the true steady-state plasma concentration $(C_p)_{ss}$. Therefore, it is accurate to state that the true steady-state plasma concentration will be attained only at time infinity.

The true steady-state plasma concentration of a drug is constant for a given infusion rate and is obtained as time approaches infinity. We know, by definition, that when $t = \infty$; $C_p = (C_p)_{ss}$. Hence, Eq. 10.3 takes the following form:

$$(C_p)_{ss} = \frac{Q}{VK}(1 - e^{-Kt_\infty}) \qquad (10.4)$$

However, e^{-Kt_∞}, by definition, is zero. Hence Eq. 10.4 becomes:

$$(C_p)_{ss} = \frac{Q}{VK}(1 - 0)$$

or

$$(C_p)_{ss} = \frac{Q}{VK} \qquad (10.5)$$

or

$$(C_p)_{ss} VK = Q \qquad (10.6)$$

Equations 10.5 and 10.6 clearly indicate that the infusion rate (Q) required to attain and then maintain the desired steady-state plasma concentration is determined by the desired plasma concentration and the systemic clearance of a drug. In addition, the systemic clearance of a drug being a constant, there is a directly proportional relationship between the desired steady-state plasma concentration and the infusion rate required for attaining this concentration.

• What will be the slope of a plot of steady-state plasma concentration against infusion rate?
• How would you compare this plot with the plot of the area under the plasma concentration versus time curve [$(AUC)_0^\infty$] against the administered dose following the administration of a

drug by intravenous bolus or extravascular routes?

- Do you detect any common thread or commonality between the two graphs?

A dimensional analysis of Eqs 10.5 and 10.6 will be help us to understand the unit(s) accompanying the value of infusion rate:

- Unit for concentration $(C_p)_{ss}$ is mass per volume, e.g. $mg\,mL^{-1}$.
- Unit for clearance will be volume per unit time, e.g. $mL\,h^{-1}$.
- So Q will be $mg\,mL^{-1} \times mL\,h^{-1}$, or $mg\,h^{-1}$.

If a body weight basis is used, this would become $mg\,mL^{-1} \times mL\,h^{-1}\,kg^{-1}$, or $mg\,h^{-1}\,kg^{-1}$.

We know from a previous discussion that $K = 0.693/t_{1/2}$ (Eq. 3.12). Substitution for K in Eq. 10.5 will yield:

$$(C_p)_{ss} = \frac{Q}{(V)\left(\frac{0.693}{t_{1/2}}\right)} = \frac{(Q)(t_{1/2})}{(V)(0.693)} \qquad (10.7)$$

Since the apparent volume of distribution, elimination rate constant, and elimination half

life $(t_{1/2})$ are constants for a given drug administered to a particular patient, the absolute value of steady-state plasma concentration is determined only by the rate of infusion. For instance, if the rate of infusion is increased by a factor of two, the steady-state plasma concentration will also increase by a factor of two (linear pharmacokinetics). However, it is important to recognize that the time at which this steady state is attained is independent of the rate of infusion. In other words, doubling the infusion rate will not allow the steady-state condition to be achieved faster (Fig. 10.8).

"Practical" steady-state concentration

A "practical" steady-state concentration has been reached when plasma concentration of a drug in the blood is within 5% of true steady-state plasma concentration. Alternatively, we may say that a "practical" steady-state concentration has been reached when the plasma concentration of a drug in the blood represents 95% or greater of the true steady-state plasma concentration.

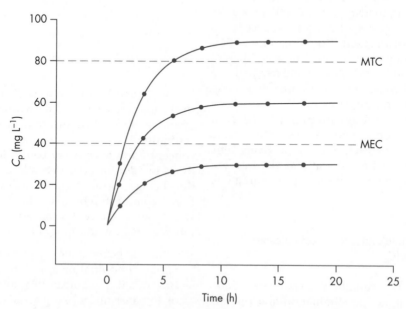

Figure 10.8   Concentration (C_p) versus time data following the administration of a drug as an intravenous infusion at different rates. MTC, minimum toxic concentration; MEC, minimum effective concentration.

Please note that the time required to reach "practical" steady-state condition is always equal to $4.32t_{1/2}$ of that drug. For example, let us assume we wish to attain a plasma concentration of $10\,\mu g\,mL^{-1}$ at true steady state; that is, the chosen infusion rate yields a true steady-state plasma concentration of $10\,\mu g\,mL^{-1}$. Therefore, $10\,\mu g\,mL^{-1} \times 0.95 = 9.5\,\mu g\,mL^{-1}$ is the "practical" steady-state concentration and it will occur at $4.32t_{1/2}$.

Let us assume that the desired true steady-state plasma concentration of the same drug is $20\,\mu g\,mL^{-1}$; that is, the chosen infusion rate (twice the infusion rate of the first example) yields a true steady-state plasma concentration of $20\,\mu g\,mL^{-1}$. Therefore, $20\,\mu g\,mL^{-1} \times 0.95 = 19.0\ \mu g\,mL^{-1}$ is the "practical" steady-state concentration and it will occur at the same time (i.e. $4.32t_{1/2}$) since the same drug is being infused.

If the elimination half life of the drug is $2\,h$, it will take $2 \times 4.32 = 8.64\,h$ to attain the "practical" steady-state condition. If the elimination half life of the drug is $10\,h$, it will be $43.2\,h$ before the "practical" steady-state condition is attained. Therefore, if a drug has a long half life (for example, the elimination half life of digoxin is approximately is 40–$50\,h$ and for phenobarbital is approximately 90–$110\,h$) and such a drug is administered to a patient using the single infusion approach, it may take a long time (approximately 7 and 15 days for digoxin and phenobarbital, respectively) before drug concentration is at a level that produces the desired effect; consequently, this may not be a suitable approach if the intention is to attain and then maintain the desired plasma concentration rapidly. By comparison, if a drug has a short elimination half life ($30\,min$ to $2\,h$), it is possible to attain and then maintain the desired plasma concentration in approximately 2–$8\,h$ using this approach. Furthermore, it is accurate to state that the time required to attain the "practical" steady-state condition may vary for different drugs (assuming, of course, that elimination half lives for these drugs are different); however, the number of elimination half lives required to attain the "practical" steady-state condition will always be same for every drug and in every patient, normal as well as renally impaired.

Why does it take 4.32 half lives to reach "practical" steady state?

Plasma concentration at any time following the administration of a single infusion can be described by the following equation, Eq. 10.3:

$$(C_p)_t = \frac{Q}{VK}(1 - e^{-Kt})$$

For a true steady-state condition, since the value of e^{-Kt} at time infinity is zero, Eq. 10.3 reduces to Eq. 10.5:

$$(C_p)_{ss} = \frac{Q}{VK}$$

If Eq. 10.3 is divided by Eq. 10.5, the following is obtained:

$$f_{ss} = \frac{(C_p)_t}{(C_p)_{ss}} = \frac{\frac{Q}{VK}(1 - e^{-Kt})}{\frac{Q}{VK}}$$

where, f_{ss} is the fraction of the true steady state achieved.

Thus,

$$f_{ss} = \frac{(C_p)_t}{(C_p)_{ss}} = (1 - e^{-Kt}) \qquad (10.8)$$

Since $K = 0.693/t_{1/2}$, substitution for K in Eq. 10.8 yields:

$$f_{ss} = \frac{(C_p)_t}{(C_p)_{ss}} = \left(1 - e^{-(0.693)\left(\frac{t}{t_{1/2}}\right)}\right)$$

If the ratio of $t/t_{1/2}$ is designated N, the number of elimination half lives, then

$$f_{ss} = \frac{(C_p)_t}{(C_p)_{ss}} = \left(1 - e^{-(0.693)(N)}\right) \qquad (10.9)$$

or

$$1 - f_{ss} = e - 0.693N$$

or

$$e - 0.693N = 1 - f_{ss} \text{ and } -0.693N = \ln(1 - f_{ss})$$

Then

$$N = \frac{\ln(1-f_{ss})}{-0.693} \tag{10.10}$$

Equation 10.10 is important since it allows us to determine the number of elimination half lives of a drug required to attain a given fraction of the true steady state. It should be clear from Eq. 10.10 that the number of elimination half lives required to attain a given fraction of steady state will always be the same, regardless of the value of the elimination half life of the drug, the infusion rate chosen and whether the drug was administered to normal or renally impaired subjects.

How would the profile of the fraction of true steady state achieved against the number of elimination half-lives look on rectilinear co-ordinates? Please keep it in mind that the value of fraction of the true steady state achieved will become equal to one as time approaches infinity.

If we wish to know the number of half lives required to reach the "practical" steady-state condition (i.e. $f_{ss} = 0.95$),

$$N = \frac{\ln(1-0.95)}{-0.693} = \frac{\ln(0.05)}{-0.693}$$

$\ln 0.05 = -2.9957$

Therefore, $N = -2.9957/-0.693 = 4.32$ half lives.

From this calculation, it should be clear that, if we infuse the drug at a constant rate up until a time equal to 4.32 half lives of the drug, the plasma concentration obtained will represent 95% of the true steady-state concentration, regardless of the chosen infusion rate, chosen drug and whether the subject has normal elimination or impaired elimination. Please note that the number of elimination half lives required to attain a fraction (in this example, 0.95) of true steady state will remain unaffected by the infusion rate, the drug chosen and the subject.

The time required to attain a fraction of steady state ($Nt_{1/2}$) will be different for each drug and in normal and renally impaired subjects since the elimination half life for each drug may be different and the elimination half life of the same drug will be different in normal and in renally impaired subjects.

Table 10.1 The relationship between the fraction of steady state plasma concentration (f_{ss}) and the number of elimination half lives (N) required for attaining that fraction of steady state

f_{ss}	N
0.10	0.15
0.50	1.00
0.75	2.00
0.875	3.00
0.95	4.32
0.99	6.65
1.00	∞

By employing Eq. 10.10, the number of elimination half lives of a drug required to attain a fraction of steady state can be determined. Table 10.1 provides this information.

The table indicates that if a drug is infused up to a time equal to one half life of the drug, the plasma concentration at that time will always, under any condition in any subject for any drug, represent 50% ($f_{ss} = 0.5$) of the true steady-state concentration for the chosen infusion rate. If the drug is infused up to two half lives, the plasma concentration will represent 75% of true steady-state concentration ($f_{ss} = 0.75$). If the infusion rate is doubled, the ratio of plasma concentration at time t to steady-state plasma concentration will remain unchanged.

Please note that in $N = t/t_{1/2}$, t represents a time at which we know the plasma concentration value and/or the time when we have stopped infusing the drug. In essence, this relationship ($N = t/t_{1/2}$) permits the transformation of a time into a number of half lives of the drug if the elimination half life of the drug is known. It is very important to recognize that:

$$f_{ss} = \frac{(C_p)_t}{(C_p)_{ss}}$$

The practical utility of these equations can be examined using some real numbers. Figure 10.9 depicts the plasma concentration versus time profile following the administration of a drug as an intravenous infusion.

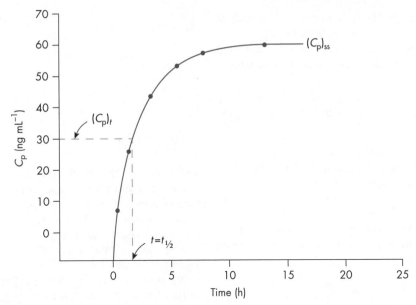

Figure 10.9 Plasma concentration (C_p) versus time profile following the administration of a drug as an intravenous infusion. ss, steady state.

The plasma concentration at 2 h [$(C_p)_t$] is $5 \mu g\,mL^{-1}$, and this represents 50% (i.e. $f_{ss} = 0.5$) of the true steady-state concentration. Use the equation:

$$f_{ss} = \frac{(C_p)_t}{(C_p)_{ss}}$$

and rearranging gives $(C_p)_{ss} = (C_p)_t/f_{ss} = 5 \mu g\,mL^{-1}/0.5 = 10 \mu g\,mL^{-1}$, the true steady-state concentration. In this example, a plasma concentration of $5 \mu g\,mL^{-1}$ occurs at 2 h since this concentration represents 50% of true steady-state concentration. The elimination half life of this drug is 2 h.

Instantaneous and continuous steady state

It takes $4.32t_{1/2}$ (in time units) of a constant infusion of a drug before a "practical" steady-state condition is attained. For example, if the half life of a drug is 2 h then it will take 8.44 h (4.32×2) before the "practical" steady-state condition is reached. Therefore, for a drug with a long half life, it will take a considerable amount of time before the "practical" steady-state condition is reached.

Life-threatening situations in the hospital setting will often demand that the desired plasma concentration of the drug (of course, always within its therapeutic range) is attained instantaneously and then is maintained for a long duration.

This may be accomplished by administering a loading intravenous bolus dose (D_L) concomitant with the commencement of the infusion rate.

The loading dose is an intravenous bolus dose. However, in this instance, unlike the case of a single, isolated intravenous bolus dose considered in Ch. 3, the loading dose is immediately followed by the commencement of an intravenous infusion at constant rate. The intravenous bolus dose permits us to attain the desired plasma concentration at time $= 0$ and the concomitant constant infusion allows us to maintain this concentration.

We know from Eq. 10.2 that:

$$X = \frac{Q}{K}(1 - e^{-Kt})$$

This represents the mass of drug in the body at a time from the infusion alone. We also know that:

$$X = X_0 e^{-Kt} \tag{10.11}$$

This represents the mass of drug in the body at any time from the intravenous bolus.

If an intravenous bolus of drug is administered at the time an intravenous infusion of the drug is started, then:

$$(X)_t = \frac{Q}{K}(1 - e^{-Kt}) + X_0 e^{-Kt} \qquad (10.12)$$

where X_0 is the loading dose (D_L) and $(X)_t$ is the total amount (or mass) of drug in the body at any time from both bolus and infusion.

Equation 10.12 represents the mass of drug in the body at any time as a result of the combination of intravenous bolus and intravenous infusion. Equation 10.12 can be modified in terms of concentration:

$$(C_p)_t = \frac{Q}{VK}(1 - e^{-Kt}) + \frac{D_L}{V}e^{-Kt} \qquad (10.13)$$

where $\frac{Q}{VK}(1 - e^{-Kt})$ will yield the contribution to the total plasma concentration at time t owing to the infusion administered at rate Q, and $\frac{D_L}{V}e^{-Kt}$ will yield the contribution to the total plasma concentration at time t owing to the intravenous bolus loading dose, D_L.

Equation 10.5 showed that $(C_p)_{ss} = Q/VK$. Hence, substituting for the term Q/VK in Eq. 10.13 with the term $(C_p)_{ss}$ from Eq. 10.5 will yield the following equation:

$$(C_p)_t = (C_p)_{ss}(1 - e^{-Kt}) + \frac{D_L}{V}e^{-Kt}$$

Using the above equation for total plasma drug concentration at any time from both bolus and infusion, and requiring that the total plasma drug concentration from bolus and infusion at time infinity be equal to the total plasma drug concentration from bolus and infusion at time zero, the following equation is obtained:

$$(C_p)_{ss}(1 - e^{-K(\infty)}) + \frac{D_L}{V}(e^{-K(\infty)})$$

$$= (C_p)_{ss}(1 - e^{-K(0)}) + \frac{D_L}{V}(e^{-K(0)})$$

$$\text{Therefore}: (C_p)_{ss}(1 - 0) + \frac{D_L}{V}(0)$$

$$= (C_p)_{ss}(1 - 1) + \frac{D_L}{V}(1)$$

and

$$(C_p)_{ss} = \frac{D_L}{V} \qquad (10.14)$$

or

$$D_L = V(C_p)_{ss} \qquad (10.15)$$

where $(C_p)_{ss}$ is the desired plasma concentration of a drug at steady state (e.g mg mL^{-1}); D_L is the intravenous bolus loading dose (e.g. mg or mg kg^{-1}); and V is the the apparent volume of distribution of the drug (e.g. mL; mL kg^{-1})

The dimensional analysis of Eqs 10.14 and 10.15 will be as follows:

V has units of volume (e.g. mL) and $(C_p)_{ss}$ has units of mass per unit volume (e.g. mg mL^{-1}). So D_L will have units of mass (e.g. mg or mg kg^{-1}).

Please attempt to show a plot of $(C_p)_{ss}$ against D_L (on rectilinear paper). What information can be obtained from the slope of this plot?

From Eq. 10.5, $(C_p)_{ss} = Q/VK$, and rearranging gives

$$(C_p)_{ss} V = Q/K \qquad (10.16)$$

However, since $(C_p)_{ss} V = D_L$ (Eq. 10.15), substituting for the term $(C_p)_{ss} V$ in Eq. 10.16 will yield:

$$D_L = Q/K \qquad (10.17)$$

where D_L is the loading dose; K is the the elimination rate constant; and Q is the infusion rate.

Dimensional analysis of Eq. 10.17 may be performed as follows:

$$D_L = \frac{Q}{K} = \frac{\text{mg h}^{-1}}{\text{h}^{-1}} \text{ or } \frac{\text{mg kg}^{-1}\text{h}^{-1}}{\text{h}^{-1}}$$

So D_L will be in units of weight (e.g. mg, mg kg^{-1}).

Please consider a rectilinear plot of loading dose (D_L) against infusion rate (Q) (Eq. 10.17). What information can be obtained from the slope of the plot?

Equations 10.14, 10.15 and 10.17 clearly suggest that the computation of the loading dose necessary to attain the desired plasma concentration of a drug instantaneously requires the knowledge of two fundamental pharmacokinetic parameters of a drug: the apparent volume of distribution and/or the elimination half life.

The selection of an equation (either Eq. 10.15 or Eq. 10.17) to determine the loading dose of a drug, by comparison, solely depends upon the available information. Equation 10.15 requires the knowledge of the apparent volume of distribution of the drug and the desired plasma concentration. Equation 10.17 requires knowledge of the infusion rate necessary to maintain the desired plasma concentration of the drug and of the elimination half life of the drug.

Since $K = 0.693/t_{1/2}$ (Eq. 3.12), substituting for K in Eq. 10.17 gives:

$$D_L = \frac{Q}{0.693/t_{1/2}}$$

or

$$D_L = \frac{Qt_{1/2}}{0.693} \tag{10.18}$$

Equation 10.18 suggests that the loading dose is determined by the proposed infusion rate and the patient's elimination half life and rate constant.

Should the patient manifest renal impairment for a drug eliminated by the kidneys, the infusion rate required to maintain the desired steady-state plasma concentration will be smaller and, please note, the elimination rate constant will also be smaller by an identical amount; therefore, the ratio of infusion rate over elimination rate constant remains unaffected. This simply suggests, therefore, that it is vitally important to adjust (lower) the infusion rate of drug in a renally impaired subject. However, adjustment in the loading dose is neither necessary nor required. This statement can further be supported upon careful examination of Eq. 10.15, which clearly suggests that the

adjustment in the loading dose of a drug is necessary only when the apparent volume of distribution of a drug changes. (This may happen in some disease states and/or owing to other abnormalities.) In summary, it is accurate to state that an adjustment in the infusion rate is always necessary and required if there is a change in the systemic clearance $[(Cl)_s]$ of a drug; however, adjustment in the loading dose is necessary only if there is a change in the apparent volume of distribution of a drug.

Figures 10.10 and 10.11, respectively, show the predicted and real plasma concentration versus time profiles following the administration of a drug as an intravenous bolus loading dose immediately followed by an infusion.

In Fig. 10.11, the plasma concentration versus time profile shows a trough. This might be attributed to an elapse in time between the completion of an intravenous bolus loading dose and the commencement of the infusion rate. The magnitude of the nadir observed in the plasma concentration versus time profile will be influenced by the elapsed time and the elimination half life of the drug. However, there is no bolus/infusion combination for a two-compartment drug that will produce a total plasma drug concentration that is constant over time; the profile will have peaks and/or nadirs. This, therefore, could be an alternative explanation for the deviation from a horizontal line in Fig. 10.11.

The salt form correction factor (S): its utility in pharmacokinetics

Although the concept of "salt value" (also called the salt form correction factor) and its utility in pharmacokinetics is being introduced at this point, it should be remembered that its use is not restricted only to the administration of drug by intravenous infusion. The salt value of a drug must always be taken into consideration, when applicable, while calculating the dose of drug, regardless of how the drug is administered; this includes intravenous single bolus dose (Ch. 3), extravascular routes (Ch. 6), and other future topics such as multiple dosing.

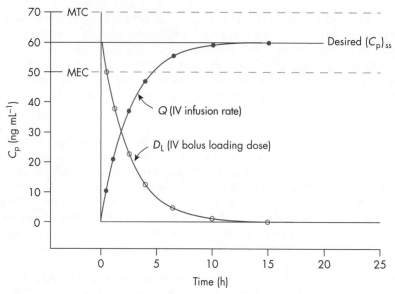

Figure 10.10 Predicted or theoretical plasma concentration (C_p) versus time profile following the administration of a drug as an intravenous bolus loading dose (D_L) immediately followed by an infusion at rate Q. MTC, minimum toxic concentration; MEC, minimum effective concentration; ss, steady state.

Administration of drugs frequently requires that drug be soluble in an aqueous medium to facilitate its administration. This is particularly true when drugs are administered intravenously. Drugs used intravenously or otherwise are very often insoluble in aqueous solvent, presenting a practical difficulty of preparing an aqueous solution. This necessitates the use a salt form of the drug that is soluble in aqueous solvent. The molecular weight of the salt is different from that of its corresponding free acid or free base. This requires the use of the salt form correction factor in the calculation of the final dose of the drug, whether by intravenous bolus, intravenous infusion, or extravascular routes. The following are some examples:

- aminophylline: (salt value of 0.8 to 0.85) is the ethylenediamine salt of theophylline
- procainamide HCl: (salt value of 0.87) is a salt of a weak base procainamide
- phenytoin sodium: (salt value of 0.92) is a sodium salt of phenytoin, a weak acidic compound
- phenobarbital sodium: (salt value of 0.90) is a sodium salt of phenobarbital, a weak acidic drug
- primidone (Mysoline): salt value of 1.00
- lidocaine HCl: (salt value of 0.87) is a salt of lidocaine, a weak basic drug.

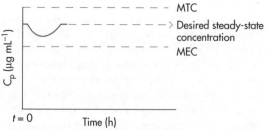

Figure 10.11 Observed (real) plasma concentration (C_p) versus time profile (rectilinear plot) following the administration of a drug as an intravenous bolus loading dose immediately followed by an infusion. MTC, minimum toxic concentration; MEC, minimum effective concentration.

Please note that it is the free acid or free base of a therapeutic agent that provides the pharmacological effect. For instance, when procainamide hydrochloride is administered to a patient, it is procainamide (free base) that is responsible for its pharmacological effect and not the hydrochloride part of the molecule. The pharmacokinetic parameters reported in the literature are obtained by measuring the free acid or base of a particular drug.

Example of the use of the salt form correction factor

Theophylline is relatively insoluble in an aqueous vehicle and, so, there is a practical difficulty in the administration of theophylline in that form. Therefore, aminophylline, which is the water-soluble salt (salt value of 0.8 to 0.85) of theophylline, is used. In this example, the salt value suggests that 100 mg aminophylline will provide 80–85 mg of theophylline. In other words, if the calculated loading dose required for attaining the desired theophylline plasma concentration instantaneously is 80 mg, then 100 mg of aminophylline must be administered. Failure to take into consideration the salt value, in this example, will result in 20% error.

For the purpose of illustration, assume that we have calculated the required intravenous bolus dose and infusion rate of theophylline to be 100 mg and 10 mg h^{-1}, respectively, to attain and then maintain the desired steady-state theophylline plasma concentration.

Calculation of the loading dose

100 mg theophylline/0.85 (salt value) = 117.64 mg aminophylline as loading dose.
Therefore, 117.64 mg of aminophylline (salt value 0.85) is equivalent to 100 mg theophylline.

Calculation of infusion rate

Analogously, calculations for the infusion rate are performed:

10 mg h^{-1} theophylline/0.85 (salt value) = 11.764 mg h^{-1} aminophylline for the infusion rate.

Therefore, 11.764 mg aminophylline (salt value 0.85) is equivalent to 10 mg theophylline.

Other examples of drugs where the salt value is used

Quinidine

Quindine is used in the treatment of atrial fibrillation and other cardiac arrhythmias and is available in three forms:

- quindine sulfate: salt value of 0.82
- quinidine gluconate: salt value of 0.62
- quinidine polygalacturonate: salt value of 0.62.

It is important to realise that for this drug, use of the quinidine gluconate salt without use of the salt form correction factor can introduce a 38% error in the dose and, consequently, in the drug plasma concentration.

Naproxen

Anyone working in a pharmacy may be familiar with the example of naproxen, where two products use different forms:

- Naprosyn (naproxen): available in tablet dosage form of 250, 375 and 500 mg strengths
- Anaprox (naproxen sodium): available in tablet dosage form of 275 and 550 mg strengths.

The different forms mean that 275 mg naproxen sodium (salt of a weak acid) is equivalent to 250 mg of naproxen (free acid) and 550 mg is equivalent to 500 mg of naproxen. These products are not interchangeable; however, they are considered pharmaceutical alternatives (see Ch. 7).

Omeprazole

Is the over-the-counter product Prilosec OTC the same as the prescription product Prilosec? Or is it, in fact, a different salt? (Answer: both products are the free-acid of omeprazole; both products are delayed-release formulations; Prilosec OTC is in tablet form, while Prilosec is in capsule form; Prilosec *suspension* is the magnesium salt of omeprazole.)

Iron-containing products

Examples of over-the-counter iron products include:

- ferrous sulfate: 325 mg tablet will provide 65 mg of elemental iron
- ferrous gluconate: 325 mg tablet will provide 38 mg of elemental iron
- ferrous fumarate: 325 mg tablet will provide 106 mg of elemental iron.

Wagner's method for rapid attainment of steady state

Returning to the intravenous infusion, another method can be used to obtain a steady state rapidly (please note steady state is not achieved instantaneously by this method). Wagner's method uses two different infusion rates (Q_1 and Q_2). Unlike the method described above, there is no intravenous bolus administration of drug in this method.

When no intravenous bolus dose is administered concomitantly with an intravenous infusion, rapid steady state can be obtained by manipulation of the infusion rates. This method has two stages.

1. The drug is infused first at a (higher) infusion rate (Q_1) for a time equal to the half life of the particular drug.
2. At time $t = t_{1/2}$, the infusion rate is changed to a second (slower) rate (Q_2), which controls the steady-state concentration.

Hence, in this method:

- the first infusion rate is always greater than the second infusion rate and this allows the desired concentration to be reached at a time equal to the elimination half life of the drug;
- the first infusion rate becomes a means of arriving at the second infusion rate and it is the second infusion rate that maintains and controls the steady-state plasma concentration until the cessation of infusion.

$$(C_p)_T = \frac{Q_1(1 - e^{-KT})}{VK} \tag{10.19}$$

where T is the time at which first infusion rate (Q_1) is changed to the second infusion rate (Q_2),

which determines and controls the steady-state plasma concentration, $(C_p)_{ss}$.

$$(C_p)_{ss} = \frac{Q_2}{VK} \tag{10.20}$$

Rearrangement of Eq. 10.19 yields:

$$Q_1 = \frac{(C_p)_T VK}{(1 - e^{-KT})}$$

Rearrangement of Eq. 10.20 yields:

$$Q_2 = (C_p)_{ss} VK$$

Equating $(C_p)_T$ with $(C_p)_{ss}$ and taking the ratio of Q_1 to Q_2 (Eqs 10.19 and 10.20) gives:

$$\frac{Q_1}{Q_2} = \frac{(C_p)_T VK}{(1 - e^{-KT})} \times \frac{1}{(C_p)_{ss} VK}$$

$$= \frac{1}{(1 - e^{-KT})} \tag{10.21}$$

The conceptual understanding of Eq. 10.21 is vital not only for the understanding of the theory and rationale behind the use of two infusion rates to attain and then maintain the desired plasma concentration of a drug but also for the understanding of calculations of loading dose and maintenance dose (D_M) when drugs are administered as an intravenous bolus and extravascularly in multiple doses (discussed in Ch. 11).

Next Eq. 10.21 is used and it is assumed that T (the time up to which the drug is infused at a first infusion rate, Q_1) is equal to the elimination half life of the drug. In other words, the drug is administered at the first infusion rate up until $t = t_{1/2}$, so $T = t_{1/2}$. Therefore, the term T in Eq. 10.21 can be substituted with $t_{1/2}$:

$$\frac{Q_1}{Q_2} = \frac{1}{(1 - e^{-Kt_{1/2}})} \tag{10.22}$$

However, since $t_{1/2} = 0.693/K$, this can then replace $t_{1/2}$ in Eq. 10.22:

$$\frac{Q_1}{Q_2} = \frac{1}{(1 - e^{-K(0.693/K)})} = \frac{1}{(1 - e^{-0.693})}$$

And, since $e^{-0.693} = 0.5$:

$$Q_1 = 2 \times Q_2; \quad \text{or} \quad Q_2 = Q_1/2 \tag{10.23}$$

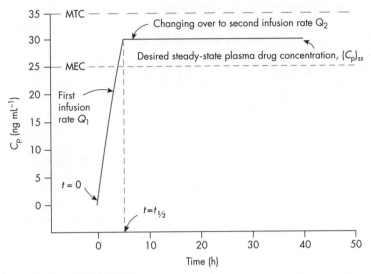

Figure 10.12 Typical plasma concentration (C_p) versus time profile following the administration of a drug by two infusion rates (Q_1 and Q_2). $t_{1/2}$, half life of drug; other abbreviations as in Fig. 10.10.

Equation 10.23 is important for understanding the concept of using two infusion rates to attain and then maintain the desired plasma concentration of a drug. It is equally important to recognize that the first infusion rate, Q_1, should never be allowed to produce drug plasma concentration at a toxic concentration. Figure 10.12 illustrates the plasma concentration versus time profile obtained by administering a drug by two infusion rates.

Some important comments on Wagner's method of using two infusion rates

1. The ratio of first infusion rate over second infusion rate (i.e. Q_1/Q_2) will always be equal to 2 if the time at which the first infusion rate is changed to second infusion rate is equal to the elimination half life of the drug. The elimination half life for each drug may be different and, therefore, the time at which the first infusion rate is changed to the second infusion rate will differ for each drug or, for that matter, in the same subject if there is evidence of renal or hepatic impairment (which can decrease the value of K).

2. If a drug is administered as a single intravenous infusion (Q), it requires the administration of a drug continuously for greater than three to four half lives of the drug before the drug concentration can attain the therapeutic range. If the drug is administered as an intravenous bolus concomitantly with an intravenous infusion, the desired drug plasma concentration is attained immediately and then maintained up to the time of cessation of the infusion.

3. If the drug is administered by choosing two infusion rates (Q_1 and Q_2), the ratio of the two infusion rates will determine the time at which the desired plasma concentration is attained. If the ratio is equal to 2, the desired plasma concentration will be attained at a time equal to the elimination half life of the drug. The greater the ratio of the two infusion rates the sooner is the attainment of the desired drug plasma concentration; conversely, the smaller the ratio of two infusion rates (the smallest possible ratio can be 1, when Q_1 and Q_2 are identical) the longer is the time required to attain the desired plasma concentration. Table 10.2 illustrates the relationship between the time (in terms of number of elimination half lives) at which the first infusion rate should be changed to the

Table 10.2 Relationship between the ratio of two infusion rates and the time at which a switch over to the second infusion is required in order to attain and maintain the desired plasma concentration

Time (No. of half lives) to change to second infusion rate (Q_2)	Ratio of first (Q_1) to second infusion rates (Q_1/Q_2)	Second infusion rate (Q_2)
$0.5 \times t_{1/2}$	3.41	$Q_1/3.41$
$1.0 \times t_{1/2}$	2.00	$Q_1/2.00$
$2.0 \times t_{1/2}$	1.31	$Q_1/1.31$
$3.0 \times t_{1/2}$	1.14	$Q_1/1.14$
$4.32 \times t_{1/2}$	1.06	$Q_1/1.06$
∞	1.00	$Q_1/1.0$ ($Q_1 = Q_2$)

second infusion rate and the ratio of the first infusion rate to the second infusion rate. How would a profile look if numbers from column 2 (the ratio of first infusion rate to second infusion rate) were plotted against the numbers from column 1 (the time in terms of elimination half lives at which the first infusion rate is changed over to second infusion rate)?

4. When Wagner's method is employed, it is important to note that the second infusion rate will remain the same for the maintenance of a desired plasma concentration of a drug, regardless of the time at which the first infusion rate was changed over to the second infusion rate. In other words, the change in the ratio of two infusion rates is a consequence of a change in the value of only the first infusion rate.

5. If it is required that a different plasma concentration of the same drug is attained, but at the same time T, and then it is maintained, both infusion rates will be different; however, the ratio of two calculated infusion rates will be identical.

Example of the use of Wagner's method

A procainamide plasma concentration of $6\,\mu g\,mL^{-1}$ is required to be reached and maintained by employing Wagner's method. So two infusion rates must be calculated.

The elimination half of procainamide is $3\,h$ and the apparent volume of drug distribution is $2000\,mL\,kg^{-1}$ body weight. The systemic clearance is equal to $462\,mL\,kg^{-1}\,h^{-1}$.

If we wish to reach and maintain a procainamide plasma concentration of $6\,\mu g\,mL^{-1}$ by employing Wagner's method, determine the two infusion rates involved.

The elimination half life of procainamide is 3 hours and the apparent volume of drug distribution is $2000\,mL\,kg^{-1}$ body weight. The systemic clearance is equal to $462\,mL\,kg^{-1}h^{-1}$.

The simplest process is first to calculate the *second* (maintenance) infusion rate Q_2.

$$Q_2 = (C_p)_{SS}^{target} VK = (C_p)_{SS}^{target}(Cl)$$
$$= (6\,\mu g\,mL^{-1})(462\,mL\,kg^{-1}\,h^{-1})$$
$$= 2.77\,mg\,kg^{-1}\,h^{-1}$$

Then calculate the *first* (loading) infusion rate

$$Q_1 = 2 \times Q_2 = (2)\,(2.77\,mg\,kg^{-1}\,h^{-1})$$
$$= 5.54\,mg\,kg^{-1}h^{-1}.$$

As discussed, the first infusion at rate Q_1 will attain the target plasma procainamide level of $6\,\mu g\,mL^{-1}$ at $t=t_{1/2}$. It is critically important that this high rate infusion be replaced by the lower rate infusion Q_2 at a time equal to one drug half life. Otherwise, plasma drug levels will rise well above the target level, likely causing toxicity.

The salt value (0.87) is then used to calculate the infusion rates for procainamide HCl:

Q_1 (the first infusion rate) will be
5.54 mg kg^{-1} h^{-1}/0.87 = 6.637 mg kg^{-1} h^{-1}
× of procainamide HCl.

Q_2 (the second infusion rate) will be $0.5 \times Q_1$
= 3.183 mg kg^{-1} h^{-1} of procainamide HCl.

In this example, the infusion of procainamide HCl is initiated at a rate of 6.367 mg kg^{-1} h^{-1} and the drug is infused for 3 h (one half life of the drug). At 3 h, the infusion is switched to the second infusion rate of 3.183 mg kg^{-1} h^{-1}.

It is important to be aware that failure to switch to the second infusion rate at the determined time will produce a value for the drug plasma concentration that differs from the desired one; similarly, failure to change the rate to the second infusion rate will yield a drug plasma concentration that is higher than intended. In this example, the procainamide plasma concentration would be 12 µg mL^{-1} at true steady state – and the therapeutic range for procainamide is 4–8 µg mL^{-1}. As a good future pharmacist, provider and a firm believer of principles of pharmaceutical care, would you want to commit a mistake of this nature?

The first infusion rate will enable the desired procainamide plasma concentration of 6 µg mL^{-1} to be reached in this patient at 3 h, and the second infusion rate will maintain the procainamide plasma concentration at that level (6 µg mL^{-1}) until the cessation of the second infusion rate.

In this example, please note, if it is desired to attain a higher procainamide plasma concentration at a given time (3 h in this example), the first and second infusion rates will be higher; however, the ratio of two infusion rates will remain unaffected. If, however, it desired to attain the same procainamide plasma concentration (i.e. 6 µg mL^{-1}) sooner than 3 h (i.e. sooner than one half life of the drug), the ratio of first to second infusion rates will be greater, solely because the first infusion rate will be increased.

10.4 Sampling blood following cessation of infusion

Figure 10.13 shows the setup for monitoring elimination of drug from plasma following the discontinuation of a constant rate intravenous infusion.

This is described by the differential equation:

$$\left(\frac{-dX}{dt}\right)_{t'} = K(X)_{t'} \tag{10.24}$$

and

$$t' = t - T$$

where t', the time following the cessation of infusion; $(X)_{t'}$ is the mass of drug in the blood at time t'; and T is the time at which the infusion was stopped (note that this could be any time: 5 min, 10 min, 30 min, one half life of the drug, 7 h, etc.).

Equation 10.24 is essentially the same as Eq. 1.17 (p. 15). In essence, once the infusion is stopped, there is no drug entering the blood and the drug present in the blood follows a mono-exponential decline that is identical to that seen for an intravenous bolus injection. Equation 10.24, when integrated, becomes

$$(X)_{t'} = (X)_T e^{-kt'} \tag{10.25}$$

Figure 10.13   Setup for the rate of elimination of drug from plasma and the plasma drug concentration following the discontinuation of a constant rate intravenous infusion.

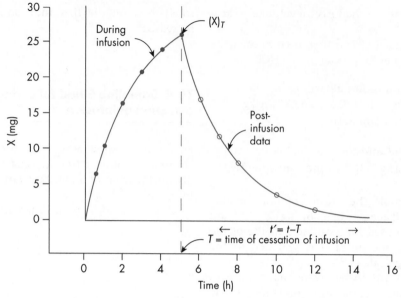

Figure 10.14 A typical profile of the amount of drug in blood against time following the administration of a drug by an intravenous infusion, showing amounts of drug in blood before and after cessation of the infusion.

where $(X)_{t'}$ is the mass or amount of drug in the blood at time t', in the post-infusion period; $(X)_T$ is the mass or amount of drug in the body at the time of cessation of infusion; K is the first-order elimination rate constant and t' is the time in the post-infusion period $(t - T)$.

Equation 10.25 is virtually identical to Eq. 1.18 (p. 15) and, therefore, the profile will look similar to that for intravenous bolus administration (Fig. 10.14).

Figure 10.15, where the post-infusion section follows Eq. 10.25, also suggests that the mass of drug in the blood/body declines monoexponentially with time following the cessation of infusion.

Please note the amount of drug in the blood, the plasma concentration of a drug and the rate of elimination of drug at the time of cessation of infusion will depend on the infusion rate as well as the time of cessation of the infusion (see Figs 10.14 and 10.15).

The higher the infusion rate and longer the duration of infusion, the higher will be the amount of drug, the concentration of drug

and the rate of elimination. And, of course, following the attainment of the true steady-state condition, for a chosen infusion rate, there will be no further change in any of these values.

10.5 Use of post-infusion plasma concentration data to obtain half life, elimination rate constant and the apparent volume of distribution

Since $X/V = C_p$ (from Eq. 3.6), Eq. 10.25 can be modified in terms of concentration:

$$(C_p)_{t'} = (C_p)_T e^{-kt'} \tag{10.26}$$

Figure 10.16 is a plot of concentration versus time in the post-infusion period.

(a)

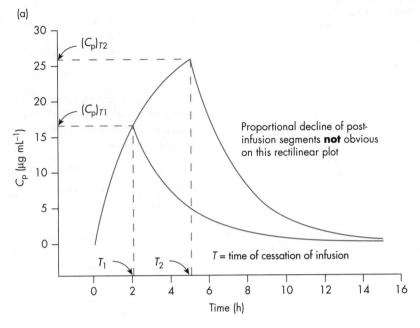

(b)

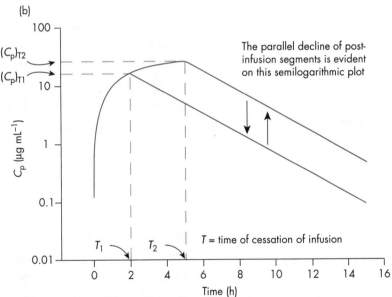

Figure 10.15 Typical profiles of the plasma concentration (C_p) against time following the administration of a drug by an intravenous infusion when the infusion is stopped at two different times: (a) rectilinear plot; (b) semilogarithmic plot.

The following conclusions may be drawn from Figures 10.14 to 10.16:

1. The elimination half life and the elimination rate constant can be determined by employing methods described above.

2. By definition, the intercept is $(C_p)_T = (X)_T / V$; this approach, however, is not a practical way to determine apparent volume of distribution (V) since we do not know the value of $(X)_T$.

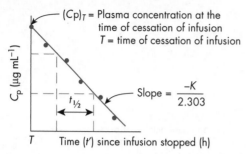

- $(C_p)_T$ = Plasma concentration at the time of cessation of infusion
- T = time of cessation of infusion
- Slope = $\dfrac{-K}{2.303}$

Figure 10.16 Plasma concentration (C_p) versus time profile following the cessation of infusion (i.e. post-infusion).

3. The absolute values of $(C_p)_T$ and $(X)_T$, and, therefore, the value of the rate of elimination are time dependent.
4. In general, if there is no loading dose:

$$(C_p)_T = \frac{Q(1 - e^{-KT})}{VK} \qquad (10.27)$$

However, when T approaches infinity, Eq. 10.27 reduces to Eq. 10.5:

$$(C_p)_T = (C_p)_{ss} = \frac{Q}{VK}$$

Method for obtaining the volume of distribution

Rearranging Eq. 10.27 as follows:

$$V = \frac{Q(1 - e^{-KT})}{(C_p)_T K}$$

When $T = \infty$, $(C_p)_T = (C_p)_{ss}$, then:

$$V = \frac{Q}{(C_p)_{ss} K}$$

When $T = t$,

$$V = \frac{Q(1 - e^{-Kt})}{(C_p)_t K}$$

Example of use of post-infusion plasma concentration data

Table 10.3 and Figs 10.17 and 10.18 show plasma concentrations during and after the infusion period when a drug was infused at a constant infusion rate ($40\,\text{mg h}^{-1}$) for 12 h while Figure 10.19 shows post-infusion concentrations.

Half life, elimination rate constant and the apparent volume of distribution from the post-infusion data and by the graphical method

$t_{1/2} = 1.7\,\text{h}$ and $K = 0.693/1.7\,\text{h} = 0.407\,\text{h}^{-1}$.

For the apparent volume of distribution, it is assumed here, solely for the purpose of demonstrating how to compute the apparent volume of distribution from the appropriate equation, that the true steady-state plasma concentration is $9.6\,\text{mg L}^{-1}$. This assumption can be justified by the fact that the time of cessation of the infusion, 12 h in this example, is substantially more than 7.34 h ($4.32 t_{1/2}$ of the drug). Therefore, the

Table 10.3 Plasma concentrations during and after infusion of a drug at a constant infusion rate of $40\,\text{mg h}^{-1}$ for 12 h

Time (h)	Concentration (mg L^{-1})
During infusion	
1.0	3.30
2.0	5.40
4.0	7.60
6.0	8.70
8.0	9.30
10.0	9.60
12.0 (=T)	**9.50**
Post-infusion ($t' = t - T$)	
2.0	4.10
4.0	1.80
6.0	0.76
8.0	0.33
10.0	0.14

t', time following the cessation of infusion; T, time infusion stopped.

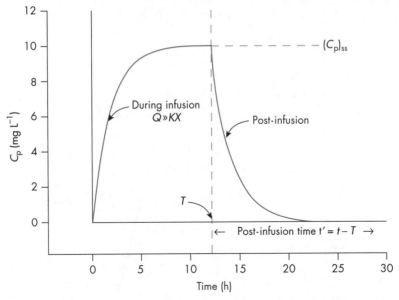

Figure 10.17 Plasma concentration (C_p) versus time during and post-infusion (rectilinear plot). T, time of cessation of infusion; t', time since the infusion was stopped; ss, steady state.

difference between the theoretical true steady-state plasma concentration $(C_p)_{ss}$ and the observed plasma concentration $(9.6\,\mathrm{mg\,L^{-1}})$ at the time of cessation of infusion (12 h) is insignificant in this example and will not introduce a serious error in the estimation of this parameter. Then,

$$(C_p)_{ss} = \frac{Q}{VK}$$

or

$$V = \frac{Q}{(C_p)_{ss}K}$$

$$V = \frac{40\,\mathrm{mg\,h^{-1}}}{(9.6\,\mathrm{mg\,L^{-1}})(0.407\,\mathrm{h^{-1}})}$$

$$= \frac{40\,\mathrm{mg\,h^{-1}}}{3.9\,\mathrm{mg\,L^{-1}\,h^{-1}}} = 10.25\,\mathrm{L}$$

One can also obtain the volume of distribution by the use of the following approach:

$$V = \frac{Q(1 - e^{-KT})}{(C_p)_T K}$$

$T = 4\,\mathrm{h}$, if the infusion had been stopped at 4 h and $(C_p)_T = 7.6\,\mathrm{mg\,L^{-1}}$, which is the plasma concentration that corresponds to $T = 4\,\mathrm{h}$. Then,

$$V = \frac{40\,\mathrm{mg\,h^{-1}}}{(7.6\,\mathrm{mg\,L^{-1}})(0.407\,\mathrm{h^{-1}})}(1 - e^{-0.407(4)})$$

$$= \frac{40\,\mathrm{mg\,h^{-1}}}{3.093\,\mathrm{mg\,L^{-1}\,h^{-1}}}(1 - e^{-1.628})$$

Since $e^{-1.628} = 0.1959$,

$$V = 12.932\,\mathrm{L} \times (1 - 0.1959)$$
$$= 12.932 \times 0.8041 = 10.39\,\mathrm{L}$$

The small difference observed in the apparent volume of distribution obtained with the two approaches is attributed to the assumption made in the first approach.

Calculating the steady state plasma concentration

$$(C_p)_{ss} = \frac{Q(t_{1/2})}{V(0.693)}$$

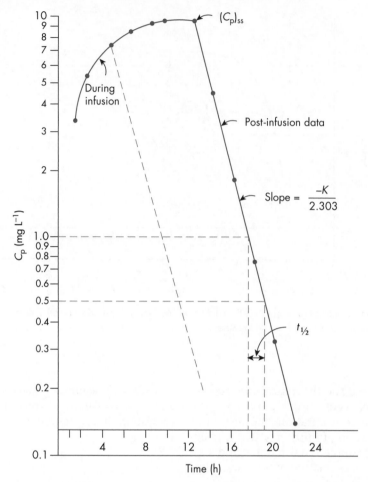

Figure 10.18   Plasma concentration (C_p) versus time during and post-infusion (semilogarithmic plot). K, elimination constant; ss, steady state.

$$(C_p)_{ss} = \frac{(40 \text{ mg h}^{-1})(1.7 \text{ h})}{10.25 \text{ L} (0.693)} = \frac{68 \text{ mg}}{7.103 \text{ L}}$$
$$= 9.57 \text{ mg L}^{-1}$$

Calculating infusion rate

$$Q = \frac{(C_p)_{ss}(V)(0.693)}{t_{1/2}}$$

$$Q = \frac{(9.57 \text{ mg L}^{-1})_{ss}(10.25 \text{ L})(0.693)}{1.7 \text{ h}}$$

$$= \frac{67.178 \text{ mg}}{1.7 \text{ h}} = 39.98 \text{ mg h}^{-1}$$

10.6 Rowland and Tozer method

The Rowland and Tozer method allows the elimination half life and elimination rate constant to be calculated for an administered drug by using plasma concentration–time data obtained during the infusion period (i.e. plasma concentration values in the post-infusion period are not required).

Plot the difference between the steady-state plasma concentration and the observed plasma concentration in Table 10.4 (i.e. $(C_p)_{ss} - (C_p)_{obs}$) versus time on semilogarithmic paper (values

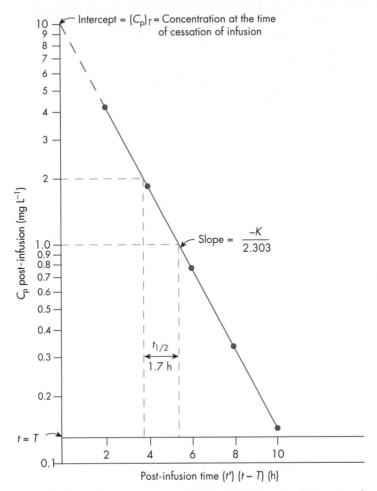

Figure 10.19   Plasma concentration (C_p) versus time post-infusion (semilogarithmic plot). T, time of cessation of infusion; t', time since the infusion was stopped; K, elimination constant; ss, steady state.

Table 10.4   Steady state and observed plasma concentration of a drug during infusion

Time during infusion (h)	$(C_p)_{obs}$ (mg L^{-1})	$(C_p)_{diff}$ (mg L^{-1})
1.00	3.3	6.25
2.00	5.4	4.15
4.00	7.6	1.95
6.00	8.7	0.85
8.00	9.3	0.25
10.0	**9.55** (average of 10 and 12 h samples)	–

$(C_p)_{obs}$, observed plasma concentration; $(C_p)_{diff}$, difference in plasma concentration between steady state and observed, $(C_p)_{ss} - (C_p)_{obs}$.

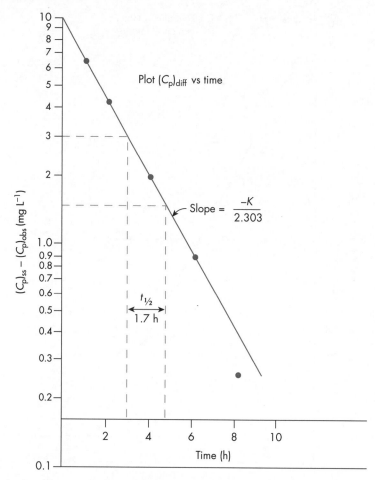

Figure 10.20   Rowland and Tozer method. Data from Table 10.4 is plotted. $(C_p)_{ss} - (C_p)_{obs}$, the difference between plasma concentration at steady state and that observed during the infusion. $t_{1/2}$, half life of drug; K, elimination constant. See text for further details.

from column 3 against values from column 1) (Fig. 10.20).

The elimination half life and elimination rate constant are calculated by the methods described above. Please note that this method will yield an accurate estimate of parameters provided that the drug is infused up until such time that the "practical" steady-state condition has been exceeded (i.e. the time of cessation of infusion is greater than $4.32t_{1/2}$ of the drug). In this example, that criterion has been met (12 h represents approximately seven half lives of drug).

Problem set 4

Problems for Chapter 10

Question 1

Table P4.1 gives the plasma concentrations (C_p) obtained after the intravenous infusion of 13 mg min^{-1} of a drug, which is eliminated exclusively by urinary excretion. The infusion was terminated at 2 h.

Plot the data and, using the plot, determine the following.

a. The elimination half life ($t_{1/2}$).
b. The elimination rate constant (K).
c. The apparent volume of distribution (V).
d. The true steady-state plasma concentration, ($C_p)_{ss}$.
e. The 'practical' steady-state plasma concentration and time it takes to reach the 'practical' steady-state condition.

Table P4.1

Time (h)	Plasma concentrations, (μg mL^{-1})
0.5	37.50
1.0	56.30
1.5	65.60
2.0	70.30
2.5	35.20
3.0	17.70
3.5	8.70
4.0	4.40
5.0	1.10

f. The loading dose (D_L) necessary to reach the true steady-state plasma concentration instantaneously.
g. The infusion rate (Q).
h. The true steady-state plasma concentration values following the administration of drug at the infusion rates of 15 and 20 mg min^{-1}.
i. The loading doses necessary to attain the instantaneous steady-state concentrations for the infusion rates in (h).

Question 2

Following an intravenous injection of 10 mg propranolol, McAllister (1976) found the values of the elimination rate constant (K) and the apparent volume of distribution (V) to be 0.00505 ± 0.0006 min^{-1} and 295 ± 53 L, respectively (mean $\pm$SD for six patients). These values were then used to calculate the loading dose (D_L) and infusion rate (Q) necessary to instantly obtain and then continuously maintain propranolol plasma concentrations of 12, 40 and 75 ng mL^{-1}.

a. What were his calculated values of D_L and Q?
b. What is the relationship between the loading dose (D_L) and the infusion rate (Q)?

Problem-solving exercise

Procainamide is used for the treatment of ventricular tachyarrhythmia. It is administered intravenously, orally and intramuscularly, and its therapeutic range is 4–8 μg mL^{-1}. When administered intravenously, a water-soluble salt, procainamide hydrochloride, is used to prepare an aqueous solution:

- therapeutic range $= 4$–8 mg L^{-1}

- elimination half life $(t_{1/2}) = 3$ h (in healthy subjects)
- apparent volume of distribution $(K) = 2$ L kg^{-1} (in healthy subjects)
- % excreted in urine $= 65\%$
- % metabolite (N-acetylprocainamide) $= 35\%$
- Salt value $= 0.87$

It is necessary to administer procainamide, as an intravenous infusion, to control arrhythmias in a patient (100 kg) admitted into a hospital. The desired 'practical' and true steady-state procainamide plasma concentrations are determined to be 5.7 and 6.0 µg mL^{-1}, respectively.

1. Determine the infusion rate (Q) of procainamide hydrochloride required to attain the 'practical' and true steady-state procainamide plasma concentrations, $(C_p)_{ss}$, of 5.7 and 6.0 µg mL^{-1}, respectively.

2. Determine the time it will take to attain the 'practical' steady-state condition in this subject.

   It is desired to attain the steady-state procainamide plasma concentration of 6 µg mL^{-1} instantaneously.

3. What would be the desired loading dose (D_L) of procainamide hydrochloride?

4. Determine the rate of elimination (KX) of procainamide at true steady-state condition and compare your answer with the chosen infusion rate.

   If it is desired to attain and then maintain the true steady-state procainamide plasma concentration $(C_p)_{ss}$ of 8 mg L^{-1} in this subject. In answering questions 5–8, make some important observations with regard to parameters that change as a result of change in the infusion rate and parameters that remain unaffected by it.

5. Determine the infusion rate (Q) required (think of linear kinetics).

6. Determine the 'practical' steady-state procainamide plasma concentration, $(C_p)_{ss}$, for the calculated infusion rate.

7. Determine the time required for attaining the 'practical' steady-state plasma concentration.

8. Determine the rate of elimination (KX) at true steady-state condition.

9. Show the profile (rectilinear coordinates) of rate of elimination at steady state against the infusion rate.

10. Show the profile (rectilinear coordinates) of 'practical' and true steady-state plasma concentrations against the infusion rate.

11. In a patient with renal impairment, the elimination half life $(t_{1/2})$ of procainamide is reported to be 14 h.

    Determine the loading dose (D_L) and infusion rate (Q) of procainamide HCl necessary to attain and then maintain the steady-state procainamide plasma concentration of 6 µg mL^{-1}.

12. Show the profile (rectilinear paper) of infusion rate necessary to attain a true steady-state plasma concentration against the systemic clearance or against the degree of renal impairment.

13. Show the profile (rectilinear paper) of loading dose necessary to attain a true steady-state plasma concentration instantaneously against the systemic clearance or against the degree of renal impairment (assuming that apparent volume of drug distribution remains unaffected).

14. In a patient with cardiac failure and shock and the renal impairment, the apparent volume of distribution and the elimination half life $(t_{1/2})$ of procainamide are reported to be 1.5 L kg^{-1} and 14 h, respectively.

    Determine the loading dose (D_L) and infusion rate (Q) of procainamide HCl necessary to attain and then maintain the steady-state procainamide plasma concentration of 6 µg mL^{-1}.

15. The administration of procainamide hydrochloride at a constant rate of 2.1241 mg kg^{-1} h^{-1} yielded the procainamide plasma concentration of 4 mg L^{-1} and 2.74 mg L^{-1} at $t = \infty$ and 5 h, respectively.

    Determine the loading dose (D_L) of procainamide hydrochloride necessary to attain a procainamide plasma concentration of 7 mg L^{-1} instantaneously.

16. It is necessary to administer procainamide by using two intravenous infusion rates (i.e. Q_1 and Q_2) to control arrhythmias in a patient (100 kg) admitted into a hospital. It is desired to attain and then maintain the procainamide plasma concentration of

$8\,\mu g\,mL^{-1}$. The elimination half life ($t_{1/2}$) of procainamide in this subject is reported to be 4 h and the apparent volume of distribution (V) is $2000\,mL\,kg^{-1}$.

Calculate two infusion rates (i.e. Q_1 and Q_2), and the time (t) at which the first infusion rate (Q_1) would be changed to the second infusion rate (Q_2).

17. What will be the true steady-state plasma concentration of procainamide should this change over be forgotten?

Answers

This problem set provides plasma concentration versus time data following the administration of a drug at a constant infusion rate. The following are our answers; your answers may differ for reasons discussed in earlier problem sets.

Question 1 answer

a. $t_{1/2} = 0.5\,h$.
b. $K = 1.386\,h^{-1}$.
c. Since the true steady-state plasma concentration is not known, plasma concentration at 2 h can be used with the intravenous infusion equation that describes the plasma concentration versus time data, We determined $V = 7504.70\,mL$ (7.504 L).
d. Employing the following values in the equation for the determination of steady-state plasma concentration yields the true $(C_p)_{ss}$.

$Q = 780\,000\,\mu g\,h$
$V = 7.504\,L$
$K = 1.386\,h^{-1}$
$Cl_s = 10\,401.51\,mL\,h^{-1}$.

Calculated true $(C_p)_{ss} = 74.99\,\mu g\,mL^{-1}$.

Please note that $(C_p)_{ss}$ is influenced by the chosen infusion rate as well as the systemic clearance of a drug (renally impaired patients).

e. By definition, the *'practical'* steady-state concentration is the plasma concentration when time is equal to 4.32 half lives of the drug and it is 95% of the true steady-state plasma concentration. In this example, therefore:

$74.99\,\mu g\,mL^{-1} \times 0.95 = 71.24\,\mu g\,mL^{-1}$.

The 'practical' steady-state plasma concentration occurs at 2.16 h (half life is 0.5 h; therefore, $4.32 \times 0.5\,h = 2.16\,h$). Note that the number of elimination half lives required to attain the 'practical' steady-state concentration will remain unaffected by the chosen in fusion rate.

f. The loading dose required to reach true steady-state plasma concentration of $74.99\,\mu g\,mL^{-1}$ instantaneously can be determined by employing either of two equations:

$$D_L = (C_p)_{ss} \times V$$
$$D_L = 74.99\,\mu g\,mL^{-1} \times 7504.70\,mL$$
$$D_L = 56277.45\,\mu g\,(562.77\,mg).$$

Alternatively,

$$D_L = \frac{Q}{K}$$
$$Q = 780\,000\,\mu g\,h^{-1}$$
$$K = 1.386\,h^{-1}$$
$$D_L = \frac{780\,000\,\mu g\,h^{-1}}{1.386\,h^{-1}}$$
$$D_L = 562770.56\,\mu g\,(562.77\,mg).$$

If a higher plasma concentration was required, the desired loading dose will also be higher.

g. $(C_p)_{ss} = \dfrac{Q}{VK}$

$Q = (C_p)_{ss} \times VK$
$VK = Cl_s = 10\,401.51\,mL\,h^{-1}$
Desired $(C_p)_{ss} = 74.99\,\mu g\,mL^{-1}$
$Q = 74.99\,\mu g\,mL^{-1} \times 10\,401.51\,mL\,h^{-1}$
$Q = 780\,009.23\,\mu g\,h^{-1}\,(780.009\,mg\,h^{-1}$
or $13.00\,mg\,min^{-1})$.

h. $(C_p)_{ss} = \dfrac{Q}{VK}$

$Q = 15\,mg\,min^{-1} = 900\,mg\,h^{-1}$
$V = 7.504\,L$
$K = 1.386\,h^{-1}$
$VK = 10401.51\,mL\,h^{-1}$
$(C_p)_{ss} = \dfrac{900\,000\,\mu g\,h^{-1}}{10\,401.51\,mL\,h^{-1}} = 86.52\,\mu g\,mL^{-1}.$

Using an identical approach, true $(C_p)_{ss} = 115.36\,\mu g\,mL^{-1}$ for the infusion rate of 20 mg min^{-1} (1200 mg h^{-1}). Plotting a graph of true $(C_p)_{ss}$ against Q values used in this example will enable determination of the systemic clearance of the drug

i. The loading doses required to attain the true $(C_p)_{ss}$ values of 86.52 and 115.36 $\mu g\,mL^{-1}$ can be calculated by two approaches.

$$D_L = (C_p)_{ss} \times V$$

$$D_L = 86.52\,\mu g\,mL^{-1} \times 7504.70\,mL$$
$$= 649306.64\,\mu g\ (649.30\,mg).$$

Alternatively,

$$D_L = \frac{Q}{K}$$

$$Q = 900.00\,mg\,h^{-1}$$
$$K = 1.386\,h^{-1}$$

$$D_L = \frac{900.00\,mg\,h^{-1}}{1.386\,h^{-1}} = 649.35\,mg.$$

Question 2 answer

To attain and maintain $12\,\mu g\,L^{-1}$ requires $D_L = 3.54\,mg$ and $Q = 17.877\,\mu g\,min^{-1}$.

For $40\,\mu g\,L^{-1}$, D_L and Q need to be 3.333 times the values needed for $12\,\mu g\,L^{-1}$ and for $75\mu g\,L^{-1}$ D_L and Q need to be 6.25 times the values required for $12\,\mu g\,L^{-1}$ or 1.875 times the values required for $40\,\mu g\,L^{-1}$. If the graph of D_L against Q, calculated above, is plotted, a useful pharmacokinetic parameter of the drug may be obtained: the reciprocal of the slope of this graph will be the first-order elimination rate constant.

Problem-solving exercise answer

From the data given the following can be calculated:

- elimination rate constant $(K) = 0.693\,h^{-1}/3\,h = 0.231\,h^{-1}$
- systemic clearance $Cl_s = VK = 2.0\,L\,kg^{-1} \times 0.231\,h^{-1} = 0.462\,L\,kg^{-1}h^{-1}$
- renal clearance $Cl_r = K_u V = 0.3003\,L\,kg^{-1}h^{-1}$
- metabolic (or non-renal) clearance $Cl_m = K_m V = 0.1617\,L\,kg^{-1}h^{-1}$.

1. The calculations below are for attaining the true $(C_p)_{ss}$ of $6.0\,\mu g\,mL^{-1}$.

$$(C_p)_{ss} = \frac{Q}{VK}$$

$$Q = (C_p)_{ss} \times VK$$

$$Q = 6\,\mu g\,mL^{-1} \times 462\,mL\,kg^{-1}h^{-1}$$
$$= 2.772\,mg\,kg^{-1}h^{-1}\ (2772\,\mu g\,kg^{-1}h^{-1})$$
of procainamide.

Using the salt value,

$$\frac{2772\,\mu g\,kg^{-1}h^{-1}}{0.87} = 3186.20\,\mu g\,kg^{-1}h^{-1}$$
procainamide HCl.

Alternatively,

$$(C_p)_{ss} = \frac{Q}{VK}$$

$$(C_p)_{ss} \times VK = Q\ \text{(infusion rate)}$$

$$V = 2.0\,L\,kg^{-1} \times 100\,kg\ \text{(patient's weight)}$$
$$V = 200\,L$$
$$Cl_s = VK = 200\,L \times 0.231\,h^{-1} = 46.2\,L\,h^{-1}$$
$$Q = 6\,\mu g\,mL^{-1} \times 200\,000\,mL \times 0.231\,h^{-1}$$
$$= 277\,200\,\mu g\,h^{-1}\ (277.20\,mg\,h^{-1})$$
of procainamide.

Using the salt value:

$$Q = \frac{277.20\,mg\,h^{-1}}{0.87}$$
$$= 318.62\,mg\,h^{-1}\text{ of procainamide HCl.}$$

2. The infusion rate of 318.62 mg h^{-1} (3.186 mg h^{-1} kg^{-1}) of procainamide hydrochloride will provide a 'practical' steady-state procainamide plasma concentration of $5.7\,\mu g\,mL^{-1}$ at 4.32 times the half life of the drug and a true steady-state procainamide plasma concentration of $6\,\mu g\,mL^{-1}$ at $t = \infty$.

Time to attain the practical $(C_p)_{ss}$
$$= 4.32 \times 3\,h$$
$$= 12.96, \text{ or approximately } 13\,h$$

Please note that once the infusion is commenced at a constant rate of 277.2 mg h^{-1} (or 2.772 mg kg^{-1}h^{-1}) at time 3 h (i.e. one half life of the drug), 6 h (i.e. 2 half lives of the drug), 9 h (i.e. 3 half lives of the drug) and at 12.96 h (i.e. 4.32 half lives of the drug) the plasma procainamide concentrations of 3, 4.5, 5.27 and $5.7 \, \mu g \, mL^{-1}$, respectively, are attained. And, of course, the true steady-state plasma concentration of $6 \, \mu g \, mL^{-1}$ is attained at $t = \infty$. For this infusion rate, the true $(C_p)_{ss}$ of 6 $\mu g \, mL^{-1}$ represents fraction of steady state (f_{ss}) = 1. The C_p of $3 \, \mu g \, mL^{-1}$ (at $t = 3$ h or one half life of the drug) represents f_{ss} of 0.5 (i.e. 50%) of true $(C_p)_{ss}$. The C_p of $4.5 \, \mu g \, mL^{-1}$ (at $t = 6$ h or two half lives of the drug) represents f_{ss} of 0.75 (i.e. 75%) of true $(C_p)_{ss}$. The C_p of $5.27 \, \mu g \, mL^{-1}$ (at $t = 9$ h or three half lives of the drug) represents f_{ss} of 0.875 (i.e. 87.5%) of true $(C_p)_{ss}$. The C_p of $5.70 \, \mu g \, mL^{-1}$ (at $t = 12.96$ h or 4.32 half lives of the drug) represents f_{ss} of 0.95 (i.e. 95%) of true $(C_p)_{ss}$.

If the infusion rate (Q) is changed, the plasma procainamide concentration at any time will change (directly proportional); however, the f_{ss} value and the number of half lives required to attain a given f_{ss} will remain unchanged.

3. Loading dose (D_L) is given by:

$$D_L = (C_p)_{ss} V$$
$$D_L = 6 \, \mu g \, mL^{-1} \times 2000 \, mL \, kg^{-1}$$
$$D_L = 12\,000 \, \mu g \, kg^{-1} \text{ procainamide}$$

For the 100 kg patient,

$$D_L = 1200\,000 \, \mu g = 1200 \, mg \text{ procainamide}$$

Using the salt value,

$$D_L = \frac{(12 \, mg \, kg^{-1} \text{ procainamide}) \times (100 \, kg \text{ body weight})}{0.87}$$
$$= \frac{1200 \, mg \text{ procainamide}}{0.87}$$
$$= 1379 \, mg \text{ procainamide HCl}$$

Alternatively,

$$D_L = \frac{Q}{K}$$
$$D_L = \frac{2.772 mg \text{ procainamide} \, kg^{-1} h^{-1}}{0.231 h^{-1}}$$
$$= 12 \, mg \, kg^{-1} \text{ procainamide}$$
$$= \frac{12 \, mg \, kg^{-1} \text{ procainamide}}{0.87}$$
$$= 13.79 \, mg \, kg^{-1} \text{ procainamide HCl}$$

For the 100 kg patient,

$$D_L = 1379 \, mg \text{ procainamide HCl}.$$

4. Only at time infinity is the rate of elimination (KX) is equal to the rate of infusion (Q)

$$Q = KX_{ss}$$

where X_{ss} is the mass or amount of drug in the blood at true steady state.

Now $X_{ss} = (C_p)_{ss} V$

For this example,

$$X_{ss} = 6 \, \mu g \, mL^{-1} \times 200\,000 \, mL$$
$$X_{ss} = 120\,0000 \, \mu g = 1200 \, mg$$

The rate of elimination $= KX_{ss} = 0.231 \, h^{-1}$ $\times 1200 \, mg = 277.20 \, mg \, h^{-1}$ procainamide.

$$Q = 2.772 \, mg \, kg^{-1} h^{-1} \times 100 \, kg$$
$$= 277.20 \, mg \, h^{-1}.$$

This proves that at true steady-state condition, the rate of elimination is equal to the infusion rate.

5. $(C_p)_{ss} = \dfrac{Q}{VK}$

$$Q = (C_p)_{ss} \times VK$$
$$Q = 8 \, \mu g \, mL^{-1} \times 462 \, mL \, kg^{-1} h^{-1}$$
$$= 3.696 \, mg \, kg^{-1} h^{-1} \, (3696 \, \mu g \, kg^{-1} h^{-1})$$
of procainamide.

Using the salt value

$$Q = \frac{3696 \, \mu g \, kg^{-1} h^{-1}}{0.87}$$
$$Q = 4248.27 \, \mu g \, kg^{-1} h^{-1}$$
$$(4.248 \, mg \, kg^{-1} h^{-1}) \text{ of procainamide HCl.}$$

Alternatively. Since the concentration of $8 \, \mu g \, mL^{-1}$ is 1.333 times the concentration of $6 \, \mu g \, mL^{-1}$, the infusion rate of procainamide HCl required to attain procainamide plasma concentration of $8\,\mu g\,mL^{-1}$ should also be 1.333 times the concentration required to attain a procainamide plasma concentration of $6\,\mu g\,mL^{-1}$ (linear kinetics), that is 3.186 $mg\,kg^{-1}\,h^{-1} \times 1.333 = 4.247\,mg\,kg^{-1}h^{-1}$.

6. By definition, the 'practical' steady-state concentration represents 95% of the true state plasma concentration: $8\,\mu g\,mL^{-1} \times 0.95 = 7.6$ $\mu g\,mL^{-1}$.Please note that this concentration is 1.333 times the corresponding plasma concentration for the infusion rate of $3.186\,mg$ $kg^{-1}\,h^{-1}$ of procainamide HCl.

7. The time required to attain the 'practical' steady-state concentration is always $4.32 \times t_{1/2}$ of the drug, regardless of the chosen infusion rate. Therefore, time required to attain the 'practical' steady-state condition is $4.32 \times 3\,h = 12.96\,h$, or $13\,h$.

8. The rate of elimination at true steady-state condition is always equal to the rate of infusion. Therefore, the rate of elimination $(KX) = X_{ss} \times K = Q$.

$X_{ss} = (C_p)_{ss} \times V$
$X_{ss} = 8\,\mu g\,mL^{-1} \times 200\,000\,mL$
$X_{ss} = 1\,600\,000\,\mu g$
rate of elimination $= 1\,600\,000\,\mu g$
  $\times 0.231\,h^{-1} = 369\,600\,\mu g\,h^{-1}$
  $(369.6\,mg\,h^{-1})$.
$Q = 3696\,\mu g\,kg^{-1}\,h^{-1}\,(3.696\,mg\,kg^{-1}\,h^{-1})$
of procainamide.

For the patient of 100 kg weight,

$Q = 3.696\,mg\,kg^{-1}\,h^{-1} \times 100\,kg$
$= 369.6\,mg\,h^{-1}$.

Please note that the this rate of elimination is 1.33 times the one for steady-state concentration of $6\,\mu g\,mL^{-1}$.

9. Figure P4.1 gives the profile (rectilinear paper) of rate of elimination at steady state against the infusion rate.

10. Figure P4.2 shows the profile of 'practical' and true steady-state plasma concentrations against the infusion rate.

11. Calculations of loading dose

$D_L = (C_p)_{ss}V$

$D_L = 6\,mg\,L^{-1} \times 2\,L\,kg^{-1} = 12\,mg\,kg^{-1}$ procainamide, which is equivalent to $12/0.87 = 13.79\,mg\,kg^{-1}$ procainamide HCl.

$D_L = \dfrac{Q}{K}$

$D_L = \dfrac{0.594\,mg\,\text{procainamide}\,kg^{-1}\,h^{-1}}{0.0495h^{-1}}$

$D_L = 12\,mg\,kg^{-1}$ of procainamide
$D_L = 13.79\,mg\,kg^{-1}$ procainamide HCl

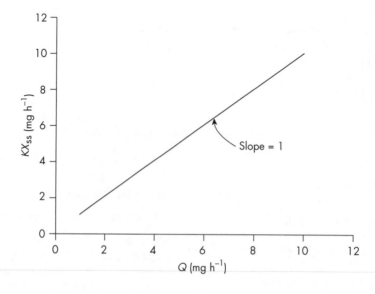

Figure P4.1

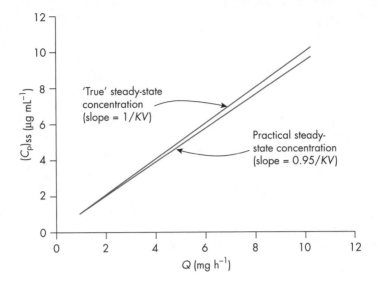

Figure P4.2

It can be seen that loading dose of procainamide HCL required to attain an identical procainamide plasma concentration is the same in both normal and renally impaired subjects.

Infusion rate:

$$(C_p)_{ss} = \frac{Q}{VK}$$

$$Q = (C_p)_{ss} \times VK$$
$$Q = 6 \, \text{mg L}^{-1} \times 2 \, \text{L kg}^{-1} \times 0.0495 \, \text{h}^{-1}$$
$$= 0.594 \, \text{mg kg}^{-1} \, \text{h}^{-1} \text{ of procainamide.}$$

This is provided by 0.682 mg kg^{-1} h^{-1} of procainamide HCl. If this infusion rate in a renally impaired subject (0.682 mg kg^{-1} h^{-1}) is compared with that in a normal subject (3.186 mg kg^{-1}h^{-1}; given in question 1 above) to attain the identical procainamide plasma concentration(6 mg L^{-1}), it can be seen that the infusion rate is reduced in the renally impaired subject.

12. Figure P4.3 gives the profile of infusion rate necessary to attain a true steady-state plasma concentration against the systemic clearance which is inversely related to the degree of renal impairment.

13. Figure P4.4 gives the profile of loading dose necessary to attain a true steady-state plasma concentration instantaneously against the systemic clearance or against the degree of renal impairment (assuming that apparent volume of drug distribution remains unaffected).

14. In cardiac failure and shock, the apparent volume of distribution of procainamide may decrease to as low as 1.5 L kg^{-1}.

    Loading dose:

$$D_L = (C_p)_{ss} V$$

$$(C_p)_{ss} = \frac{Q}{VK}$$

$$D_L = 6 \, \mu\text{g mL}^{-1} \times 1500 \, \text{mL kg}^{-1}$$

$$D_L = 9000 \, \mu\text{g kg}^{-1} \, (9.00 \, \text{mg kg}^{-1})$$
$$\text{of procainamide.}$$

This is provided by 10.344 mg kg^{-1} of procainamide HCl.

$$D_L = \frac{Q}{K}$$

$$D_L = \frac{512 \, \mu\text{g kg}^{-1} \, \text{h}^{-1} \text{ procainamide HCl}}{0.0495 \text{h}^{-1}}$$

$$D_L = 10344.80 \, \mu\text{g kg}^{-1} \, (10.344 \, \text{mg kg}^{-1})$$
$$\text{of procainamide HCl.}$$

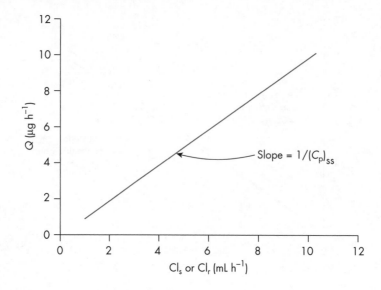

Figure P4.3

Infusion rate:

$$(C_p)_{ss} = \frac{Q}{VK}$$

$Cl_s = VK = 1500\ \text{mL kg}^{-1} \times 0.0495\ \text{h}^{-1}$
$Cl_s = 74.25\ \text{mL kg}^{-1}\,\text{h}^{-1}$
$Q = (C_p)_{ss} \times VK$
$Q = 6\ \mu\text{g mL}^{-1} \times 74.25\ \text{mL kg}^{-1}\,\text{h}^{-1}$
$\quad = 445.5\ \mu\text{g kg}^{-1}\,\text{h}^{-1}$ of procainamide.

This is provided by $512.068\ \mu\text{g kg}^{-1}\text{h}^{-1}$ of procainamide HCl.

Since the apparent volume of distribution and the elimination half life of the drug were affected in this subject, it will be necessary to adjust the infusion rate as well as the loading dose (D_L) of the drug.

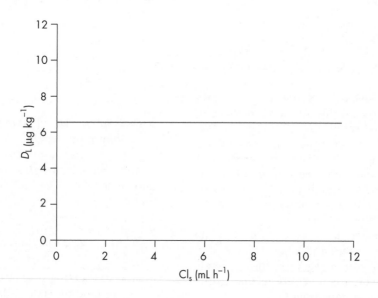

Figure P4.4

15. $D_L = (C_p)_{ss} V$

or

$$D_L = \frac{Q}{K}$$

In order to use these two equations, either the apparent volume of distribution or the elimination rate constant must be known.

$$\frac{Q}{(C_p)_{ss}} = VK = \text{systemic clearance}$$

and

$$N = \frac{\ln(1 - f_{ss})}{-0.693} = t/t_{1/2}$$

This, therefore, requires determination of f_{ss}:

$$f_{ss} = \frac{(C_p)_t}{(C_p)_{ss}} = \frac{2.74 \text{ mg L}^{-1}}{4 \text{ mg L}^{-1}} = 0.685$$

$$N = \frac{\ln(1 - f_{ss})}{-0.693} = \frac{\ln(1 - 0.685)}{-0.693} = \frac{-1.1551}{-0.693}$$

$N = 1.666$, which means that 5 h represents $1.666 \times t_{1/2}$ of the drug.

$N = t/t_{1/2}$; rearrangement yields $t_{1/2} = t/N$. $t_{1/2} = 5 \text{ h}/1.666 = 2.999 \text{ h}$

$$K = \frac{0.693}{2.999} = 0.231 \text{ h}^{-1}$$

Since kinetics are linear,

$$Q = \left(\frac{7}{4}\right)(2.1241 \text{ mg kg}^{-1}\text{h}^{-1})$$
$$= 3.7171 \text{ mg kg}^{-1}\text{h}^{-1}$$

$$D_L = \frac{Q}{K} = \frac{3.7171 \text{ mg kg}^{-1}\text{h}^{-1}}{0.231\text{h}^{-1}}$$
$$= 16.091 \text{mg kg}^{-1}$$

16. The first infusion rate allows the desired plasma concentration to be obtained at the elimination half life ($t_{1/2}$) of the drug, while the second infusion rate permits this concentration to be maintained. When an infusion is run for one drug half life, the plasma concentration (C_p) is always equal to $0.5f_{ss}$. Therefore, the concentration of $8 \mu\text{g mL}^{-1}$ occurring at the time $= 4$ h (at one half life of a drug) represents one half of the concentration that would occur if infusion Q_1 were continued indefinitely. (This, in fact, should not be done because the plasma procainamide concentration would reach a toxic level.). If the high-rate infusion Q_1 were allowed to be continued indefinitely, $(C_p)_{ss}$ would become:

$$(C_p)_{ss} = \frac{C_p}{f_{ss}} = \frac{8 \mu\text{g mL}^{-1}}{0.5}$$

$(C_p)_{ss} = 16 \mu\text{g mL}^{-1}$. This is a toxic concentration and, therefore, is *not* a target concentrations. This is why Q_1 is run only for a time equal to one drug half life before it is converted to the low-rate infusion Q_2.

$$Q_1 = (C_p)_{ss} \times VK$$
$$Q_1 = 16 \mu\text{g mL}^{-1} \times 2000 \text{ mL kg}^{-1}$$
$$\times 0.17325 \text{ h}^{-1} = 5544 \mu\text{g kg}^{-1}\text{h}^{-1}$$
of procainamide.

This is provided by

$$= \frac{5544 \mu\text{g kg}^{-1}\text{h}^{-1}}{0.87} = 6372.413 \mu\text{g kg}^{-1}\text{h}^{-1}$$
of procainamide HCl.

The second infusion rate $(Q_2) = {}^1/_2 \times (Q_1) = 3186.20 \mu\text{g kg}^{-1}\text{h}^{-1}$ of procainamide HCl.

In this example, Q_1 can be initiated at $6.372 \text{ mg kg}^{-1}\text{h}^{-1}$ and continued for 4 h (one half life of the drug). At 4 h, the infusion is changed over to Q_2 of $3.186 \text{ mg kg}^{-1}\text{h}^{-1}$.

17. Failure to change over to the second infusion rate will result in a procainamide plasma concentration of $16 \mu\text{g mL}^{-1}$ at true steady state. The therapeutic range for this drug is 4–$8 \mu\text{g mL}^{-1}$.

11

Multiple dosing: intravenous bolus administration

Objectives

Upon completion of this chapter, you will have the ability to:

- use the Dost ratio to transform a single dose equation into a multiple dose equation
- calculate plasma drug concentration at any time t following the nth intravenous bolus dose of a drug
- calculate peak, trough and average steady-state plasma drug concentrations
- explain the role of dose (X_0) and dosing interval (τ) in the determination of average steady-state drug concentration
- design a dosage regimen that will yield the target average steady-state plasma concentration in a particular patient
- explain and calculate the accumulation ratio (R)
- explain and calculate drug concentration fluctuation at steady state (Φ)
- calculate the number of doses, n, required to reach a given fraction of steady-state (f_{ss})
- calculate the number of elimination half lives (N) required to reach a given fraction of steady state
- calculate loading and maintenance intravenous bolus doses.

11.1 Introduction

Some drugs, such as analgesics, hypnotics and antiemetics, may be used effectively when administered as a single dose. More frequently, however, drugs are administered on a continual basis. In addition, most drugs are administered with sufficient frequency that measurable and, often, pharmacologically significant concentrations of drug remain in the body when a subsequent dose is administered.

For drugs administered in a fixed dose and at a constant dosing interval (e.g. 250 mg every 6 h), the peak plasma concentration following the second and succeeding doses of a drug is higher than the peak concentration following the administration of the first dose. This results in an accumulation of drug in the body relative to the first dose. Additionally, at steady state, the plasma concentration of drug during a dosing interval at any given time since the dose was administered will be identical.

When a drug is administered on a continual basis, the rate and extent of accumulation is a function of the relative magnitudes of the dosing interval and the half life of the drug.

A single intravenous bolus dose (one compartment)

Figure 11.1 illustrates a typical plasma concentration versus time profile following the administration of a single intravenous bolus dose of a drug that follows first-order elimination and one-compartment distribution.

Two equations, introduced in earlier chapters, describe the data points over time after an intravenous bolus dose:

$$X = X_0 e^{-Kt} \tag{11.1}$$

and

$$C_p = (C_p)_0 e^{-Kt} \tag{11.2}$$

At $t=0$, $X=X_0$ and $C_p=(C_p)_0$ (i.e. highest or maximum or peak plasma concentration, or intercept of the concentration versus time plot) and, at $t=\infty$, $X=0$ and $C_p=0$.

Multiple dosing concepts

Under the condition illustrated in Fig. 11.2, plasma concentration of a drug at a given time will be identical following the administration of the first, second, third and all subsequent doses as long as the administered dose (X_0) remains unchanged and the time between subsequent doses is very long (greater than seven or eight elimination half lives). This is because there is essentially no drug accumulation in the body; in other words, there is no drug left in the body from previous doses.

In reality, however, most therapeutic agents (antihypertensive agents, antianxiety medications, antiepileptics and many more) are administered at finite time intervals. For drugs administered in a fixed dose and at a constant dosing interval (e.g. 250 mg every 6 h), the peak plasma level (highest plasma concentration), following the administration of second and each succeeding dose of a drug, is higher than the peak concentration following the administration of the first dose (Fig. 11.3). This phenomenon is the consequence of drug accumulation in the body relative to the first dose. Additionally, at steady state, the plasma concentration of drug at any given point in time during the dosing interval will be identical.

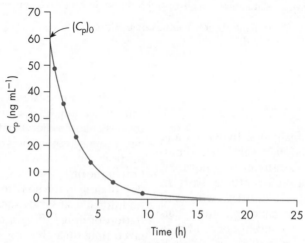

Figure 11.1   A typical plasma concentration (C_p) versus time profile for a single intravenous bolus dose of a drug that follows first-order elimination and has one compartment distribution. (C_p)$_0$: the initial and highest plasma concentration attained (the y-axis intercept of the concentration versus time plot).

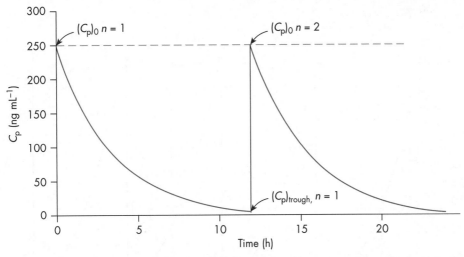

Figure 11.2   Plasma concentration (C_p) versus time profile following the administration of dose of a drug as an intravenous bolus ($n = 1$). Please note that the second identical dose ($n = 2$) was administered after a long interval. (It is assumed that the interval is > 10 half lives of drug and, therefore, there is an insignificant amount of drug left in the blood from the first dose.)

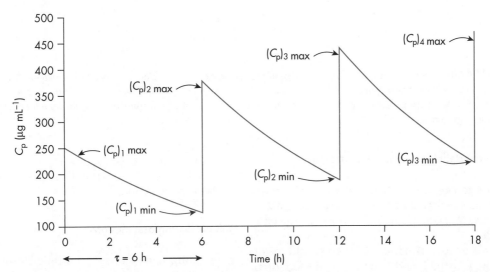

Figure 11.3   Plasma concentration (C_p) versus time profile following the administration by intravenous bolus of identical doses of a drug (1–4) at identical dosing intervals (τ). Please note that peak plasma concentration or, for that matter, the plasma concentration at any given time for the second, the third and subsequent doses are higher than for the first dose (because of drug accumulation). min, minimum; max, maximum.

Following the administration of a number of doses (theoretically an infinite number of doses, and practically greater than seven or eight doses) of a suitable but identical size and at a suitable but identical dosing interval, the condition is reached where the administration of a chosen dose (X_0) and dosing interval (τ) will provide, at steady state, all concentrations within the therapeutic range of a drug (Fig. 11.4)

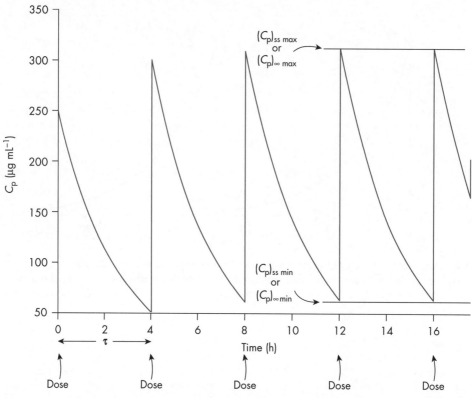

Figure 11.4   Plasma concentration (C_p) versus time profile following the administration of an identical intravenous bolus dose of a drug at an identical dosing interval (τ). Please note that the steady-state (ss) peak plasma concentrations are identical. Similarly, the steady-state plasma concentrations at any given time after the administration of a dose are identical. min, minimum; max, maximum.

Important definitions in multiple dosing

Dosage regimen.   The systematized dosage schedule for a drug therapy, or the optimized dose (X_0) and dosing interval (τ) for a specific drug.

Drug accumulation (R).   The build up of drug in the blood/body through sequential dosing.

Steady-state condition.   Steady state is achieved at a time when, under a given dosage regimen, the mass (amount) of drug administered (for intravenous) or absorbed (for extravascular route), is equal to the mass (amount) of drug eliminated over a dosing interval.

Loading dose (D_L).   A single intravenous bolus dose administered in order to reach steady-state condition instantly.

Maintenance dose (D_m).   The dose administered every dosing interval to maintain the steady-state condition.

Multiple dosing assumptions

In obtaining expressions for multiple dosing, the following theoretical assumptions or suppositions are made, though they may not always be valid.

1. Linear pharmacokinetics applies; that is, the rate process obeys passive diffusion and first-order elimination kinetics (please review first-order process).
2. Tissues can take up an infinite amount of drug, if necessary.
3. The apparent volume of distribution (V), elimination half life ($t_{1/2}$) and the elimination rate

constant (K) are independent of the number of administered doses.
4. The time interval (τ [tau]) between dosing or successive doses is constant.
5. The administered dose (X_0) is equal at each successive time interval.

It should be noted that, in practice, some of the assumptions may not be valid for some drugs (e.g. salicylate, ethanol, phenytoin), for which capacity-limited kinetics (i.e. non-linear kinetics) may apply.

Before proceeding further on this important topic and for the purpose of simplifying complex-looking equations into more manageable and practical equations, we will reiterate the significance of the term e^{-Kt}, which has been so ubiquitous in this text. Please note that when $t=0$, $e^{-Kt}=1$ and when $t=\infty$, $e^{-Kt}=0$. Furthermore, it is of paramount importance to recognize that the size of the dose administered, dosing interval and the concept of measuring dosing interval in terms of the number of elimination half lives (N) of a drug play a pivotal role in assessing, computing, evaluating and examining numerous parameters that are salient features accompanying multiple-dosing pharmacokinetics.

It is also worth mentioning here that the pharmacokinetic parameters obtained following the administration of a single dose of a drug, intra- or extravascularly, may prove to be helpful while tackling some equations in multiple-dosing pharmacokinetics. This includes the intercepts of the plasma concentration versus time data, the systemic clearance and the absolute bioavailability of a drug, when applicable.

11.2 Useful pharmacokinetic parameters in multiple dosing

The following parameters are of importance.

1. The Dost ratio (r).
2. The (amount and) concentration of drug in the body at any time t during the dosing interval following administration of the nth (i.e. first dose, second dose, third dose, fourth dose, etc.) dose of a drug as an intravenous bolus or by an extravascular route.

3. The maximum and minimum (amount and) concentration

$$[(C_{p_n})_{\max} \text{ and } (C_{p_n})_{\min}]$$

of a drug in the body, following the administration of dose of a drug as an intravenous bolus or by an extravascular route.
4. The steady-state plasma concentrations [$(C_p)_\infty$]: attained only after administration of many doses (generally more than seven or eight).
5. The maximum and minimum plasma concentrations at steady state [$(C_p)_{\infty\max}$ and $(C_p)_{\infty\min}$] following administration of a drug as an intravenous bolus or by an extravascular route.
6. The "average" steady-state plasma concentration, $(\bar{C}_p)_{ss}$, for an intravenous bolus dose and for an extravascular dose.
7. Drug accumulation (R), determined by different methods, for an intravenous bolus and extravascular route.
8. Fluctuation (Φ), determined following the administration of drug as an intravenous bolus.
9. Number of doses (n) required to attain a given fraction of steady state (f_{ss}), following the administration of drug as an intravenous bolus or by an extravascular route.
10. Calculation of loading (D_L) and maintenance dose (D_m) for both intravenous bolus and extravascular routes.

The Dost ratio (r)

The Dost ratio permits the determination of the amount and/or the plasma concentration of a drug in the body at any time t (range, $t=0$ to $t=\tau$) following the administration of the nth (i.e. second dose, third dose, fourth dose, etc.) dose by intravascular and/or extravascular routes. In other words, this ratio will transform a single dose equation into a multiple-dosing equation.

$$r = \frac{1 - e^{-nK\tau}}{1 - e^{-K\tau}} \tag{11.3}$$

where r is the Dost ratio (named after a German scientist who developed this equation); n is the number of administered doses (range from 1 to ∞); K is the the first-order elimination rate constant; and τ is the the dosing interval (i.e. 4 h, 6 h, 8 h, etc.).

Use of the dost ratio for intravenous bolus administration (one compartment)

Inserting the Dost ratio (i.e. Eq. 11.3) between the terms X_0 and e^{-Kt} of Eq. 11.1 ($X = X_0 e^{-Kt}$) or between $(C_p)_0$ and e^{-Kt} of Eq. 11.2 ($C_p = (C_p)_0 e^{-Kt}$) yields equations that permit the determination of the amount and/or plasma concentration of a drug in the body at any time, t, following administration of the nth dose.

$$(X_n)_t = \frac{X_0(1 - e^{-nK\tau})}{(1 - e^{-K\tau})} e^{-Kt} \qquad (11.4)$$

Since $X/V = C_p$ and dose$/V = (C_p)_0$, following substitution for $(X_n)_t$ with the concentration term $(C_p)_n$ and X_0 with $(C_p)_0$, Eq. 11.4 becomes:

$$(C_{p_n})_t = \frac{(C_p)_0(1 - e^{-nK\tau})}{(1 - e^{-K\tau})} e^{-Kt} \qquad (11.5)$$

In Eqs 11.4 and 11.5, X_0 is the the administered dose; $(C_p)_0$ is the the initial plasma concentration (dose$/V$); n is the nth dose; K is the the elimination rate constant; τ is the the dosing interval; and t is the time since the nth dose was administered.

The following important comments will help in understanding the underlying assumptions and the practical uses of Eqs 11.4 and 11.5.

1. There are two terms in Eqs 11.4 and 11.5 that will simplify these two equations into more practical equations: $e^{-nK\tau}$ and e^{-Kt}.
2. When $n = 1$ (i.e. administration of the first dose), Eqs 11.4 and 11.5 will simplify or collapse into equations for a single dose (i.e. $X = X_0 e^{-Kt}$ [Eq. 11.1] or $C_p = (C_p)_0 e^{-Kt}$ [Eq. 11.2]).
3. When $n = \infty$ (i.e. administration of many doses; generally more than eight or nine), the term $1 - e^{-nK\tau}$ of Eqs 11.4 and 11.5 approaches a value of 1 and, therefore "vanishes" from these equations.

4. It is important to note that, in multiple-dosing kinetics, $t \geq 0$ and $t \leq \tau$ (a value between dosing interval) following the administration of the dose.

For example, if a dose is administered every 8 h, time values will be between 0 and 8 h; $t = 0$ represents the time at which the dose is administered and $t = 8$ h represent τ. For the second and subsequent doses, therefore, we start again from time 0 to 8 h. Therefore, t in multiple dose pharmacokinetics is the time since the latest (nth) dose was given.

Equations 11.4 and 11.5 permit us to determine the amount and the concentration of drug, respectively, at a time (from 0 to τ) following administration of the nth dose (first, second, third dose, fourth, etc.).

We know from general mathematical principles and previous discussions that at $t = 0$, $e^{-Kt} = 1$, and the plasma concentration (C_p) at this time is the highest plasma concentration or maximum plasma concentration $(C_p)_{max}$. Therefore, Eqs 11.4 and 11.5 reduce to:

$$(X_n)_{max} = \frac{X_0(1 - e^{-nK\tau})}{(1 - e^{-K\tau})} \qquad (11.6)$$

$$(C_{p_n})_{max} = \frac{(C_p)_0(1 - e^{-nK\tau})}{(1 - e^{-K\tau})} \qquad (11.7)$$

In Eq. 11.6, the term $(X_n)_{max}$ represents the maximum amount of drug in the body following administration of the nth dose (or an intravenous bolus, this will always occur at $t = 0$).

In Eq. 11.7, the term $(C_{p_n})_{max}$ represents the maximum plasma concentration of a drug in the body following the administration of the nth dose. (Again, for an intravenous bolus this will always occur at $t = 0$.)

When time is equal to τ (i.e. $t = \tau$), the body will display the minimum amount,

$$(X_n)_{min},$$

and/or the minimum plasma concentration,

$$(C_{p_n})_{min},$$

of a drug. Therefore, Eqs 11.4 and 11.5 reduce to:

$$(X_n)_{min} = \frac{X_0(1 - e^{-nK\tau})}{(1 - e^{-K\tau})} e^{-K\tau} \qquad (11.8)$$

$$(C_{p_n})_{min} = \frac{(C_p)_0(1 - e^{-nK\tau})}{1 - e^{-K\tau}} e^{-k\tau} \qquad (11.9)$$

In Eq. 11.8, the term $(X_n)_{min}$ represents the minimum amount of a drug in the body following administration of the nth dose. (This will always occur at $t = \tau$, regardless of the route of administration.)

In Eq. 11.9, the term $(C_{p_n})_{min}$ represents the minimum plasma concentration of a drug in the body following administration of the nth dose (it will also always occur at time, $t = \tau$). Please note that this concentration is referred to, in clinical literature, as the "trough" plasma concentration. Please note that the only difference between Eqs 11.6 and 11.8 (for expressing the amount) and Eqs 11.7 and 11.9 (for expressing the concentration) is the term $e^{-K\tau}$. This simply reflects the time of occurrence of the maximum and minimum amount (or concentration) of drug in the body as illustrated in Fig. 11.5.

Steady-state plasma concentration

The steady-state condition is attained following the administration of many doses (when n is a high number) of a drug (i.e. $n \approx \infty$). When n approaches infinity, the value for the term $e^{-nK\tau}$ approaches 0; and therefore $1 - e^{-nK\tau} \approx 1.0$ in Eqs 11.4 and 11.5 and X_n and C_{p_n} become equal to X_∞ and $(C_p)_\infty$, respectively.

$$(X_\infty)_t = \frac{X_0}{(1 - e^{-K\tau})} e^{-Kt} \qquad (11.10)$$

In Eq. 11.10, the term $(X_\infty)_t$ represents the amount of drug in the body at any time t (i.e. between $t > 0$ and $t < \tau$) following the attainment of steady state. This will occur only after the administration of many doses.

$$(C_{p_\infty})_t = \frac{(C_p)_0}{(1 - e^{-K\tau})} e^{-Kt} \qquad (11.11)$$

In Eq. 11.11, the term $(C_{p_\infty})_t$ represents the plasma concentration of drug in the body at any time t (i.e. between $t > 0$ and $t < \tau$) following the

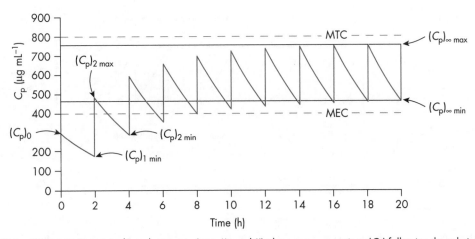

Figure 11.5 Maximum (max; peak) and minimum (min; "trough") plasma concentrations (C_p) following the administration of an identical intravenous bolus dose of a drug at an identical dosing interval. MTC, minimum toxic concentration; MEC, minimum effective concentration.

attainment of steady state. This will occur following the administration of many doses.

At this time, you are urged to consider the similarity between equations for a single intravenous bolus dose (Ch. 3) and multiple doses of intravenous bolus. You may notice an introduction of the term $1 - e^{-nK\tau}$ in the denominator. Otherwise, everything else should appear to be identical.

Equation 11.11 permits the determination of plasma concentration at any time ($t = 0$ to $t = \tau$), following the attainment of steady state. Please note that $(C_p)_0$ is the initial plasma concentration (dose/V) that can be obtained following the administration of a single dose. Therefore, if we know the dosing interval and the elimination half life of a drug, we can predict the steady-state plasma concentration at any time t (between 0 and τ) (Fig. 11.6).

The maximum and minimum plasma concentrations at steady state

For drugs administered intravenously, the maximum and minimum steady-state plasma concentrations will occur at $t = 0$ and $t = \tau$, respectively, following the administration of many doses (i.e. n is large). Equation 11.11 may be used to determine the steady-state maximum and minimum plasma concentrations as follows:

$$(C_{p_\infty})_{max} \quad \text{or} \quad (C_{p_{ss}})_{max} = \frac{(C_p)_0}{(1 - e^{-K\tau})}$$

$$(11.12)$$

In Eq. 11.12, the term $(C_{p_\infty})_{max}$ or $(C_{p_{ss}})_{max}$ represents the maximum plasma concentration of a drug in the body at the steady-state condition (i.e. following the administration of many doses). This maximum will occur only at $t = 0$ (immediately after administration of the latest bolus dose) since $e^{-Kt} = 1$, when $t = 0$).

$$(C_{p_\infty})_{min} \quad \text{or} \quad (C_{p_{ss}})_{min} = \frac{(C_p)_0}{(1 - e^{-K\tau})} e^{-K\tau}$$

$$(11.13)$$

In Eq. 11.13, the term $(C_{p_\infty})_{min}$ or $(C_{p_{ss}})_{min}$ represents the minimum or trough plasma concentration of a drug at steady-state condition (i.e. following the administration of many doses and when time since the latest dose, t, is equal to τ). Since Eq. 11.12,

$$\frac{(C_p)_0}{(1 - e^{-K\tau})} = (C_{p_\infty})_{max}$$

substituting from Eq. 11.12 for the term $(C_{p_\infty})_{max}$ or $(C_{p_{ss}})_{max}$ in Eq. 11.13 yields the following equation:

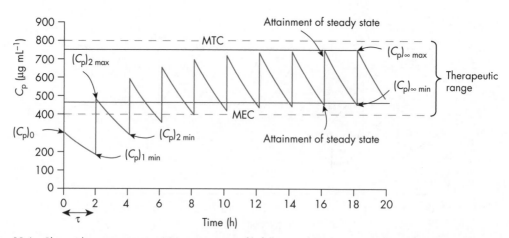

Figure 11.6 Plasma drug concentration (C_p) versus time profile following the intravenous bolus administration of many equal doses at an identical dosing interval (τ). In this representation, the dosing regimen has been designed so that the plasma drug concentrations will fall within the therapeutic range at steady state.

$$(C_{p_\infty})_{\min} \quad \text{or} \quad (C_{p_{ss}})_{\min} = (C_{p_\infty})_{\max} e^{-K\tau}$$

$$(11.14)$$

Please note the importance of Eqs 11.12, 11.13 and 11.14 in multiple-dosing pharmacokinetics following the administration of drug as an intravenous bolus dose.

Equation 11.12 permits determination of maximum plasma concentration at steady state. A careful examination of Eq. 11.12 clearly suggests that peak steady-state concentration for a drug is influenced by the initial plasma concentration, the elimination rate constant and, more importantly, the dosing interval. And, since the administered dose is identical and the elimination rate constant is a constant for a given patient receiving a particular drug, the maximum plasma concentration at steady state is influenced only by the dosing interval. Therefore, more frequent administration (i.e. a smaller τ value) of an identical dose of a drug will yield a higher maximum plasma concentration at steady state. Conversely, less frequent administration (i.e. greater τ value) of an identical dose of a drug will yield a smaller maximum plasma concentration at steady state.

Equations 11.13 and 11.14 permit determination of the minimum or trough plasma concentration at steady state. A careful examination of the equation clearly suggests that the minimum or trough plasma concentration for a drug is influenced by the initial plasma concentration, the elimination rate constant and, more importantly, the dosing interval. Since the administered dose is identical and the elimination rate constant is a constant, the minimum plasma concentration at steady state is influenced only by the dosing interval.

Administration of an identical dose of a drug more frequently (i.e. a smaller τ value) will yield a higher minimum plasma concentration at steady state. Conversely, administration of the same dose of a drug less frequently (i.e. a greater τ value) will yield a smaller minimum plasma concentration at steady state.

If the dosing interval is very long (greater than seven or eight half lives of a drug, or infinity), what will be the maximum and minimum plasma concentrations at time infinity following the administration of an identical dose intravenously?

Please consider the following profiles:

1. Maximum or peak plasma concentration at steady state against the number of administered doses.
2. Minimum or trough plasma concentration at steady state against the number of administered doses.
3. Maximum or peak plasma concentration against the number of administered doses.
4. Minimum or trough plasma concentration against the number of administered doses.
5. Maximum or peak plasma concentration at steady state against the dosing interval.
6. Minimum or trough plasma concentration at steady state against the dosing interval.

Figure 11.7 shows the plasma concentration versus time profile following attainment of steady state for a drug administered by multiple intravenous bolus injections.

The "average" plasma concentration at steady state

A parameter that is very useful in multiple dosing is the "average" plasma concentration at steady state, $(\overline{C}_p)_{ss}$. Please note that the term average is in the quotation marks to signify that it does not carry the usual meaning (i.e. arithmetic mean). Although not an arithmetic average, this plasma concentration value will fall between the maximum and minimum steady-state plasma concentration values. This "average" concentration is the one desired therapeutically for patients on a regular dosage regimen. The parameter can be defined as:

$$(\overline{C}_p)_{ss} = \frac{\int_0^\tau C_{p_\infty} dt}{\tau}$$

$$(11.15)$$

where $\int_0^\tau C_{p_\infty} dt$ is the area under the plasma concentration time curve at steady state during dosing interval (τ). (i.e. between $t=0$ and $t=\tau$).

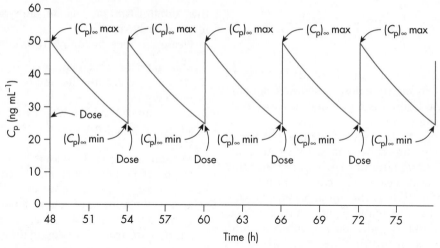

Figure 11.7 Plasma concentration (C_p) versus time profile following the attainment of steady-state condition for a drug administered by multiple intravenous bolus injections.

It may be shown that integration of Eq. 11.11, following substitution for $(C_p)_0$ with X_0/V, from $t=0$ to $t=\tau$ yields:

$$\frac{\int_0^\tau C_{p_\infty} dt}{\tau} = \frac{X_0}{VK} \qquad (11.16)$$

Substitution of X_0/VK from Eq. 11.16 for the term $\int_0^\tau C_{p_\infty} dt$ in Eq. 11.15 yields:

$$(\overline{C}_p)_{ss} = \frac{X_0}{VK\tau} \qquad (11.17)$$

where X_0 is the the administered dose; V is the the apparent volume of distribution; K is the the elimination rate constant; and τ is the the dosing interval.

Equation 11.17 indicates that knowing the apparent volume of distribution and the elimination rate constant of a drug, or the systemic clearance of a drug (all parameters obtained from a single intravenous bolus dose of a drug), the "average" plasma concentration of a drug at steady state following the intravenous administration of a fixed dose (X_0) at a constant dosing interval can be predicted. Furthermore, it should also be clear from Eq. 11.17 that only the size of the dose and the dosing interval need to be

adjusted to obtain a desired "average" steady-state plasma concentration, since apparent volume of distribution, the elimination rate constant and systemic clearance are constant for a particular drug administered to an individual subject.

It should be noted that the "average" plasma concentration, obtained by employing Eqs 11.15 or 11.17, is neither the arithmetic nor the geometric mean of maximum and minimum plasma concentrations at infinity. Rather, it is the plasma concentration at steady state, which, when multiplied by the dosing interval, is equal to the area under the plasma concentration–time curve $(AUC)_0^\tau$ (i.e. from $t=0$ to $t=\tau$).

$$(\overline{C}_p)_{ss}\tau = \int_0^\tau C_{p_\infty} dt \qquad (11.18)$$

Therefore, from geometric considerations, "average" concentration must represent some plasma concentration value between the maximum and the minimum plasma concentrations at infinity.

The proximity between the values of the "average" steady-state concentration and the arithmetic mean of the maximum and the minimum plasma concentrations at infinity is solely influenced by the chosen dosing interval. The smaller the dosing interval (i.e. more frequent administration of a dose), the greater will be the proximity between the "average" steady-state concentration and the arithmetic mean of the maximum and the minimum plasma concentrations at infinity.

From Ch. 4, we know that:

$$\int_0^{\infty} C_p dt = (AUC)_0^{\infty} \qquad (11.19)$$

and

$$(AUC)_0^{\infty} = \frac{Dose}{Cl_s} = \frac{Dose}{VK} \qquad (11.20)$$

By substitution for $(AUC)_0^{\infty}$ in Eq. 11.19, we obtain:

$$\int_0^{\infty} C_p dt = \frac{X_0}{VK} \qquad (11.21)$$

Equation 11.21 and Eq. 11.16 both equal X_0/VK. Therefore, Eq. 11.21 for $(AUC)_0^{\infty}$ (following the administration of a single intravenous bolus dose) is equivalent to Eq. 11.16, an equation for $(AUC)_0^{\tau}$ during dosing interval at steady state. Therefore, $(AUC)_0^{\tau}$ at steady state is equivalent

to the total area under the curve following a single dose (Fig. 11.8 and 11.9).

This allows us to calculate the "average"-plasma concentration of a drug at steady state from a single dose study by employing the following equation:

$$(\overline{C}_p)_{ss} = \frac{\int_0^{\infty} C_p dt}{\tau} \qquad (11.22)$$

And since $dose/VK = (AUC)_0^{\infty}$ following the administration of a single intravenous bolus dose, substituting for the term $dose/VK$ in Eq. 11.17 with the term $(AUC)_0^{\infty}$ yields the following equation:

$$(\overline{C}_p)_{ss} = \frac{(AUC)_0^{\infty}}{\tau} \qquad (11.23)$$

Please note, Eqs 11.22 and 11.23 do not require the calculation or the knowledge of the apparent volume of distribution, the elimination rate constant or the dose given every dosing interval. These equations, however, do assume that apparent volume of distribution, the elimination rate constant and the dose are constants over the entire dosing period. In Eq. 11.23, please note that the term $(AUC)_0^{\infty}$ is the area under the plasma concentration time curve following the administration of a single dose. Therefore, the dosing

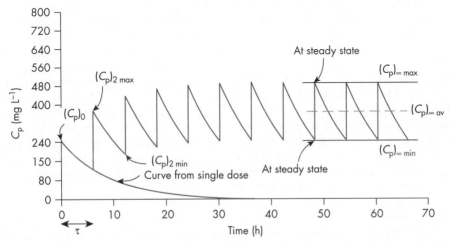

Figure 11.8 Plasma concentration (C_p) versus time profile following the administration of a single dose and multiple doses of a drug as intravenous bolus. min, minimum; max, maximum; av, average.

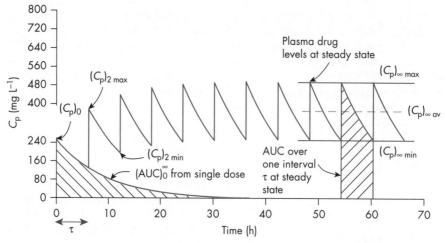

Figure 11.9 Plasma concentration (C_p) versus time profile following the administration of multiple intravenous bolus doses of a drug. min, minimum; max, maximum; av, average; τ, dosing interval.

interval is the only factor that influences the "average" steady-state concentration for a specified dose in a particular individual.

More frequent administration of an identical dose, therefore, will yield a higher "average" steady-state concentration.

Important comments on "average" steady state concentration

Regardless of the route of drug administration, the "average" plasma concentration at steady state is influenced by the dose administered, the fraction of the administered dose that reaches the general circulation (for extravascular routes), the systemic clearance of the drug and the chosen dosing interval.

In a normal subject, systemic clearance of a drug is constant and it is presumed to be independent of the dose administered and the route of administration; therefore, it will not play any role in influencing the "average" steady-state concentration. The "average" steady-state plasma concentration will be influenced by the three remaining parameters: the dose administered, the chosen dosing interval and the absolute bioavailability (F), when applicable.

The "average" plasma concentration is always directly proportional to the dose administered (linear pharmacokinetics). The term dosing interval is in the denominator of Eq. 11.17. Therefore, the larger the dosing interval, the lower will be the "average" steady-state plasma concentration (assuming, of course, the dose remains unchanged). If, however, the ratio of dose over dosing interval is maintained constant, the "average" steady-state concentration will remain unchanged. For example, administration of a 400 mg dose of a drug at every 8 h (i.e. 50 mg h^{-1}) or the administration of 200 mg dose at every 4 h (i.e. 50 mg h^{-1}) will provide identical "average" steady-state plasma concentrations.

When a drug is administered by an extravascular route, it must be remembered that the fraction of the administered dose reaching the general circulation, or absolute bioavailability, plays an influential role (see Ch. 12). In addition, since the absolute bioavailability of a drug is influenced by the route of drug administration, the chosen dosage form and the formulation of a chosen dosage form, administration of the same dose of the same drug is likely to provide different "average" steady-state concentration. This, of course, assumes that the systemic clearance of a drug is not affected by any of these factors and the dosing interval is identical.

In renally impaired subjects, there will be a decrease in the systemic clearance of a drug eliminated by the kidneys; and, therefore, the normal dosage regimen of that drug will provide higher "average" steady-state concentration (Eq. 11.17).

This, therefore, requires adjustment in the dosage regimen. The dosage adjustment, in turn, can be accomplished by three approaches.

1. Administration of a smaller dose at a normal dosing interval.
2. Administration of a normal dose at a longer dosing interval (i.e. decreasing the frequency of drug administration).
3. A combination of both (i.e. administration of a smaller dose less frequently).

Please consider the following profiles.

1. "Average" concentration at steady state against the administered dose.
2. "Average" concentration at steady state against the systemic clearance (for a fixed dosage regimen).
3. "Average" concentration at steady state against the dosing interval.
4. "Average" concentration at steady state against the number of half-lives in a dosing interval.

11.3 Designing or establishing the dosage regimen for a drug

The following approach is recommended for the purpose of designing or establishing the dosage regimen for a drug:

1. Know the therapeutic range and/or the effective concentration range for the drug.
2. Select the desired or targeted "average" steady-state plasma concentration. It is a common practice to choose the mean of the therapeutic range of the drug as a starting desired "average" steady-state plasma concentration. For example, if the therapeutic range is 10–30 $mg\,L^{-1}$, choose 20 $mg\,L^{-1}$ as the targeted "average" steady-state concentration.
3. Use Eq. 11.17 (for an intravenous bolus administration):

$$(\overline{C}_\mathrm{p})_{ss} = \frac{X_0}{VK\tau}$$

Rearrange Eq. 11.17

$$(\overline{C}_\mathrm{p})_{ss} VK = \frac{X_0}{\tau}$$

4. Select the dosing interval (it is a safe and good practice to start with a dosing interval equal to the drug's elimination half life).
5. Using this dosing interval, and rearranging the equation in Step 3, calculate the dose (X_0) needed to attain the desired "average" steady-state concentration.

$$(\overline{C}_\mathrm{p})_{ss} VK\tau = X_0$$

$\mu g\,mL^{-1} \times mL\,h^{-1} \times h = dose$ (μg)   or
$\mu g\,mL^{-1} \times mL\,kg^{-1}h^{-1} \times h = dose$ ($\mu g\,kg^{-1}$).

6. Round off the number for the calculated dose and the chosen dosing interval. For example, a calculated dose of 109.25 mg may be rounded off to the nearest whole number of the commercially available product (i.e. 100 or 125 mg), whichever is more practical. The half life of 4.25 h may be rounded off to 4 h.
7. Using the rounded numbers for the dose and dosing interval, calculate the "average" steady-state concentration, peak steady-state concentration and trough steady-state concentration.
8. Make sure, by performing calculations, that the calculated peak steady-state concentration is below the minimum toxic concentration and calculated trough steady-state concentration is above the minimum effective concentration.
9. If necessary, make small adjustments (fine tuning) in the dose and dosing interval.

While designing the optimum and practical dosage regimen for a drug administered extravascularly, the approach and steps involved are identical; however, it is important to take into consideration the absolute bioavailability of drug, which may vary depending upon the dosage form, route of drug administration and the formulation (see Ch. 12).

11.4 Concept of drug accumulation in the body (R)

As mentioned in the introduction to this chapter, the administration of a drug in a multiple dose regimen will always result in the accumulation of drug in the body. The extent of accumulation (R) of a drug may be quantified in several ways.

Calculation of drug accumulation from the "average" plasma concentration

During any dosing interval, the "average" plasma concentration of a drug may be defined as:

$$(\overline{C}_p)_n = \frac{\int_0^\tau C_{p_n} dt}{\tau}$$

where $\int_0^\tau C_{p_n} dt$ is the area under the plasma concentration time curve during the nth dosing interval.

Integrating Equation 11.5 from $t=0$ to $t=\tau$, following substituting of dose/V for $(C_p)_0$, yields:

$$\int_0^\tau C_{p_n} dt = \frac{X_0}{VK}[1 - e^{-nK\tau}] \tag{11.24}$$

This is the same as:

$$(\overline{C}_p)_n = \frac{X_0}{VK\tau}[1 - e^{-nK\tau}] \tag{11.25}$$

However, Eq. 11.17

$$\frac{X_0}{VK\tau} = (\overline{C}_p)_{ss}$$

Substitution for the term $X_0/VK\tau$ (Eq. 11.17) into Eq. 11.25 gives:

$$(\overline{C}_p)_n = (\overline{C}_p)_{ss}[1 - e^{-nK\tau}] \tag{11.26}$$

Rearrangement of Eq. 11.26 yields:

$$\frac{(\overline{C}_p)_n}{(\overline{C}_p)_{ss}} = [1 - e^{-nK\tau}] \tag{11.27}$$

When $n=1$ (i.e. following the administration of the first dose), Eq. 11.27 becomes

$$\frac{(\overline{C}_p)_1}{(\overline{C}_p)_{ss}} = [1 - e^{-K\tau}] \tag{11.28}$$

The inverse ratio, $(C_p)_{ss}/(C_p)_1$, may be defined as an accumulation factor (R); hence,

$$\frac{(\overline{C}_p)_{ss}}{(\overline{C}_p)_1} = \frac{1}{1 - e^{-K\tau}} \tag{11.29}$$

From the knowledge of the elimination rate constant and/or the elimination half life of a drug and the dosing interval, the extent to which a drug would accumulate in the body following a fixed dosing regimen can be computed by employing Eq. 11.29.

Use of other ratios to calculate drug accumulation

We know that the minimum amount of drug in the body, following the administration of a first intravenous dose, can be obtained by using the equation below:

$$(X_1)_{min} = X_0 e^{-KT} \tag{11.30}$$

In concentration terms (since $X = VC_p$), Eq. 11.30 becomes:

$$(C_{p_1})_{min} = \frac{X_0}{V}e^{-K\tau} = (C_p)_0 e^{-K\tau} \tag{11.31}$$

We also know that $(X_1)_{max} = X_0 = $ dose.

$$(C_{p_1})_{max} = \frac{X_0}{V} = (C_p)_0 \tag{11.32}$$

We also know from Eqs 11.12 and 11.13 that

$$(C_{p_\infty})_{max} = \frac{(C_p)_0}{(1 - e^{-K\tau})}$$

and

$$(C_{p_\infty})_{min} = \frac{(C_p)_0}{(1 - e^{-K\tau})}e^{-K\tau}$$

The ratio of $(C_{p\infty})_{min}$ to $(C_{p1})_{min}$, (i.e. Eq. 11.13 to Eq. 11.31) and $(C_{p\infty})_{max}$ to $(C_{p1})_{max}$, (i.e. Eq. 11.12 to Eq. 11.32) yields an accumulation factor (R):

$$R = \frac{(C_{p\infty})_{min}}{(C_{p_1})_{min}} = \frac{\frac{(C_p)_0}{(1-e^{-K\tau})}e^{-K\tau}}{(C_p)_0 e^{-K\tau}} = \frac{1}{1-e^{-K\tau}}$$

(11.33)

Analogously,

$$R = \frac{(C_{p\infty})_{max}}{(C_{p_1})_{max}} = \frac{\frac{(C_p)_0}{(1-e^{-K\tau})}}{(C_p)_0} = \frac{1}{1-e^{-K\tau}}$$

(11.34)

Thus, a comparison of "average" concentration, minimum concentration and maximum plasma concentrations of a drug following the administration of the first dose and at steady state provides an insight into the extent to which a drug would be expected to accumulate upon multiple-dosing administrations.

Important comments on drug accumulation

As mentioned in the introduction, the administration of a drug on a multiple dose regimen will result in accumulation of drug in the body. The drug accumulation, indeed, is an indelible and salient feature of multiple-dosing pharmacokinetics.

It is important to understand that the numerical value for drug accumulation (i.e. for R), either calculated or reported, simply indicates how high the plasma concentration will be at steady state compared with the first dose of the drug at a comparable time within the dosage regimen.

For example, calculated or reported value of $R=2$ simply suggests that the peak plasma concentration at steady state will be twice the peak plasma concentration for the first dose. Analogously, the minimum plasma concentration at steady state will be two times as high as the minimum plasma concentration for the first dose. An R value of 2 also means that the "average" plasma concentration at steady state will be twice the "average" plasma concentration for the first dose. This is applicable for an intravenous bolus of drug. Therefore, knowledge of the calculated or reported R value permits prediction of the

peak, trough or "average" plasma concentrations at steady state from the knowledge of maximum, minimum or "average" plasma concentration for the first dose. Furthermore, knowledge of the R value may also provide useful information about the chosen dosing interval.

Careful examination of three equations (Eqs 11.29, 11.33 and 11.34) clearly indicates that, regardless of the method employed, drug accumulation solely depends on the dosing interval, since the elimination rate constant is a constant for a drug. Furthermore, Eqs 11.29, 11.33 and 11.34 suggest that the quantification of drug accumulation requires knowledge of the elimination rate constant of a drug and the dosing interval. The dosing interval can be measured in terms of the number of elimination half lives. Please attempt to find answers for the following questions:

- Will the administered dose of a drug affect drug accumulation? How will the profile (rectilinear paper) of drug accumulation against administered dose look?
- What will be the lowest value for drug accumulation? (Hint: if the dosing interval is equal to infinity, what will be value for R? Substitute for the term τ with ∞ in Eqs 11.29, 11.33 and 11.34.)
- What will be the profile (rectilinear paper) of drug accumulation against dosing interval look like?
- What will be the profile (rectilinear paper) of drug accumulation against dosing interval in terms of the number of half lives look like?
- If the subsequent doses are administered at a time equal to one half life of the drug, what will be the accumulation factor? In other words, if the dosing interval is equal to one half life of the drug, what will be the value of the accumulation factor? Will the drug accumulation be higher if the frequency of drug dosing is greater?

Calculation of drug accumulation

If the elimination half life of a drug is 24 h, for example,

$$K = 0.693/24 = 0.028875\,h^{-1} \approx 0.029\,h^{-1}$$

If a dose of this drug is administered every 24 h (i.e. $\tau = 24$ h or one half life of the drug), Eqs. 11.29, 11.33, and 11.34,

$$R = \frac{1}{1 - e^{-K\tau}}$$

$$R = \frac{1}{1 - e^{-(0.029\ \text{h}^{-1})(24\ \text{h})}} = 2.0$$

If, however, a dose is administered more frequently (i.e. every 6 h, or $\tau = 6$ h or in this example, 25% of one half life of a drug), there will be greater accumulation of the drug, Eqs. 11.29, 11.33, and 11.34:

$$R = \frac{1}{1 - e^{-K\tau}}$$

$$R = \frac{1}{1 - e^{-(0.029\ \text{h}^{-1})(6\ \text{h})}} = 6.25$$

Therefore, in this example, if the subsequent doses are administered at a 24 h interval (i.e. dosing interval equals one half life of the drug), the peak steady-state concentration, the trough steady-state concentration and the "average" steady-state concentration will be twice the corresponding plasma concentration for the first dose. Is it accurate to say that if the peak plasma concentration at steady state is twice the peak plasma concentration for the first dose then the dosing interval represents the half life of the drug?

If the subsequent doses are administered more frequently (every 6 h or $\tau = 0.25 t_{1/2}$) the peak steady-state concentration, the trough steady-state concentration and the "average" steady-state concentration will be 6.25 times as high as the corresponding plasma concentration for the first dose. This is simply the consequence of the phenomenon of drug accumulation.

From calculations provided here, it is accurate to state that the failure to follow the dosage regimen (prescribed dose at a prescribed dosing interval) of a drug can result in serious consequences. Therefore, it is important that patients in your pharmacy, and/or a family member, follow the prescribed directions scrupulously, particularly for drugs that manifest a narrow therapeutic range and a long elimination half life. From your pharmacy experience, you may be aware that some patients tend to take selected

Table 11.1 The relationship between drug accumulation (R) and the dosing interval (τ) in terms of number of elimination half life of a drug

No. elimination half lives in a dosing interval	Drug accumulation, or R value
0.25	6.24
0.5	3.41
1.0	2.00
2.0	1.33
3.0	1.14
4.0	1.07
∞	1.00

therapeutic agents (generally controlled substances) more frequently than directed by a prescriber because of a "feel good" philosophy.

Please compare Eqs 11.29, 11.33 and 11.34, with Eqs 10.21 and 10.22 (intravenous infusion chapter) for a remarkable similarity.

By employing any one of the equations (i.e. Eqs 11.29, 11.33, and 11.34) and using dosing interval in terms of number of elimination half lives, one can construct a table (Table 11.1) illustrating the relationship between the dosing interval and drug accumulation.

11.5 Determination of fluctuation (Φ): intravenous bolus administration

Fluctuation (Φ) is simply a measure of the magnitude of variation in, or the differences between, the peak and trough plasma concentrations at steady state or, by some definitions, the peak and "average" plasma concentrations at steady state.

Fluctuation, therefore, is simply a measure of the ratio of the steady-state peak or maximum plasma concentration to the steady-state minimum or trough plasma concentration of a drug or the ratio of the peak or maximum steady-state concentration to the "average" plasma concentration at steady state for the chosen dosage regimen.

The observed or calculated fluctuation for a dosage regimen of a drug also depends solely on the chosen dosing interval and, like drug accumulation, it is also expressed by using the concept of a numerical value.

A high fluctuation value indicates that the ratio of the steady-state peak or maximum concentration to the trough or minimum concentration is large. Conversely, a low fluctuation value suggests that the ratio of these concentrations is small. Ideally, it is preferable to have a smaller ratio (i.e. smaller Φ value) of maximum to minimum concentration at steady state, as illustrated in Fig. 11.10.

Calculation of fluctuation factor

By comparison of maximum concentration with minimum concentration at steady state

Eq. 11.12

$$(C_{p_\infty})_{max} \quad \text{or} \quad (C_{p_{ss}})_{max} = \frac{(C_p)_0}{(1 - e^{-K\tau})}$$

Eq. 11.13

$$(C_{p_\infty})_{min} \quad \text{or} \quad (C_{p_{ss}})_{min} = \frac{(C_p)_0}{(1 - e^{-K\tau})} e^{-K\tau}$$

Divide $(C_{p_{ss}})_{max}$ by $(C_{p_{ss}})_{min}$ (i.e. Eq. 11.12 by Eq. 11.13)

$$\frac{(C_{p_\infty})_{max} \text{ or } (C_{p_{ss}})_{max}}{(C_{p_\infty})_{min} \text{ or } (C_{p_{ss}})_{min}} = \frac{\frac{(C_p)_0}{(1 - e^{-K\tau})}}{\frac{(C_p)_0}{(1 - e^{-K\tau})} e^{-K\tau}} = \frac{1}{e^{-K\tau}}$$

(11.35)

If the dosing interval (τ) in Eq. 11.35 is expressed in terms of number (N) of elimination half lives ($t_{1/2}$), $N = \tau / t_{1/2}$ or $\tau = N t_{1/2}$.

However, $K = 0.693 / t_{1/2}$; therefore, $\tau = 0.693 N / K$.

Substitute for τ and K in Eq. 11.35 gives:

$$\Phi = \frac{(C_{p_{ss}})_{max}}{(C_{p_{ss}})_{min}} = \frac{1}{e^{-\left(\frac{0.693}{t_{1/2}}\right)(N)(t_{1/2})}} = \frac{1}{e^{-(0.693)(N)}}$$

(11.36)

Equation 11.35 indicates that when N is small (i.e. dosing is more frequent), the range of drug concentrations is smaller (i.e. the difference between the maximum and minimum plasma concentrations, at steady state, will be smaller).

Hence, frequent dosing (smaller dose), if practical, is preferred over less-frequent larger doses in order to avoid a toxicity problem at steady state.

Table 11.2 shows that more frequent dosing (i.e. smaller N value) results in smaller ratio of maximum to minimum steady-state plasma concentrations.

Compare the accumulation and fluctuation values when the dosing interval is equal to one half life of the drug. Plot the graph of fluctuation against the dosing interval.

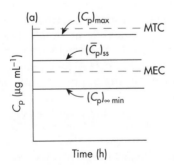

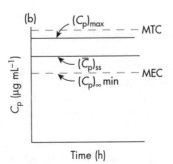

Figure 11.10   Plasma concentration (C_p) versus time plot illustrating high (a) and low (b) fluctuation (Φ) values following the attainment of the steady-state condition. min, minimum; max, maximum; MTC, minimum toxic concentration; MEC, minimum effective concentration.

By comparison of maximum concentration at steady state with "average" plasma concentration at steady state

Eq. 11.12

$$(C_{p_\infty})_{max} \quad \text{or} \quad (C_{p_{ss}})_{max} = \frac{(C_p)_0}{(1 - e^{-K\tau})}$$

and Eq. 11.17

$$(\overline{C}_p)_{ss} = \frac{X_0}{VK\tau}$$

Since dose$/V = (C_p)_0$,

$$\frac{(C_{p_{ss}})_{max}}{(\overline{C}_p)_{ss}} = \frac{\frac{(C_p)_0}{(1-e^{-K\tau})}}{\frac{(C_p)_0}{K\tau}} = \frac{K\tau}{(1-e^{-K\tau})}$$

However, since $\tau = Nt_{1/2}$ and $K = 0.693/t_{1/2}$, substitution for τ and K gives:

$$\frac{(C_{p_{ss}})_{max}}{(\overline{C}_p)_{ss}} = \frac{\left(\frac{0.693}{t_{1/2}}\right)(N)(t_{1/2})}{1 - e^{-\left(\frac{0.693}{t_{1/2}}\right)(N)(t_{1/2})}} = \frac{(0.693)(N)}{1 - e^{-(0.693)(N)}}$$

$$(11.37)$$

Equation 11.37 gives the ratio of the maximum to "average" steady-state drug concentrations when there are N elimination half lives. The equation also indicates that the more frequent the dosing (N is smaller), the smaller is the ratio between the maximum and "average" drug concentration.

Important comments on drug fluctuation

It is clear from Eqs 11.36 and 11.37 and Table 11.2 that drug fluctuation, just as for drug accumulation, is simply a function of dosing interval and the elimination half life or elimination rate constant of a drug. Since the elimination half life and rate constant are constant for a particular drug administered to an individual patient, fluctuation is influenced only by the dosing interval. It should be clear from Table 11.2 that the more frequent the dosing of a drug, the smaller is the

Table 11.2 Relationship between drug fluctuation $(\Phi)^a$ and the dosing interval (τ) in terms of number of elimination half life of a drug

No. elimination half lives in a dosing interval	Drug fluctuation
0.5	1.41
1.0	2.0
2.0	4.0
3.0	8.0

^{a} Drug fluctuation is the ratio of peak and trough plasma concentrations at steady state.

fluctuation (i.e. the smaller the difference between peak and trough concentrations at steady state and peak and "average" concentrations at steady state). Therefore, ideally and if practical and convenient for the patient, it is better to administer a smaller dose of a drug more frequently than a larger dose less frequently. In reality, however, convenience and practicality may prevail over what is ideal.

Let us take an example of metoprolol, a beta-blocker. It is better to administer 50 mg every 12 h rather than 100 mg every 24 h. If possible and practical, however, 25 mg every 6 h is even better.

The "average" steady-state plasma concentration of metoprolol from a 100 mg dose every 24 h, a 50 mg dose every 12 h or a 25 mg dose every 6 h will be identical; however, 25 mg every 6 h will provide peak, trough and "average" concentrations that are much closer to each other than can be achieved with 50 mg every 12 h or 100 mg every 24 h. By employing this more frequent dosing approach, one can optimize the dosage regimen in such a manner that, at steady state, all plasma concentration values will be in the therapeutic range of the drug; in other words, following the attainment of the steady-state condition, plasma concentration will remain in the therapeutic range as long as the patient follows the prescribed dosage regimen scrupulously.

11.6 Number of doses required to reach a fraction of the steady-state condition

The number of doses required to attain a given fraction of the steady-state condition may be calculated as follows, Eq. 11.5:

$$(C_{p_n})_t = \frac{(C_p)_0(1 - e^{-nK\tau})}{(1 - e^{-K\tau})} e^{-Kt}$$

where $(C_{p_n})_t$ is the plasma concentration at time t after the nth dose.

For steady state (i.e. after administration of many doses), Equation 11.5 becomes Eq. 11.11:

$$(C_{p_\infty})_t = \frac{(C_p)_0}{(1 - e^{-K\tau})} e^{-Kt}$$

where $(C_{p_\infty})_t$ is the steady-state plasma concentration at time t.

Take the ratio of $(C_{p_n})_t$ to $(C_{p_\infty})_t$:

$$\frac{(C_{p_n})_t}{(C_{p_\infty})_t} = \frac{\frac{(C_p)_0(1 - e^{-nK\tau})}{(1 - e^{-K\tau})} e^{-Kt}}{\frac{(C_p)_0}{(1 - e^{-K\tau})} e^{-Kt}} = f_{ss} = 1 - e^{-nK\tau}$$

(11.38)

where f_{ss} is the fraction of the steady state.

As $N = \tau/t_{1/2}$ or $\tau = Nt_{1/2}$, and $K = 0.693/t_{1/2}$, τ and K in Eq. 11.38 can be substituted:

$$\frac{(C_{p_n})_t}{(C_{p_\infty})_t} = f_{ss} = 1 - e^{-\frac{(n)(0.693)(N)(t_{1/2})}{t_{1/2}}}$$

$$f_{ss} = 1 - e^{-0.693nN}$$

$$\ln(f_{ss} - 1) = -0.693nN$$

or

$$n = -\ln(1 - f_{ss})/0.693N \qquad (11.39)$$

where n is the number of doses required to reach a given fraction of the steady-state (f_{ss}) condition and N is the number of elimination half lives in the dosing interval.

Using Eq. 11.39, one can calculate the number of doses required to attain a fraction of steady-state concentration (Table 11.3).

Table 11.3 indicates that the more frequent the dosing (smaller N value or smaller dosing interval), the greater the number of doses required to reach a given fraction of steady-state condition.

11.7 Calculation of loading and maintenance doses

It may take a long time and the administration of many doses (over seven or eight) before the desired "average" steady-state drug concentration is attained. Therefore, an intravenous bolus loading dose (D_L) may be administered to obtain an instant steady-state condition. The calculated loading dose should be such that that, at time τ after its administration, the plasma concentration of drug is the desired minimum plasma concentration at steady state, that is:

Table 11.3   Relationship between the numbers (n) of doses required to attain a desired fraction of steady state (f_{ss}) and the dosing interval in terms of number of elimination half lives (N)

f_{ss}	n				
	$N = 0.5$	$N = 1.0$	$N = 2.0$	$N = 3.0$	$N \neq n$
0.50	2.00	1.00	0.50	0.33	1.00
0.90	6.64	3.32	1.66	1.11	3.32
0.95	8.64	4.32	2.16	1.44	4.32
0.99	13.29	6.64	3.32	2.21	6.64

$$(C_{p_{ss}})_{min} = \frac{D_L}{V} e^{-K\tau} \qquad (11.40)$$

From Eq. 11.13 we know that:

$$(C_{p_{ss}})_{min} = \frac{X_0}{V} \frac{e^{-K\tau}}{(1 - e^{-K\tau})}$$

where X_0 is the intravenous bolus maintenance dose (D_m).

Equating Eqs 11.40 and 11.13, therefore, yields:

$$\frac{D_L}{V} e^{-K\tau} = \frac{D_M}{V} \frac{e^{-K\tau}}{(1 - e^{-K\tau})}$$

Upon simplification and rearrangement,

$$\frac{D_L}{D_M} = \frac{V e^{-K\tau}}{V(1 - e^{-K\tau})e^{-K\tau}} = \frac{1}{1 - e^{-K\tau}} \qquad (11.41)$$

Substituting for τ and K using $\tau = N t_{1/2}$ and $K = 0.693/t_{1/2}$ gives:

$$\frac{D_L}{D_M} = \frac{1}{1 - e^{-\left(\frac{0.693}{t_{1/2}}\right)(N)(t_{1/2})}} = \frac{1}{1 - e^{-(0.693)(N)}}$$

$$(11.42)$$

Equations 11.41 and 11.42 provide the ratio of loading dose to maintenance dose required to attain the steady-state condition instantaneously when there are N elimination half lives in a dosing interval (τ). Furthermore, Eq. 11.42 indicates that the more frequent the dosing (i.e. smaller N value or τ), the larger is the loading dose required compared with the maintenance dose (i.e. the greater is the ratio of D_L/D_m) in order to attain the instantaneous steady-state condition.

From Table 11.4, it is clear that if we wish to attain immediately the desired steady-state concentration for a drug dosed at an interval equal to half the elimination half life of the drug, the loading dose required will be 3.41 times the maintenance dose of the drug. If the dosing interval is equal to the half life of the drug, the loading dose will be twice the maintenance dose.

Figure 11.11 illustrates a typical plasma concentration versus time profile following the administration of a series of single maintenance

Table 11.4 Relationship between the ratios of loading dose to maintenance dose required to attain the steady-state condition and the dosing interval in terms of number of elimination half lives (N)

N	Ratio loading dose/maintenance
0.5	3.41
1.0	2.00
2.0	1.33
3.0	1.14

doses and administration of a loading dose followed by a series of maintenance doses.

11.8 Maximum and minimum drug concentration at steady state

For an intravenous bolus, the maximum drug concentration occurs at $t = 0$ after a dose at steady state, and the minimum drug concentration occurs at $t = \tau$ (i.e. one dosing interval after the dose is given).

At time t after a dose is given at steady state:

$$(C_{p_\infty})_t = \frac{X_0}{V} \frac{e^{-Kt}}{(1 - e^{-K\tau})}$$

When $t = 0$, $e^{-Kt} = 1.0$ and:

$$(C_{p_\infty})_{max} = (C_{p_{ss}})_{max} = \frac{X_0}{V(1 - e^{-K\tau})} \qquad (11.43)$$

When $t = \tau$,

$$(C_{p_\infty})_{min} = (C_{p_{ss}})_{min} = \frac{X_0 e^{-K\tau}}{V(1 - e^{-K\tau})} \qquad (11.44)$$

Subtracting $(C_{p_{ss}})_{min}$ from $(C_{p_{ss}})_{max}$ (i.e. Eq. 11.44 from Eq. 11.43) gives:

$$(C_{p_{ss}})_{max} - (C_{p_{ss}})_{min}$$

$$= \frac{X_0}{V(1 - e^{-K\tau})} - \frac{X_0 e^{-K\tau}}{V(1 - e^{-K\tau})} = \frac{X_0 - X_0 e^{-K\tau}}{V(1 - e^{-K\tau})}$$

$$= \frac{X_0(1 - e^{-K\tau})}{V(1 - e^{-K\tau})} = \frac{dose}{V} = (C_p)_0$$

$$(11.45)$$

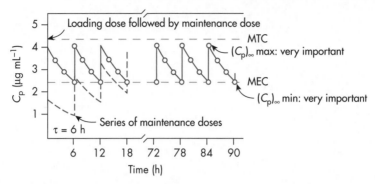

Figure 11.11   A plot of plasma concentration (C_p) versus time following repetitive intravenous bolus administration of a drug. The figure demonstrates the plasma level resulting from either a series of maintenance doses (dashed line) or an initial loading dose followed by a series of maintenance doses (continuous line). min, minimum; max, maximum; MTC, minimum toxic concentration; MEC, minimum effective concentration; τ, dosing interval.

where $(C_p)_0$ is the peak concentration from the initial intravenous bolus dose.

However, VC_p is the mass of drug in the body, X. Hence,

$$(X_{ss})_{max} - (X_{ss})_{min} = \text{dose} = X_0 \qquad (11.46)$$

Equations 11.45 and 11.46 clearly indicate that, at steady state, the difference between max-imum and minimum concentrations or peak and trough concentrations is equal to the initial plasma concentration or maximum plasma concentration following the administration of the first dose. Furthermore, this confirms that, at steady state, the amount or the mass of drug leaving the body during one dosing interval is equal to the administered dose.

12

Multiple dosing: extravascular routes of drug administration

Objectives

Upon completion of this chapter, you will have the ability to:

- calculate plasma drug concentration at any time t following the nth extravascular dose of drug
- calculate the peak time after a dose at steady state, t'_{max}, and the concentration at this time, $(C_p)_{\infty max}$
- calculate peak, trough and "average" steady-state plasma drug concentrations
- calculate the accumulation ratio (R)
- calculate drug concentration fluctuation at steady state (Φ)
- calculate the number of doses (n) required to reach a given fraction of steady state (f_{ss})
- calculate the number of elimination half lives (N) required to reach a given fraction of steady state
- calculate loading and maintenance extravascular (including oral) doses
- use interconversion equations to convert an existing dose of drug to the dose required when changing between loading, maintenance, intravenous bolus, and/or oral doses.

12.1 Introduction

Unlike intravascular dosage forms, in which a solution of drug is injected (usually by the intravenous route) into the systemic circulation, extravascular dosage forms are not immediately delivered into the systemic circulation. Extravascular dosage forms such as oral, intramuscular, subcutaneous and transdermal patches are meant to deliver drug to the systemic circulation; however, this systemic delivery is not instantaneous. Therefore, the pharmacokinetic equations require a term reflecting an absorption process. In order to understand multiple oral dosing, one must first review the pharmacokinetics for a single extravascular dose of drug.

A single extravascular dose (one compartment)

From the profile presented in Fig. 12.1 and from Ch. 6 (Eqs 6.5 and 6.6), we know the following two equations:

$$(X)_t = \frac{K_a F X_0}{K_a - K}[e^{-Kt} - e^{-K_a t}] \tag{12.1}$$

$$(C_p)_t = \frac{K_a F X_0}{V(K_a - K)}[e^{-Kt} - e^{-K_a t}] \tag{12.2}$$

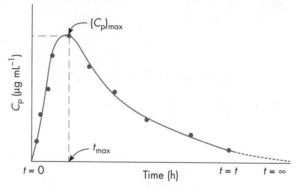

Figure 12.1 A typical plasma concentration (C_p) versus time profile for a drug that follows first-order elimination, one-compartment distribution and is administered as a single dose of drug by an extravascular route. $(C_p)_{max}$, peak plasma concentration; t_{max}, peak time.

At $t = 0$ and $t = \infty$, $X = 0$ and $C_p = 0$; and at $t = t_{max}$ (i.e. peak time), $X = (X)_{max}$ and $C_p = (C_p)_{max}$ (i.e. peak plasma concentration or highest plasma concentration). Please note the difference between intra- and extravascular routes of drug administration with regard to the time at which the highest, or peak, plasma concentration occurs.

Multiple extravascular dosing

The vast majority of drugs administered on a continual basis are administered orally. Of these, a significant fraction yields a plasma drug concentration versus profile that can be described by a one-compartment model with first-order absorption and elimination. The equation describing the plasma concentration versus time curve following multiple dosing of a drug which is absorbed by an apparent first-order process can be arrived at as follows. We know the equation for oral administration (single dose):

$$(C_p)_t = \frac{K_a F X_0}{V(K_a - K)}[e^{-Kt} - e^{-K_a t}]$$

Multiplication of each exponential term (i.e. e^{-Kt} and $e^{-K_a t}$) by the multiple-dosing function, and setting K_i in each function equal to the rate constant for each exponential term yields:

$$(C_{p_n})_t = \frac{K_a F X_0}{V(K_a - K)}$$

$$\times \left[\frac{1 - e^{-nK\tau}}{1 - e^{-K\tau}}e^{-Kt} - \frac{1 - e^{-nK_a \tau}}{1 - e^{-K_a \tau}}e^{-K_a t}\right]$$

$$(12.3)$$

where $(C_{p_n})_t$ is the plasma concentration at time t following the administration of the nth dose; V is the apparent volume of distribution; K, the elimination rate constant; τ is the dosing interval; t is the time from $t > 0$ to $t < \tau$ during dosing interval; K_a is the apparent first-order rate constant for absorption; F is the fraction of the administered dose absorbed into the systemic circulation; and X_0 is the the administered dose.

Please note that when a drug is administered extravascularly, at $t = 0$ there is no drug in the blood. The highest or peak plasma concentration will always occur at peak time (t_{max}).

Equation 12.3 may be employed to predict the plasma concentration of drug at any time during the dosing interval following the administration of nth dose (second, third, fourth, etc) (Fig. 12.2). However, in order to make such predictions, it is essential to have knowledge of the apparent volume of distribution, the fraction of the administered dose absorbed into the systemic circulation, the apparent first-order rate constant for absorption, the intercept of the plasma concentration versus time profile following the administration of the single dose, and the elimination rate constant. Furthermore, earlier

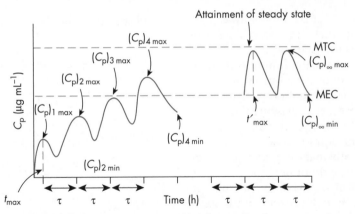

Figure 12.2 Typical plasma concentration (C_p) versus time profile following the administration of many identical doses (1–4) of a drug at an identical dosing interval (τ) by an extravascular route and the attainment of steady-state condition. min, minimum; max, maximum; MTC, minimum toxic concentration; MEC, minimum effective concentration.

discussions have shown that, for extravascularly administered drug, the peak plasma concentration will occur at the peak time and the minimum, or trough, plasma concentration will occur at $t = \tau$. It is, therefore, essential for us to know the peak time and the dosing interval for a given dosage regimen.

12.2 The peak time in multiple dosing to steady state (t'_{max})

Assuming that the fraction of each dose absorbed is constant during a multiple-dosing regimen, the time at which a maximum plasma concentration of drug at steady state occurs (t'_{max}) can be obtained by differentiating the following equation with respect to time and setting the resultant equal to 0.

$$(C_{p_\infty})_t = \frac{K_a F X_0}{V(K_a - K)}$$

$$\times \left[\frac{1}{1 - e^{-K\tau}} e^{-Kt} - \frac{1}{1 - e^{-K_a\tau}} e^{-K_a t} \right] \tag{12.4}$$

Differentiating Eq. 12.4 with respect to t yields:

$$\frac{d(C_{p_\infty})_t}{dt} = \frac{K_a F X_0}{V(K_a - K)} \left[\frac{K_a e^{-K_a t}}{1 - e^{-K_a\tau}} - \frac{K e^{-Kt}}{1 - e^{-K\tau}} \right] \tag{12.5}$$

To find $t = t'_{max}$, we set the above expression to equal zero. The result can be simplified to:

$$\frac{K_a e^{-K_a t'_{max}}}{1 - e^{-K_a\tau}} = \frac{K e^{-K t'_{max}}}{1 - e^{-K\tau}} \tag{12.6}$$

Further rearrangement and simplification of Eq. 12.6 yields:

$$t'_{max} = \frac{2.303}{K_a - K} \log \left(\frac{K_a}{K} \frac{1 - e^{-K\tau}}{1 - e^{-K_a\tau}} \right) \tag{12.7}$$

The peak time following the administration of a single extravascular dose is obtained by employing the following equation (equivalent to Eq. 6.15):

$$t_{max} = \frac{2.303 \log (K_a / K)}{K_a - K} \tag{12.8}$$

Please consider the differences between Eqs 12.7 and 12.8.

Subtracting Eq. 12.7 from Eq. 12.8 yields:

$$t_{max} - t'_{max} = \frac{2.303}{K_a - K} \log \left(\frac{1 - e^{-K_a\tau}}{1 - e^{-K\tau}} \right) \tag{12.9}$$

Since the right side of Eq. 12.9 is always positive, it is apparent that the maximum plasma concentration at steady state occurs at an earlier time than that following the administration of a single dose. Furthermore, the time at which the maximum plasma concentration is observed following the first dose (i.e. t_{max}) is often the time at which the plasma is sampled after the administration of subsequent doses to assess peak plasma concentration. Mathematical principles clearly suggest that this would not be a sound practice since the time at which a maximum plasma concentration occurs is not constant until steady state is attained.

12.3 Maximum plasma concentration at steady state

Once the time at which maximum plasma concentration of drug occurs at steady state is known, the maximum plasma concentration at steady state can be derived by substitution of t'_{max} in the following equation, Eq. 12.4:

$$(C_{p_\infty})_t = \frac{K_a F X_0}{V(K_a - K)}$$

$$\times \left[\frac{1}{1 - e^{-K\tau}} e^{-Kt} - \frac{1}{1 - e^{-K_a\tau}} e^{-K_a t} \right]$$

Substitution of t'_{max} for t in Eq. 12.4 gives:

$$(C_{p_\infty})_{max} = \frac{K_a F X_0}{V(K_a - K)}$$

$$\times \left[\frac{1}{1 - e^{-K\tau}} e^{-Kt'_{max}} \right. \qquad (12.10)$$

$$\left. - \frac{1}{1 - e^{-K_a\tau}} e^{-K_a t'_{max}} \right]$$

A previous equation (Eq. 12.6) stated that:

$$\frac{K_a e^{-K_a t'_{max}}}{1 - e^{-K_a\tau}} = \frac{K e^{-Kt'_{max}}}{1 - e^{-K\tau}}$$

Rearrange Eq. 12.6 for the term $e^{-K_a t'_{max}}$:

$$e^{-K_a t'_{max}} = \frac{1 - e^{-K_a\tau}}{1 - e^{-K\tau}} \frac{K}{K_a} e^{-Kt'_{max}}$$

Substitution for $e^{-K_a t'_{max}}$ in Eq. 12.10, yields:

$$(C_{p_\infty})_{max} = \frac{K_a F X_0}{V(K_a - K)} \left[\frac{1}{1 - e^{-K\tau}} e^{-Kt'_{max}} \right.$$

$$\left. - \left(\frac{1}{1 - e^{-K_a\tau}} \right) \left(\frac{1 - e^{-K_a\tau}}{1 - e^{-K\tau}} \right) \left(\frac{K}{K_a} \right) e^{-Kt'_{max}} \right]$$

$$(C_{p_\infty})_{max} = \frac{K_a F X_0}{V(K_a - K)} \left[\frac{1}{1 - e^{-K\tau}} e^{-Kt'_{max}} \right.$$

$$\left. - \left(\frac{K}{K_a(1 - e^{-K\tau})} \right) e^{-Kt'_{max}} \right]$$

$$(C_{p_\infty})_{max} = \frac{K_a F X_0}{V(K_a - K)} \left(\frac{K_a - K}{K_a(1 - e^{-K\tau})} \right) e^{-Kt'_{max}}$$

$$(C_{p_\infty})_{max} = \frac{F X_0}{V} \left(\frac{1}{1 - e^{-K\tau}} \right) e^{-Kt'_{max}} \qquad (12.11)$$

Peak plasma concentration following the administration of a single extravascular dose, or the first dose, is obtained as follows:

$$(C_{p_1})_{max} = \frac{F X_0}{V} e^{-Kt_{max}} \qquad (12.12)$$

where,

$$\frac{F X_0}{V} = \left(\frac{K_a - K}{K_a} \right)(I)$$

and where I is the intercept of plasma concentration versus time profile for a single dose.

Substituting for $F X_0/V$ in Eq. 12.11 yields:

$$(C_{p_\infty})_{max} = \frac{K_a}{K_a - K}(I)\left(\frac{1}{1 - e^{-K\tau}} \right) e^{-Kt'_{max}}$$

$$(12.13)$$

Equation 12.13 permits determination of peak plasma concentration for a drug administered extravascularly provided the intercept value for an identical single dose, peak time, elimination half life and the dosing interval are known.

It will be very helpful to begin to compare Eq. 11.12 (for an intravenous bolus) and Eq. 12.13 (for extravascularly administered dose) for similarity and differences, if any, and identify the commonality between the two equations. It may be quickly apparent that the information obtained following the administration of a single dose of a drug, either intravenously or

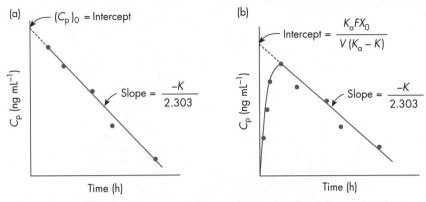

Figure 12.3 Semilogarithmic plots of plasma concentration (C_p) versus time profiles following the administration of a single dose of a drug as an intravenous bolus (a) and by an extravascular route (b). X_0, the dose; F, fraction of administered dose that is available to reach the general circulation; K_a and K, first-order absorption and elimination rate constants, respectively; V, apparent volume of distribution.

extravascularly, and the chosen dosing interval permit the prediction of maximum plasma concentrations at steady state for either route of drug administration.

For example, in Eq. 11.12 (for intravenous bolus), $(C_p)_0$ represents the intercept of the plasma concentration versus time profile following the administration of a single dose of a drug. In Eq. 12.13 (for extravascularly administered dose), we can obtain the intercept value from the plasma concentration versus time plot. In both Eqs 11.12 and 12.13, the denominator term is identical (i.e. $1 - e^{-K\tau}$). For an intravenous bolus, maximum or peak plasma concentration occurs at time 0 and, for an extravascular route, maximum concentration will occur at peak time (Fig. 12.3).

12.4 Minimum plasma concentration at steady state

Equation 12.4 states:

$$(C_{p_\infty})_t = \frac{K_a F X_0}{V(K_a - K)}$$
$$\times \left[\frac{1}{1 - e^{-K\tau}} e^{-Kt} - \frac{1}{1 - e^{-K_a\tau}} e^{-K_a t} \right]$$

Substituting τ for t in Eq. 12.4 yields:

$$(C_{p_\infty})_{\min} = \frac{K_a F X_0}{V(K_a - K)}$$
$$\times \left[\frac{1}{1 - e^{-K\tau}} e^{-K\tau} - \frac{1}{1 - e^{-K_a\tau}} e^{-K_a\tau} \right]$$
$$(12.14)$$

In the post-absorptive phase (i.e. as the term $e^{-K_a\tau}$ approaches zero), Eq. 12.14 becomes:

$$(C_{p_\infty})_{\min} = \frac{K_a F X_0}{V(K_a - K)} \left[\frac{1}{1 - e^{-K\tau}} e^{-K\tau} \right]$$
$$(12.15)$$

where,

$$\frac{K_a F X_0}{V(K_a - K)}$$

is the intercept of the plasma concentration time profile ($\mu g\, mL^{-1}$) following administration of a single dose.

The above equation allows us to calculate the trough steady-state plasma drug concentration for multiple oral dosing.

The minimum, or trough, plasma concentration following the administration of a single, or the first, dose is obtained as follows:

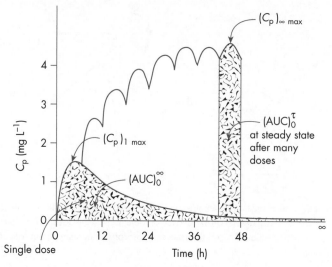

Figure 12.4 Typical plasma concentration (C_p) versus time profile following the administration of many identical doses of a drug at an identical dosing interval by an extravascular route and the attainment of steady-state condition. AUC, area under the plasma concentration versus time profile; τ, dosing interval.

$$(C_{p_1})_{min} = \frac{K_a F X_0}{V(K_a - K)} \left[e^{-K\tau} - e^{-K_a\tau} \right] \quad (12.16)$$

where,

$$\frac{K_a F X_0}{V(K_a - K)}$$

is the intercept of the plasma concentration time profile ($\mu g\, mL^{-1}$) following administration of a single dose.

In the post-absorptive phase (i.e. as the term $e^{-K_a\tau}$ approaches zero), Eq. 12.16 becomes:

$$(C_{p_1})_{min} = \frac{K_a F X_0}{V(K_a - K)} \left[e^{-K\tau} \right] = I e^{-K\tau} \quad (12.17)$$

By applying the steady-state function and by substituting I for the intercept defined above, we obtain:

$$(C_{p_\infty})_{min} = I \left(\frac{1}{1 - e^{-K\tau}} \right) e^{-K\tau} \quad (12.18)$$

which is a restatement of Eq. 12.15.

Equation 12.18 permits determination of minimum plasma concentration (i.e. trough plasma concentration) for a drug administered

extravascularly, provided we know the intercept value for an identical single dose, elimination half life, and the dosing interval. This equation assumes that we are in the post-absorption phase at τ h after the dose is given. Once again, note that trough, or minimum, plasma concentration will occur at time τ regardless of the route of drug administration.

12.5 "Average" plasma concentration at steady state: extravascular route

The "average" plasma concentration of a drug at steady state for extravascularly administered dose can be calculated from:

$$(\overline{C}_p)_{ss} = \frac{F X_0}{V K \tau} \quad (12.19)$$

It is clear from Eq. 12.19 that the "average" plasma concentration, $(\overline{C}_p)_{ss}$, is dependent on the size of the dose administered X_0, the fraction of the administered dose reaching general circulation or absorbed (F) and the dosing interval (τ). The dose is administered as a single dose every τ time units or is subdivided and administered at some fraction of τ (i.e. 600 mg once a day is equivalent to 300 mg every 12 h, which is equivalent to 150 mg every 6 h). However, upon subdividing the daily dose, the difference between the steady-state minimum and the steady-state maximum plasma concentration will usually decrease.

The only difference between Eq. 11.17 (for an intravenous solution) and Eq. 12.19 (for extravascular administration) is the incorporation of the term F, the absolute bioavailability of a drug. Should the drug be completely absorbed following extravascular administration, Eqs 11.17 and 12.19 will be exactly the same; therefore, identical "average" steady-state concentrations would be expected for an identical dosage regimen.

The area under the plasma concentration versus time curve from $t=0$ to $t=\infty$, following first-order input of a single dose, can be obtained using:

$$\int_0^\infty C_p dt = \frac{FX_0}{VK} \tag{12.20}$$

In Ch. 11, it was shown, in turn, that this is equal to the area under the plasma concentration time curve during a dosing interval, at steady state:

$$\int_0^\infty C_p dt = \frac{FX_0}{VK} = \int_0^\tau (C_{p_\infty})_t dt \tag{12.21}$$

Equation 12.21 allows,

$$\int_0^\tau (C_{p_\infty})_t dt$$

to be substituted for FX_0/VK in Eq. 12.19, yielding:

$$(\overline{C}_p)_{ss} = \frac{\int_0^\tau (C_{p_\infty})_t dt}{\tau} \tag{12.22}$$

which is the same as:

$$(\overline{C}_p)_{ss} = \frac{(AUC)_0^\tau}{\tau} \tag{12.23}$$

Equation 12.21 also allows:

$$\int_0^\infty (C_{p_\infty})_t dt$$

to be substituted for

$$\int_0^\tau (C_{p_\infty})_t dt$$

in Eq. 12.22, resulting in:

$$(\overline{C}_p)_{ss} = \frac{\int_0^\infty (C_p) dt}{\tau} \tag{12.24}$$

which is the same as:

$$(\overline{C}_p)_{ss} = \frac{(AUC)_0^\infty}{\tau} \tag{12.25}$$

Equations 12.24 and 12.25 are probably more useful for predicting

$$(\overline{C}_p)_{ss}$$

than Eqs 12.22 and 12.23, since the area under the plasma concentration versus time curve following a single dose is generally easily determined. Furthermore, estimates of the absolute bioavailability and apparent volume of distribution, which are necessary for the utilization of Eq. 12.19, are not required for this method. Comparison of Eqs 11.23 and 12.23 may be very beneficial at this time.

12.6 Determination of drug accumulation: extravascular route

The accumulation factor (R) following the administration of a drug by an extravascular route can be calculated by comparing the minimum plasma concentration of drug at steady state with the minimum plasma concentration following the first dose:

$$R = \frac{(C_{p_\infty})_{min}}{(C_{p_1})_{min}} \tag{12.26}$$

This method is relatively simple only when dealing with the situation in which each subsequent dose is administered in the post-absorptive phase of the preceding dose. This situation probably occurs for a large number of drugs, although it may not be valid for sustained-release products and for drugs that are very slowly absorbed (i.e. having a smaller difference between the absorption and the elimination rate constants owing to very slow absorption).

Equation 12.3 describes plasma drug concentration at t hours after the nth dose of a multiple oral dosing regimen:

$$(C_{p_n})_t = \frac{K_a F X_0}{V(K_a - K)}$$
$$\times \left[\frac{1 - e^{-nK\tau}}{1 - e^{-K\tau}} e^{-Kt} - \frac{1 - e^{-nK_a\tau}}{1 - e^{-K_a\tau}} e^{-K_a t}\right]$$

By setting the number of doses as $n = 1$ (first dose) and time as $t = \tau$ in Eq. 12.3, an expression for the minimum plasma concentration following the first dose, $(C_{p_1})_{min}$, can be obtained, Eq. 12.16:

$$(C_{p_1})_{min} = \frac{K_a F X_0}{V(K_a - K)} [e^{-K\tau} - e^{-K_a\tau}]$$

Similarly by setting $t = \tau$ in the following expression,

$$(C_{p_\infty})_{min}$$

may be computed. Eq. 12.4,

$$(C_{p_\infty})_t = \frac{K_a F X_0}{V(K_a - K)}$$
$$\times \left[\frac{1}{1 - e^{-K\tau}} e^{-Kt} - \frac{1}{1 - e^{-K_a\tau}} e^{-K_a t}\right]$$

When $t = \tau$, Eq. 12.14:

$$(C_{p_\infty})_{min} = \frac{K_a F X_0}{V(K_a - K)}$$
$$\times \left[\frac{1}{1 - e^{-K\tau}} e^{-K\tau} - \frac{1}{1 - e^{-K_a\tau}} e^{-K_a\tau}\right]$$

In the post-absorptive phase (i.e. as the term $e^{-K_a\tau}$ approaches zero), Eqs 12.14 and 12.16 become Eqs 12.15 and 12.17:

$$(C_{p_\infty})_{min} = \frac{K_a F X_0}{V(K_a - K)} \left[\frac{1}{1 - e^{-K\tau}} e^{-K\tau}\right]$$

$$(C_{p_1})_{min} = \frac{K_a F X_0}{V(K_a - K)} [e^{-K\tau}]$$

Hence, accumulation equals the ratio of Eq. 12.15 to Eq. 12.17:

$$R = \frac{(C_{p_\infty})_{min}}{(C_{p_1})_{min}} = \frac{\frac{K_a F X_0}{V(K_a - K)} \left[\frac{1}{1 - e^{-K\tau}} e^{-K\tau}\right]}{\frac{K_a F X_0}{V(K_a - K)} [e^{-K\tau}]}$$
$$= \frac{1}{1 - e^{-K\tau}} \tag{12.27}$$

This expression, which relies on fairly rapid absorption such that each subsequent dose is administered in the post-absorptive phase, can be readily employed to determine the extent of accumulation following extravascular administration of a drug as long as dosing interval and the elimination rate constant of the drug are available. Note the similarity between Eq. 12.27 for multiple oral dosing and Eqs 11.29, 11.33 and 11.34 for multiple intravenous bolus administration.

For slower extravascular absorption, a similar, but more detailed, derivation (not shown) provides an equation for the accumulation factor that requires no assumptions:

$$R = \frac{1}{(1 - e^{-K\tau})(1 - e^{-K_a\tau})} \tag{12.28}$$

12.7 Calculation of fluctuation factor (Φ) for multiple extravascular dosing

For an extravascular dosage for that is relatively rapidly absorbed, one may use Equation 12.29 equivalent to Equation 11.36 (for fluctuation with multiple intravenous bolus administration) to calculate fluctuation at steady state:

$$\Phi = \frac{(C_{p_{ss}})_{max}}{(C_{p_{ss}})_{min}}$$

$$= \frac{1}{e^{-\left(\frac{0.693}{t_{1/2}}\right)(N)(t_{1/2})}}$$

$$= \frac{1}{e^{-(0.693)(N)}} \qquad (12.29)$$

However, if this assumption is not justified, the following equation is required:

$$\Phi_{po} = \frac{(C_{p_{ss}})_{max}}{(C_{p_{ss}})_{min}}$$

$$= \frac{K_a - K}{K_a} \left[\frac{(e^{-Kt'_{max}})(1 - e^{-K_a \tau_{po}})}{e^{-K\tau_{po}} - e^{-K_a \tau_{po}}} \right] \qquad (12.30)$$

12.8 Number of doses required reaching a fraction of steady state: extravascular route

The time required to reach a certain fraction of the ultimate steady state following oral administration can be estimated as follows:

$$f_{ss} = \overline{C}_{p_n} / \overline{C}_{p_{ss}} \qquad (12.31)$$

where,

$$\overline{C}_{p_n} = \frac{\int_0^\tau C_{p_n} dt}{\tau} \qquad (12.32)$$

and Eq. 12.19

$$(\overline{C}_p)_{ss} = \frac{FX_0}{VK\tau}$$

From earlier discussion, Eq. 12.3

$$(C_{p_n})_t = \frac{K_a FX_0}{V(K_a - K)}$$

$$\times \left[\frac{1 - e^{-nK\tau}}{1 - e^{-K\tau}} e^{-Kt} - \frac{1 - e^{-nK_a\tau}}{1 - e^{-K_a\tau}} e^{-K_a t} \right]$$

Integration of Eq. 12.3 from $t=0$ to $t=\tau$ yields:

$$\int_0^\tau (C_{p_n})_t dt = \frac{FX_0}{VK(K_a - K)} \left[\left(\frac{1 - e^{-nK_a\tau}}{1 - e^{-K_a\tau}} \right) \frac{e^{-K_a\tau}}{K_a} \right.$$

$$- \left(\frac{1 - e^{-nK\tau}}{1 - e^{-K\tau}} \right) \frac{e^{-K\tau}}{K}$$

$$+ \left(\frac{1 - e^{-nK\tau}}{1 - e^{-K\tau}} \right) \frac{1}{K}$$

$$\left. - \left(\frac{1 - e^{-nK_a\tau}}{1 - e^{-K_a\tau}} \right) \frac{1}{K_a} \right]$$

This equation, upon rearrangement and simplification, becomes,

$$\int_0^\tau (C_{p_n})_t dt = \frac{FX_0}{VK} \left(1 + \frac{Ke^{-nK_a\tau}}{K_a - K} - \frac{K_a e^{-nK\tau}}{K_a - K} \right) \qquad (12.33)$$

However, since

$$(\overline{C}_p)_n = \frac{\int_0^\tau (C_p)_n dt}{\tau} \qquad (12.22)$$

substituting for

$$\int_0^\tau (C_p)_n dt$$

in Eq. 12.33 gives:

$$\overline{C}_{p_n} = \frac{FX_0}{VK\tau} \left(1 + \frac{Ke^{-nK_a\tau}}{K_a - K} - \frac{K_a e^{-nK\tau}}{K_a - K} \right)$$

We also know that Eq. 12.19,

$$(\overline{C}_p)_{ss} = \frac{FX_0}{VK\tau}$$

Hence,

$$f_{ss} = \frac{(\overline{C}_p)_n}{(\overline{C}_p)_{ss}}$$

$$= \frac{\frac{FX_0}{VK\tau} \left(1 + \frac{Ke^{-nK_a\tau}}{K_a - K} - \frac{K_a e^{-nK\tau}}{K_a - K} \right)}{\frac{FX_0}{VK\tau}}$$

$$= 1 + \frac{Ke^{-nK_a\tau}}{K_a - K} - \frac{K_a e^{-nK\tau}}{K_a - K} \qquad (12.34)$$

From Eq. 12.34 it is clear that the time required to reach a certain fraction of the steady-state concentration is a complex function of the absorption and elimination rate constants (i.e. K_a and K). The larger the value of the absorption rate constant relative to the elimination rate constant, the less dependent on the absorption rate constant is the time required to reach a given fraction of steady state. If $K_a \gg K$ (i.e. $K_a/K \geq 10$), Eq. 12.34 approaches:

$$f_{ss} = 1 - e^{-nK\tau} \tag{12.35}$$

Equation 12.35 can be rearranged as follows:

$$1 - f_{ss} = e^{-nK\tau}$$

$$-nK\tau = \ln(1 - f_{ss})$$

$$-n = \ln(1 - f_{ss})/K\tau \tag{12.36}$$

Since $\tau = Nt_{1/2}$ and $K = 0.693/t_{1/2}$, substitution for τ and K in Eq. 12.36 yields:

$$n = -\ln(1 - f_{ss})/0.693N \tag{12.37}$$

Equations 11.39 (for intravenous bolus) and 12.37 are identical; hence, they convey the same message. The administration of a smaller dose more frequently will require a greater number of doses to attain a given fraction of steady state (see Table 11.3). Conversely, administration of larger dose less frequently will require fewer doses to attain a given fraction of steady-state condition. Note that Eq. 12.37 is identical to Eq. 11.39 only when the absorption rate constant is much greater than the elimination rate constant and each subsequent dose is administered in the post-absorption phase.

12.9 Determination of loading and maintenance dose: extravascular route

As discussed above, an initial loading dose may be desirable since a long period of time is required to reach steady state for drugs with long half lives. The loading dose required to achieve steady-state concentrations on the first

dose may be determined by letting this initial loading dose equal X_0 in the equation for $(C_{p_1})_{\min}$ and setting this equal to X_0 in the equation. For $(C_{p_\infty})_{\min}$, Eq. 12.16:

$$(C_{p_1})_{\min} = \frac{K_a F X_0}{V(K_a - K)}[e^{-K\tau} - e^{-K_a\tau}]$$

and Eq. 12.14

$$(C_{p_\infty})_{\min} = \frac{K_a F X_0}{V(K_a - K)}$$

$$\times \left[\frac{1}{1 - e^{-K\tau}}e^{-K\tau} - \frac{1}{1 - e^{-K_a\tau}}e^{-K_a\tau}\right]$$

The goal is that $(C_{p_1})_{\min}$ from the loading dose will exactly equal $(C_{p_\infty})_{\min}$ from the multiple-dosing regimen. Hence, equating the two equations:

$$\frac{K_a F (X_0)_{D_L}}{V(K_a - K)}(e^{-K\tau} - e^{-K_a\tau})$$

$$= \frac{K_a F (X_0)_{D_M}}{V(K_a - K)}\left[\frac{e^{-K\tau}}{1 - e^{-K\tau}} - \frac{e^{-K_a\tau}}{1 - e^{-K_a\tau}}\right] \tag{12.38}$$

The equation can be rearranged as:

$$\frac{(X_0)_{D_L}}{(K_a - K)}[e^{-K\tau} - e^{-K_a\tau}]$$

$$= \frac{(X_0)_{D_M}}{(K_a - K)}\left[\frac{e^{-K\tau}}{(1 - e^{-K\tau})} - \frac{e^{-K_a\tau}}{(1 - e^{-K_a\tau})}\right] \tag{12.39}$$

which, upon simplification, becomes:

$$\frac{(X_0)_{D_L}e^{-K\tau}}{(K_a - K)} - \frac{(X_0)_{D_L}e^{-K_a\tau}}{(K_a - K)}$$

$$= \frac{(X_0)_{D_M}e^{-K\tau}}{(K_a - K)(1 - e^{-K\tau})} - \frac{(X_0)_{D_M}e^{-K_a\tau}}{(K_a - K)(1 - e^{-K_a\tau})}$$

$$(X_0)_{D_L}(e^{-K\tau} - e^{-K_a\tau})$$

$$= \frac{(X_0)_{D_M}e^{-K\tau}}{1 - e^{-K\tau}} - \frac{(X_0)_{D_M}e^{-K_a\tau}}{1 - e^{-K_a\tau}}$$

$$(X_0)_{D_L} = (X_0)_{D_M}$$

$$\times \left(\frac{e^{-K_a\tau} - e^{-(K_a+K)\tau} - e^{-K\tau} + e^{-(K_a+K)\tau}}{(1 - e^{-K_a\tau})(1 - e^{-K\tau})(e^{-K_a\tau} - e^{-K\tau})}\right)$$

Further simplification yields:

$$(X_0)_{D_L} = (X_0)_{D_M}$$

$$\times \left(\frac{(e^{-K_a\tau} - e^{-K\tau}) - e^{-(K_a+K)\tau} + e^{-(K_a+K)\tau}}{(1 - e^{-K_a\tau})(1 - e^{-K\tau})(e^{-K_a\tau} - e^{-K\tau})} \right)$$

$$(X_0)_{D_L} = (X_0)_{D_M} \left(\frac{1}{(1 - e^{-K_a\tau})(1 - e^{-K\tau})} \right)$$

$$(12.40)$$

If the maintenance dose, $(X_0)_{D_M}$, is administered in the post-absorptive phase (i.e. after the occurrence of the peak time) of the loading dose, Eq. 12.40 will collapse into Eq. 12.41, since the value of the term $e^{-K_a\tau}$ approaches zero:

$$(X_0)_{D_L} = (X_0)_{D_M} \left(\frac{1}{(1 - e^{-K\tau})} \right) \qquad (12.41)$$

In addition, irrespective of the size of the initial or loading dose, the steady-state plasma concentrations of drug ultimately reached will be the same (Fig. 12.5) since the steady-state concentration is governed by the size of the maintenance dose.

Equation 12.41 is identical to Eq. 11.41 for an intravenous bolus. Therefore, information pro-vided in Table 11.4 (p.240) will also apply for the extravascularly administered drugs provided the dose is administered in the post-absorptive phase. (In real life, that is generally the case.)

Figure 12.5 illustrates a typical plasma concentration versus time profile following the administration of a series of single maintenance doses and administration of a loading dose followed by the series of maintenance doses. In this figure, note that peak and trough concentrations at steady state are identical, regardless of the ratio of loading doses to maintenance dose (numbers 2, 3 and 4 in the figure). However, for number 3, where the ratio of loading to maintenance dose is 2 (i.e. loading dose is twice the maintenance dose), the immediate peak plasma concentration and peak plasma concentration at steady state are almost identical.

In practice, when a physician wishes to attain the desired plasma concentration of drug immediately, it is customary for the patient to be directed to take two tablets of a particular strength to start with followed by one tablet at a specific interval. This practice is valid the closer the dosing interval is to one elimination half life of the drug. Examples include penicillin VK, azithromycin (Zithromax), and many others.

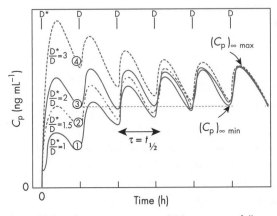

Figure 12.5 Plasma concentration (C_p) versus time following repetitive extravascular administration of a drug by either a series of maintenance doses (D) (1) or an initial loading dose followed by a series of maintenance doses (D*) (2–4). 1, series of maintenance doses (i.e. no loading dose); 2, loading dose 1.5 times maintenance dose; 3, loading dose twice maintenance dose; 4, loading dose three times the maintenance dose. τ, dosing interval; $t_{1/2}$, drug half life.

12.10 Interconversion between loading, maintenance, oral and intravenous bolus doses

Table 12.1 shows how an existing dose of a drug (eliminated by linear pharmacokinetics) can be converted to the dose required when changing between loading, maintenance, oral and/or intravenous bolus doses.

Equations 12.42 through 12.53 allow movement back and forth between loading dose (D_L), maintenance dose (D_M), an oral dose and an intravenous bolus dose.

A note of caution. Not all of these equations may be safely rearranged algebraically. Rearrangement is unnecessary as there are equations ready made for any conversion required. For example, Eq. 12.42 should not be rearranged in order to solve for $(D_M)_{IV}$ from a known $(D_M)_{oral}$. Instead, Eq. 12.43 is used, which already is in the form

Table 12.1 Interconversion chart

Equation	Comment	Equation Number
$D_M^{PO} = \dfrac{S_{IV} D_M^{IV}}{S_{PO} F_{PO}}$ for $\tau_{IV} = \tau_{PO}$	Dangerous fluctuation may occur in the PO→IV conversion direction! Use IV→PO only.	(12.42)
$D_M^{IV} = \dfrac{S_{PO} D_M^{PO} F_{PO} \tau_{IV}}{S_{IV} \tau_{PO}}$	Select τ_{IV} from Eq. 12.44	(12.43)
$\tau_{IV} = \dfrac{\ln \Phi_{ss}^{PO}}{K}$ for $\Phi_{ss}^{PO} = \Phi_{ss}^{IV}$	In order to keep the same $(\overline{C}_{p_{ss}})$, you must also adjust the dose (using Eq. 12.43, 12.47, 12.52, or 12.53 as appropriate.)	(12.44)
If $K_A > K$, $\Phi_{ss}^{PO} = \left[\dfrac{K_A - K}{K_A}\right] \left[\dfrac{e^{-K t'_{max}}}{e^{-K \tau_{PO}}}\right]$ Otherwise, $\Phi_{ss}^{PO} = \left[\dfrac{K_A - K}{K_A}\right]$		(12.45)
$\left[\dfrac{(e^{-K t'_{max}})(1 - e^{-K_A \tau_{PO}})}{e^{-K \tau_{PO}} - e^{-K_A \tau_{PO}}}\right]$ (Eq. 12.30) $t'_{max} = \dfrac{2.303}{K_a - K} \log\left(\dfrac{K_a}{K} \dfrac{1 - e^{-K\tau}}{1 - e^{-K_a \tau}}\right)$ (Eq. 12.7)		
$D_M^{PO} = \dfrac{S_{IV} D_L^{IV}(1 - e^{-K\tau})}{S_{PO} F_{PO}}$ for $\tau_{IV} = \tau_{PO}$	Dangerous fluctuation may occur in the PO→IV conversion direction! Use IV→PO only.	(12.46)
$D_L^{IV} = \dfrac{S_{PO} D_M^{PO} F_{PO} \tau_{IV}}{S_{IV}(1 - e^{-K \tau_{IV}}) \tau_{PO}}$	Select τ_{IV} from Eq. 12.44	(12.47)
$D_L^{IV} = \dfrac{V C_{max}^{ss}}{S_{IV}}$		(12.48)
$D_L^{IV} = \dfrac{D_M^{IV}}{1 - e^{-K \tau_{IV}}}$ $D_M^{IV} = D_L^{IV}(1 - e^{-K \tau_{IV}})$	Same salt form used Same salt form used	(11.41)
$D_L^{PO} = \dfrac{D_M^{PO}}{(1 - e^{-K \tau_{PO}})(1 - e^{-K_A \tau_{PO}})}$ $D_M^{PO} = D_L^{PO}(1 - e^{-K \tau_{PO}})(1 - e^{-K_A \tau_{PO}})$	Same salt form used Same salt form used	(12.49)
$D_L^{PO} = \dfrac{S_{IV} D_M^{IV}}{S_{PO} F_{PO}(1 - e^{-K\tau})(1 - e^{-K_A \tau})}$ for $\tau_{IV} = \tau_{PO}$	Dangerous fluctuation may occur in the PO→IV conversion direction! Use IV→PO only.	(12.50)
$D_L^{PO} = \dfrac{S_{IV} D_L^{IV}}{S_{PO} F_{PO}(1 - e^{-K_A \tau})}$ for $\tau_{IV} = \tau_{PO}$	Dangerous fluctuation may occur in the PO→IV conversion direction! Use IV→PO only.	(12.51)
$D_M^{IV} = \dfrac{S_{PO} D_L^{PO} F_{PO}(1 - e^{-K \tau_{PO}})(1 - e^{-K_A \tau_{PO}}) \tau_{IV}}{S_{IV} \tau_{PO}}$	Select τ_{IV} from Eq. 12.44	(12.52)
$D_M^{IV} = \dfrac{S_{PO} D_L^{PO} F_{PO}(1 - e^{-K \tau_{PO}})(1 - e^{-K_A \tau_{PO}}) \tau_{IV}}{S_{IV}(1 - e^{-K \tau_{IV}}) \tau_{PO}}$	Select τ_{IV} from Eq. 12.44	(12.53)

necessary to solve directly for $(D_M)_{IV}$. The rule of thumb is to use the equation that has the item you want to solve for isolated on the left-hand side of the equal sign. The reason for this caution is that going in the direction from a known oral regimen to a calculated intravenous regimen necessitates the calculation of a shorter dosing interval in order to control the excessive fluctuation that would otherwise occur from the multiple intravenous bolus regimen. Of course, Eq. 12.19 (which relates $(C_{ave})_{ss}$ to X_0/τ) tells us that if the interval is shortened, the dose should be decreased proportionately in order to keep $(C_{ave})_{ss}$ the same.

Equation 12.42

This is the simplest equation in this series. Going from a known, satisfactory maintenance intravenous bolus regimen to a maintenance oral regimen, we can safely keep the same dosing interval: that is set $\tau_{oral} = \tau_{IV}$. If anything, the fluctuation at steady state (Φ_{ss}) will decrease. So, it is safe with respect to toxic peaks or subtherapeutic troughs. Since the dosing interval has not been changed, we do *not* have to adjust the dose by the multiplying by a factor $[\tau_{new}/\tau_{old}]$. The only possible adjustment is in the case when the fraction of the administered oral dose reaching general circulation or absorbed (F_{oral}) is <1. In this situation, Eq. 12.42 will cause the oral dose to be larger than the intravenous bolus dose by a factor $1/F_{oral}$. Do not rearrange Eq. 12.42 algebraically to solve for $(D_M)_{IV}$ based on an existing $(D_M)_{oral}$. Instead, use Eq. 12.43, which is ready made for that purpose.

Equation 12.43

Notice that Eq. 12.43 includes two different dosing intervals: τ_{IV} in the numerator and τ_{oral} in the denominator; τ_{oral} is the known interval for a satisfactory oral dosing regimen. In order to control fluctuation for the new multiple intravenous bolus dosing regimen, it is necessary to calculate a smaller (shorter) value for τ_{IV} and then insert this value into the numerator of Eq. 12.43. Since this means that the intravenous bolus will be given more frequently, and since $(C_{ave})_{ss}$ should

be kept the same, the multiple intravenous bolus regimen needs to give less drug. This proportional adjustment is made by multiplying $(D_M)_{oral}$ by $[\tau_{IV}/\tau_{oral}]$. Of course, $(D_M)_{oral}$ is also multiplied by F_{oral}, in case this is <1, so that excessive drug is not provided by the intravenous route. Getting back to τ_{IV}; it is clear that this needs to be smaller than τ_{oral}, but how much smaller? An equation is needed that will equate fluctuation at steady state from the multiple intravenous bolus regimen to the (satisfactory) fluctuation at steady state from the multiple oral regimen. Equation 12.44 serves this purpose.

Equation 12.44

Equation 12.44 is based on $(\Phi_{ss})_{IV} = 1/(e^{-k\tau}) = e^{+k\tau}$. However, in order to use Eq. 12.44, $(\Phi_{ss})_{oral}$, the fluctuation from the existing multiple oral regimen, must be calculated. Equation 12.45 covers the situation when the absorption rate constant is at least five times the size of the elimination rate constant; Eq. 12.30 is used when this assumption is not justified.

But our work is still not done! In order to use either Eq. 12.45 or Eq. 12.30, a value for t'_{max}, the time to peak at steady state from our oral regimen, is needed. This is calculated from Eq. 12.7, for which we know values of the absorption and the elimination rate constants. Once the time to peak at steady state for the oral regimen is calculated, we can work our way backwards: t'_{max} allows calculation of $(\Phi_{ss})_{oral}$ by Eq. 12.45 or 12.30; then having a value of $(\Phi_{ss})_{oral}$ allows calculation of τ_{IV} by Eq. 12.44. Finally τ_{IV} can be inserted into Eq. 12.43 and the equation solved for the new multiple intravenous bolus maintenance dose, $(D_M)_{IV}$.

This same procedure is used to calculate τ_{IV} for use in Eqs 12.47, 12.52 and 12.53 when calculation of $(D_L)_{IV}$ from $(D_M)_{oral}$, $(D_M)_{IV}$ from $(D_L)_{oral}$, or $(D_L)_{IV}$ from $(D_L)_{oral}$, respectively, is needed.

Equation 12.46

Equation 12.46 is used to go from a known $(D_L)_{IV}$ to a $(D_M)_{oral}$. Again, this equation should not be rearranged algebraically to go in the opposite direction (instead simply use Eq. 12.47.) Notice that Eq. 12.46 first converts $(D_L)_{IV}$ to $(D_M)_{IV}$ by multiplying $(D_L)_{IV}$ by the inverse of the accumulation factor $1/R_{IV}$ (see Eq. 11.41). Equation 12.47 then adjusts for extent of oral absorption <1 by dividing the result by F_{oral}.

Equation 12.47

Equation 12.47 is used to go from a known $(D_M)_{oral}$ to a $(D_L)_{IV}$.

Equation 12.48

$(D_L)_{IV}$ can also be calculated from Eq. 12.48 provided that the volume of distribution and desired target peak plasma concentration are known. Notice that $(D_L)_{IV}$ will instantly give the same plasma drug concentration that would be achieved by giving $(D_M)_{IV}$ repeatedly until steady state.

Equation 11.41, which can be used in either direction, shows that $(D_L)_{IV}$ equals $(D_M)_{IV} \times R_{IV}$.

Equation 12.49, which also can be used in either direction, shows that $(D_L)_{oral}$ equals $(D_M)_{oral} \times R_{oral}$.

Equation 12.50

Equation 12.50 is safe to use to convert $(D_M)_{IV}$ to $(D_L)_{oral}$, but not in the opposite direction (instead use Eq. 12.52). Equation 12.50 can be thought of as first converting $(D_M)_{IV}$ to $(D_M)_{oral}$ by dividing by F_{oral}, as was done in Eq. 12.42. Next, $(D_M)_{oral}$ is converted to $(D_L)_{oral}$ by multiplying by the oral accumulation factor R_{oral}.

Equation 12.51

Equation 12.51 may be used to convert $(D_L)_{IV}$ to $(D_L)_{oral}$, but not in the opposite direction (instead use Eq. 12.53). Equation 12.51 uses Eq. 12.52 to express $(D_L)_{oral}$ in terms of $(D_M)_{IV}$ and then recognizes from Eq. 11.41 that $(D_M)_{IV} = (D_L)_{IV}/R_{IV}$. Notice that $(D_L)_{oral}$ does not simply equal $(D_L)_{IV}/F_{oral}$.

Problem set 5

Problems for Chapters 11 and 12

Question 1

A 70 kg male with a history of asthma has been admitted to the hospital for a severe acute asthmatic attack and is given 300 mg aminophylline as an intravenous bolus of the dihydrate every 8 h (dosing interval, τ) to control the attack. From prior history in this patient:

- elimination half life $(t_{1/2}) = 7$ h
- apparent volume of distribution of theophylline $(V) = 30$ L.

Aminophylline dihydrate is the ethylenediamine salt of theophylline containing two waters of hydration and 79% as active drug.

a. Calculate the maximum steady-state plasma concentration of theophylline, $(C_{p\infty})_{max}$.
b. Calculate the 'trough', or minimum, steady-state plasma concentration of theophylline, $(C_{p\infty})_{min}$.
c. Calculate the 'average' steady-state concentrations of theophylline, $(\bar{C}_p)_{ss}$ for the dosage regimen above and for a regimen in which one-half the original dose is administered at 4 h intervals.
d. What will be the theophylline plasma concentration immediately prior to the administration of the fourth dose?
e. What will be the theophylline plasma concentration immediately following the administration of the fourth dose?
f. Determine the drug accumulation factor (R), in as many ways as you can think of for the two different dosage regimens employed in (c) of this question.

g. Determine the fluctuation (Φ) for the two different dosage regimens employed in (c) of this question.
h. What is the loading-dose needed to produce an immediate steady-state concentration?
i. How long will it take to reach one half of the steady-state concentration of theophylline (i.e. $f_{ss} = 0.50$)?
j. A patient weighing 200 lb receives 520 mg theophylline per day as Tedral tablets. The drug is 100% available for absorption from the tablets, and its elimination half life and apparent volume of distribution are 4.5 h and 0.48 L kg^{-1}, respectively.
   What 'average' steady-state plasma concentration $(C_p)_{ss}$ would be obtained?

Question 2

A 60 kg patient with cardiac arrhythmias is going to be given procainamide HCl orally every 6 h. The clinical pharmacist is asked to recommend a loading and maintenance dose to achieve an 'average' steady-state concentration of $6 \mu g\,mL^{-1}$. Procainamide has:

- half life $(t_{1/2}) = 3.5$ h
- apparent volume of distribution $(V) = 1.7$ L kg^{-1}
- absolute bioavailability $(F) = 0.85$
- salt value $(S) = 0.87$
- elimination rate constant $(K) = 0.198$ h^{-1}
- absorption rate constant $(K_a) = 2.31$ h^{-1}.

a. Calculate the oral maintenance dose (D_m).
b. Calculate a maintenance intravenous bolus regimen using a dosing interval of 4 h to prevent excessive fluctuation.

257

c. Assuming that the next intravenous (maintenance) dose will be given in 4 h, calculate the loading dose (D_L) if procainamide HCl were to be administered as an intravenous bolus.

d. How long will it take to attain 97% of the 'average' steady-state concentration, $(\bar{C}_p)_{ss}$ in the absence of a loading dose?

Question 3

An antihypertensive drug is to be administered as an intravenous bolus to a patient at a dosage regimen of 1600 mg daily in four equally divided doses at equal time intervals. Drug data are:

- elimination half life ($t_{1/2}$) = 5 h
- apparent volume of distribution (V) = 68.5 L.

a. Calculate the 'average' steady-state concentration, $(\bar{C}_p)_{ss}$.

b. How long does it take to reach the steady-state?

c. What is the loading dose (D_L) required to produce an immediate steady-state concentration?

Question 4

Digitoxin is available as an oral dosage form with:

- absorption rate constant (K_a) = 1.40 h^{-1}
- elimination half life ($t_{1/2}$) = 6 days.

a. What is the accumulation factor (R) of digitoxin administered once daily?

Question 5

Acetozolamide was administered as an oral dose of 500 mg to nine patients with glaucoma. The following pharmacokinetic parameters were reported:

- absorption rate constant (K_a) = 2.20 h^{-1}
- elimination rate constant (K) = 0.180 h^{-1}
- apparent volume of distribution (V) = 14 L
- absolute bioavailability (F) = 1.

The maximum amount of acetozolamide desired in the body (minimum toxic concentration;

MTC) is 600 mg; while 10 mg L^{-1} is the minimum plasma concentration required for therapeutic effect (MEC).

a. Choose a dosage regimen for this drug. Tablets are available in 125 and 250 mg strengths.

Question 6

Elixophylline elixir contains 80 mg anhydrous theophylline per tablespoonful and drug is completely absorbed. An 88 lb female patient receives 8 tablespoonfuls of Elixophylline elixir once daily. The patient's data are:

- elimination half life ($t_{1/2}$) = 6.93 h
- apparent volume of distribution (V) = 0.50 L kg^{-1}.

Incidentally, this product also contains 20% v/v of ethanol as a co-solvent.

a. What 'average' steady-state plasma concentration, $(\bar{C}_p)_{ss}$ would be attained?

b. How much ethanol does the patient receive per day?

Question 7

Lisinopril (Zestril) is an angiotensin-converting enzyme inhibitor used for the treatment of hypertension, alone or in combination with thiazide diuretics. Reported data are (Ritschel and Kearns, 2004):

- therapeutic range = 0.025–0.04 µg mL^{-1}
- systemic clearance (Cl_s) = 8352 mL h^{-1}
- absolute bioavailability (F) = 30%.

a. Will a dosage regimen of a 20 mg Zestril tablet once daily, to a subject with hypertension provide the 'average' steady-state plasma concentration, $(\bar{C}_p)_{ss}$ necessary to control hypertension?

Question 8

Vancomycin (Vancocin) is used for serious or severe infections not treatable with other antimicrobial drugs. Reported values are (Ritschel and Kearns, 2004):

- therapeutic range $= 5–40\,\mu g\,mL^{-1}$
- elimination half life $(t_{1/2}) = 6\,h$
- apparent volume of distribution $(V) = 0.47\ L\,kg^{-1}$.

a. Will the intravenous bolus dose of $4.5\,mg\,kg^{-1}$ of vancomycin, administered repetitively every 6 h (dosing interval; τ) to a subject, provide peak, trough and 'average' steady-state vancomycin plasma concentrations $[(C_{p\infty})_{max}, (C_{p\infty})_{min}, (\bar{C}_p)_{ss}$, respectively] within the therapeutic range of the drug?

b. Using information obtained, determine the vancomycin accumulation in the subject in Question 6 (88 lb female patient) by using two different approaches.

Question 9

Bromopride (Viaben) is an antiemetic agent chemically related to metoclopromide (Reglan). Following the administration of a capsule containing 20 mg bromopride to healthy subjects, Brodie *et al.* (1986) reported:

- elimination half life $(t_{1/2}) = 2.8\,h$
- absorption half life $(t_{1/2})_{abs} = 0.575\,h$
- plasma concentration–time profile intercept (I) on the y-axis $= 44\,ng\,mL^{-1}$
- absolute bioavailability $(F) = 45\%$.

a. Determine the peak time (t_{max}) following the administration of a 20 mg capsule.
b. Determine the peak time following the administration of a 20 mg capsule repetitively at 8 h interval until the attainment of steady state (t'_{max}).
c. Determine the 'average' steady-state bromopride plasma concentrations, $(\bar{C}_p)_{ss}$ for the dosage regimens of a 10 mg capsule every 4 h and 20 mg capsule every 8 h.
d. Determine the drug accumulation factor (R) for the dosage regimens of 10 mg capsule every 6 h or a 20 mg capsule every 6 h.
e. Determine the drug accumulation for the dosage regimen of a 20 mg capsule every 4 h.

Answers

Question 1 answer

a. As salt value of aminophyliine is 0.79, 300 mg aminophylline gives a dose of 237 mg theophylline. Also,

elimination rate constant $(K) = 0.099\,h^{-1}$
initial plasma concentration,
$(C_p)_0 = Dose/V = 237\,000\,\mu g/30\,000\,mL$
$(C_p)_0 = 7.90\,\mu g\,mL^{-1}$.

For an *intravenous bolus administration*,

$$(C_{p\infty})_{max} = \frac{(C_p)_0}{1 - e^{-K\tau}}$$

$$(C_{p\infty})_{max} = \frac{7.90\,\mu g\,mL^{-1}}{1 - e^{-0.099\times8}} = \frac{7.90\,\mu g\,mL^{-1}}{1 - e^{-0.792}}$$

$$= \frac{7.90\,\mu g\,mL^{-1}}{0.5471} = 14.44\,\mu g\,mL^{-1}.$$

b. For an intravenous bolus administration,

$$(C_{p\infty})_{min} = \frac{(C_p)_0}{1 - e^{-K\tau}} \times e^{-K\tau}$$

$$(C_{p\infty})_{min} = \frac{7.90\,\mu g\,mL^{-1}}{1 - e^{-0.099(8)}} \times e^{-0.099(8)}$$

$$= 14.44\,\mu g\,mL^{-1} \times 0.45293$$

$$= 6.540\,\mu g\,mL^{-1}.$$

c. For an intravenous bolus administration,

$$(\bar{C}_p)_{ss} = \frac{Dose}{VK\tau} = \frac{X_0}{VK\tau}$$

$$(\bar{C}_p)_{ss} = \frac{237\,000\,\mu g}{(30\,000\,mL)(0.099\,h^{-1})(8\,h)}$$

$$= \frac{237\,000\,\mu g}{23\,760\,mL} = 9.975\,\mu g\,mL^{-1}.$$

For the dosage regimen of 300 mg aminophylline (237 mg theophylline) administered intravenously every 8 h, the 'average' steady-state theophylline plasma concentration is $9.975\,\mu g\,mL^{-1}$ (please note that this value is not the arithmetic mean of the peak and trough theophylline plasma concentrations). If one-half the dose (150 mg aminophylline or 118.5 mg theophylline) is administered every

$4\,h$ ($\tau = 4\,h$), the 'average' steady-state theophylline plasma concentration will be:

$$(\bar{C}_p)_{ss} = \frac{(X)_0}{VK\tau}$$

$$= \frac{118\,500\,\mu g}{(30\,000\,\text{mL})(0.099\,h^{-1})(4\,h)}$$

$$= \frac{118\,500\,\mu g}{11\,880\,\text{mL}} = 9.975\,\mu g\,\text{mL}^{-1}.$$

Please note that since the ratio of dose over dosing interval remained identical and the systemic clearance is same for the drug, the 'average' theophylline plasma concentration did not change. *Question for reflection*: Will the peak and 'trough' concentrations for this dosage regimen be the same as that of the previous dosage regimen (i.e. 300 mg every 8 h)? Consider the answer carefully.

d. The theophylline plasma concentration immediately prior to the administration of the fourth dose ($n = 4$) will be the same as the minimum or trough plasma concentration (at $t = \tau$) following the administration of the third dose, $(C_{p3})_{min}$. In this problem, $n = 3$ (third dose), $\tau = 8\,h$, $K = 0.099\,h^{-1}$ and $(C_p)_0 = 7.90\,\mu g\,\text{mL}^{-1}$.

$$(C_{pn})_{min} = \frac{(C_p)_0(1 - e^{-nK\tau})}{1 - e^{-K\tau}} \times e^{-K\tau}$$

$$(C_{p3})_{min} = \frac{7.90\,\mu g\,\text{mL}^{-1}(1 - e^{-(3)(0.099)(8)})}{1 - e^{-(0.099)(8)}}$$

$$\times e^{-(0.099)(8)}$$

$$(C_{p3})_{min} = \frac{7.90\,\mu g\,\text{mL}^{-1}(1 - e^{-2.376})}{1 - e^{-0.792}} \times e^{-0.792}$$

$$= \frac{7.90\,\mu g\,\text{mL}^{-1}(1 - 0.09292)}{1 - 0.45293} \times 0.45293$$

$$= 5.933\,\mu g\,\text{mL}^{-1}$$

e. The theophylline plasma concentration immediately after the administration of the fourth dose ($n = 4$) will be the same as the peak plasma concentration following the administration of the fourth dose, $(C_{p4})_{max}$. This occurs immediately ($t = 0$) after the fourth dose is given. In this problem, $n = 4$ (fourth dose), $\tau = 8\,h$, $K = 0.099\,h^{-1}$ and $(C_p)_0 = 7.90\,\mu g\,\text{mL}^{-1}$.

$$(C_{pn})_{max} = \frac{(C_p)_0(1 - e^{-nK\tau})}{1 - e^{-K\tau}} \times e^{-K(0)}$$

$$= \frac{(C_p)_0(1 - e^{-nK\tau})}{1 - e^{-K\tau}}$$

$$(C_{p4})_{max} = \frac{7.90\,\mu g\,\text{mL}^{-1}(1 - e^{-(4)(0.099)(8)})}{1 - e^{-(0.099)(8)}}$$

$$= \frac{7.90\,\mu g\,\text{mL}^{-1}(1 - e^{-3.1768})}{1 - e^{-0.792}}$$

$$= \frac{7.90\,\mu g\,\text{mL}^{-1}(1 - 0.04208)}{1 - 0.45293}$$

$$(C_{p4})_{max} = \frac{7.90\,\mu g\,\text{mL}^{-1}(0.95792)}{0.54707}$$

$$= 13.832\,\mu g\,\text{mL}^{-1}.$$

f. The drug accumulation factor (R) can be determined from knowledge of peak plasma concentration at steady state $(C_{p\infty})_{max}$ and peak plasma concentration following the administration of dose 1, $(C_{p1})_{max}$, of the dosage regimen; *or* the trough plasma concentration at steady state $(C_{p\infty})_{min}$ and the minimum plasma concentration for the first dose, $(C_{p1})_{min}$; *or* the 'average' plasma concentration at steady state $(C_p)_{ss}$ and the 'average' plasma concentration following the administration of the first dose, $(C_{p1})_{ss}$; *or* the elimination half life of a drug ($t_{1/2}$) and the dosing interval (τ) of the dosage regimen. For the theophylline dosage regimen of 237 mg every 8 h, we have determined:

$$(C_{p\infty})_{max} = 14.44\,\mu g/\text{mL}$$
$$(C_{p\infty})_{min} = 6.540\,\mu g\,\text{mL}^{-1}$$
$$(C_p)_{ss} = 9.975\,\mu g\,\text{mL}^{-1}.$$

Peak plasma concentration for the first dose $(C_{p1})_{max} = (C_p)_0 = 7.9\,\mu g\,\text{mL}^{-1}$ (Dose/V)
Minimum plasma concentration following the administration of the first dose, $(C_{p1})_{min}$, can be obtained as follows:

$$(C_{p1})_{min} = (C_p)_0 e^{-K\tau}$$
$$(C_{p1})_{min} = 7.9\,\mu g\,\text{mL}^{-1} \times e^{-0.099 \times 8}$$
$$(C_{p1})_{min} = 7.9\,\mu g\,\text{mL}^{-1} \times e^{-0.792}$$
$$(C_{p1})_{min} = 7.9\,\mu g\,\text{mL}^{-1} \times 0.45293$$
$$(C_{p1})_{min} = 3.578\,\mu g\,\text{mL}^{-1}.$$

$$R = \frac{(C_{p\infty})_{max}}{(C_{p1})_{max}} = \frac{\dfrac{(C_p)_0}{1-e^{-K\tau}}}{(C_p)_0} = \frac{1}{1-e^{-K\tau}}$$

or

$$R = \frac{(C_{p\infty})_{min}}{(C_{p1})_{min}} = \frac{\dfrac{(C_p)_0 e^{-K\tau}}{1-e^{-K\tau}}}{(C_p)_0 e^{-K\tau}} = \frac{1}{1-e^{-K\tau}}$$

or

$$R = \frac{(\bar{C}_p)_{ss}}{(\bar{C}_p)_{n=1}} = \frac{1}{1-e^{-K\tau}}$$

$(C_{p1})_{ss}$ can be determined from:

$$(\bar{C}_p)_{n=1} = (\bar{C}_p)_{ss}(1-e^{-K\tau})$$

$$
\begin{aligned}
(\bar{C}_p)_{n=1} &= 9.975\,\mu g\,mL^{-1}(1-e^{-(0.099)(8)}) \\
&= 9.975\,\mu g\,mL^{-1}(1-e^{-0.792}) \\
&= (9.975\,\mu g\,mL^{-1})(1-0.45293) \\
&= 5.457\,\mu g\,mL^{-1}
\end{aligned}
$$

where $(\bar{C}_p)_{n=1}$ is the 'average' steady-state plasma concentration following the administration of the first dose.

Using the available information and an appropriate equation, R can be determined in various ways as described below. Please note that, regardless of the method chosen, the value of R will be same. Moreover, it is affected only by the dosing interval and the elimination half life of a drug.

$$R = \frac{1}{1-e^{-K\tau}} = \frac{1}{1-e^{-(0.099)(8)}} = \frac{1}{1-e^{-0.792}}$$
$$= \frac{1}{1-0.45293} = 1.828$$

$$R = \frac{(C_{p\infty})_{max}}{(C_{p1})_{max}} = \frac{14.44\,\mu g\,mL^{-1}}{7.9\,\mu g\,mL^{-1}} = 1.828$$

$$R = \frac{(C_{p\infty})_{min}}{(C_{p1})_{min}} = \frac{6.540\,\mu g\,mL^{-1}}{3.578\,\mu g\,mL^{-1}} = 1.828$$

$$R = \frac{(\bar{C}_p)_{ss}}{(\bar{C}_p)_{n=1}} = \frac{9.975\,\mu g\,mL^{-1}}{5.457\,\mu g\,mL^{-1}} = 1.828$$

For the aminophylline dosage regimen of 150 mg every 4 h (i.e. 118.5 mg theophylline every 4 h), one would expect greater accumulation of drug since dosing interval (τ) is smaller. The drug accumulation can be determined by employing same methods. For example,

$$R = \frac{1}{1-e^{-K\tau}} = \frac{1}{1-e^{-(0.099)(4)}} = \frac{1}{1-e^{-0.396}}$$

$$= \frac{1}{1-0.6730} = 3.058$$

Other methods to determine R for this dosage regimen will require knowledge of $(C_{p\infty})_{max}$, $(C_{p\infty})_{min}$, $(\bar{C}_p)_{ss}$ and $(\bar{C}_{p1})_{ss}$, $(C_{p1})_{max}$ [$= (C_p)_0$] and $(C_{p1})_{min}$.

Using the methods shown above, the following values were determined for this dosage regimen:

$$
\begin{aligned}
(C_{p\infty})_{max} &= 12.079\,\mu g\,mL^{-1} \\
(C_{p\infty})_{min} &= 8.129\,\mu g\,mL^{-1} \\
(C_{p1})_{max} &= (C_p)_0 = 3.95\,\mu g\,mL^{-1} \\
(C_{p1})_{min} &= 2.658\,\mu g\,mL^{-1} \\
(\bar{C}_p)_{ss} &= 9.975\,\mu g\,mL^{-1} \\
(\bar{C}_p)_{n=1} &= 3.262\,\mu g\,mL^{-1}.
\end{aligned}
$$

Note that regardless of the method chosen, the drug accumulation factor for this dosage regimen will be 3.058.

g. Fluctuation can be determined from the knowledge of the elimination half life ($t_{1/2}$) of the drug and the dosing interval (τ) of the dosage regimen.

$$\Phi = \frac{1}{e^{-K\tau}}$$

Therefore, for the theophylline dosage regimen of 237 mg dose every 8 h,

$$\Phi = \frac{1}{e^{-(0.099)(8)}} = \frac{1}{e^{-0.792}} = \frac{1}{0.45293}$$

$$= 2.2078.$$

For the dosage regimen of 118.5 mg theophylline administrated every 4 h, the fluctuation will be smaller:

$$\Phi = \frac{1}{e^{-K\tau}} = \frac{1}{e^{-(0.099)(4)}} = \frac{1}{0.6730} = 1.485$$

The calculations in parts (f) and (g) support the theory that a smaller dose given more frequently will yield greater drug accumulation and smaller drug fluctuation.

h. It has already been determined that administration of 300 mg aminophylline (equivalent to 237 mg theophylline), every 8 h yields a peak steady-state theophylline plasma concentration of 14.44 µg mL^{-1}. The following equation allows determination of the loading dose (D_L) necessary to attain this theophylline plasma concentration instantaneously.

$$\frac{D_L}{D_m} = \frac{1}{1 - e^{-K\tau}}$$

maintenance dose $D_m = 300$ mg aminophylline (237 mg theophylline)

$\tau = 8$ h

$t_{1/2} = 7$ h

$K = 0.099$ h^{-1}

$$\frac{D_L}{D_m} = \frac{1}{1 - e^{-(0.099)(8)}} = \frac{1}{1 - e^{-0.792}}$$
$$= \frac{1}{1 - 0.45293}$$

$$D_L = D_m\left(\frac{1}{0.54707}\right) = D_m(1.8279)$$

$D_L = 300$ mg$(1.8279) = 548.37$ mg aminophylline. With a salt value of 0.79, this is equivalent to 433.2 mg theophylline.

The following approach will determine the loading dose (D_L) to attain a theophylline plasma concentration of 15.53 µg mL^{-1} instantaneously:

$$\frac{D_L}{D_m} = \frac{1}{1 - e^{-0.693(N)}}$$

where N is the number of elimination half lives in a dosing interval.
$N = \tau/t_{1/2} = 8$ h$/7$ h $= 1.1428$.

$$D_L = \frac{D_m}{1 - e^{-0.693(1.1428)}} = \frac{D_m}{1 - 0.45295}$$
$$= \frac{300 \text{ mg}}{0.54705}$$
$$= 548.395 \text{ mg aminophylline}$$

This is equivalent to 433.2 mg theophylline.

i. Time required to attain any fraction of steady state may be determined by using the following equation:

$$f_{ss} = 1 - e^{-Kt}$$
$$f_{ss} - 1 = -e^{-Kt}$$
$$K = 0.693/t_{1/2}$$
$$f_{ss} = 0.50$$
$$\ln 0.5 = -Kt$$
$$\ln 0.5 = \frac{-0.693(t)}{t_{1/2}}$$

$t/t_{1/2} = N$(number of elimination half lives required to reach a given fraction of steady state).

$$\ln 0.5 = -0.693N$$
$$-0.693/-0.693 = N = t/t_{1/2}$$
$$N = 1$$

In this example, it will take one half life (i.e. 7 h) of the drug to reach 50% of the steady-state concentration.

j. Weight of the patient $= 200$ lb $= 90.909$ kg

Administered dose $= 520$ mg $= 5.720$ mg kg^{-1}
Fraction absorbed $(F) = 100\%$ or 1.0
Dosing interval $(\tau) = 24$ h

$t_{1/2} = 4.5$ h

$K = 0.154$ h^{-1}

$V = 0.48$ L kg^{-1}

Systemic clearance: Cl$_s = VK = 6.7199$ L h^{-1} $= 0.07392$ L h^{-1} kg^{-1}.

For drugs administered extravascularly (in this example, orally),

$$(\bar{C}_p)_{ss} = \frac{F\text{Dose}}{VK\tau} = \frac{FX_0}{VK\tau}$$

$$(\bar{C}_p)_{ss} = \frac{1 \times 520\,000\,\mu g}{(43\,636\,\text{mL})(0.154\,h^{-1})(24\,h)}$$

$$= \frac{520\,000\,\mu g}{161\,278\,\text{mL}} = 3.224\,\mu g\,\text{mL}^{-1}.$$

On a body weight basis:

$$(\bar{C}_p)_{ss} = \frac{1 \times 5720\,\mu g\,kg^{-1}}{(480\,\text{mL}\,kg^{-1})(0.154\,h^{-1})(24\,h)}$$

$$= \frac{5720\,\mu g\,kg^{-1}}{1774\,\text{mL}\,kg^{-1}} = 3.224\,\mu g\,\text{mL}^{-1}.$$

The value of $(\bar{C}_p)_{ss}$ can also be found from the area under the plasma concentration versus time curve for the extravascularly administered dose of a drug:

$$(AUC)_0^\infty = \frac{FX_0}{Cl_s} = \frac{FX_0}{VK}$$

$$= \frac{1 \times 520\,000\,\mu g}{(43\,636\,\text{mL})(0.154\,h^{-1})}$$

$$= 77.38\,\mu g\,\text{mL}^{-1}\,h.$$

$$(\bar{C}_p)_{ss} = \frac{FX_0}{VK\tau}$$

For a dose administered by the extravascular route:

$$FX_0/VK = (AUC)_0^\infty$$

Substituting for FX_0/VK with the $(AUC)_0^\infty$ value in the equation above yields the 'average' plasma concentration value:

$$(\bar{C}_p)_{ss} = \frac{(AUC)_0^\infty}{\tau} = \frac{77.38\,\mu g\,\text{mL}^{-1}\,h}{24\,h}$$

$$= 3.224\,\mu g\,\text{mL}^{-1}.$$

Question 2 answer

a.
$$D_m = \frac{(\bar{C}_p)_{ss}VK\tau}{FS}$$

$$(C_p)_{ss} = \frac{FX_0}{VK\tau}$$

$$D_m = \frac{6\,\mu g\,\text{mL}^{-1} \times 102\,000\,\text{mL} \times 0.198\,h^{-1} \times 6\,h}{0.85 \times 0.87}$$

$$= \frac{727\,056\,\mu g}{0.7395} = 983.2\,\text{mg}.$$

$D_m = 983.2\,\text{mg}$ procainamide HCl orally every 6 h.

b.
$$D_m = \frac{6\,\mu g\,\text{mL}^{-1} \times 102\,000\,\text{mL} \times 0.198\,h^{-1} \times 4\,h}{1 \times 0.87}$$

$$= \frac{484\,704\,\mu g}{0.87} = 557\,\text{mg}$$

$D_m = 557\,\text{mg}$ procainamide HCl by intravenous bolus every 4 h.

c. The intravenous $D_m = 557\,\text{mg}$

$K = 0.198\,h^{-1}$
dosing interval $(\tau) = 4\,h$

$$\frac{D_L}{D_m} = \frac{1}{1 - e^{-K\tau}}$$

$$D_L = 557\,\text{mg}\left(\frac{1}{1 - e^{-(0.198)(4)}}\right)$$

$$= 557\,\text{mg}\left(\frac{1}{1 - 0.45294}\right)$$

$$= 557\,\text{mg}(1.828) = 1018\,\text{mg}.$$

In this example, therefore, administration of 1018 mg procainamide HCl as a intravenous loading dose followed by the intravenous bolus maintenance dose of 557 mg every 4 h will attain and then maintain an 'average' procainamide plasma concentration of $6\,\mu g\,\text{mL}^{-1}$.

d. Time required to attain any fraction of steady state may be determined by using the following equation:

$$f_{ss} = 1 - e^{-Kt}$$
$$f_{ss} - 1 = -e^{-Kt}$$

$$K = 0.693/t_{1/2}$$
$$f_{ss} = 0.97$$
$$(0.97 - 1) = -e^{-Kt}$$
$$\ln 0.03 = -Kt$$

$$\frac{\ln 0.03}{-K} = \frac{\ln 0.03}{-0.198\,\text{h}^{-1}} = \text{time} = t$$

$$= 17.71\,\text{h}.$$

This time is approximately 5.05 half lives of the drug.

Question 3 answer

a. For an intravenous bolus administration

$$(\bar{C}_p)_{ss} = \frac{\text{Dose}}{VK\tau} = \frac{X_0}{VK\tau}$$

In this example;
dose administered $(X_0) = 400\,\text{mg}$
dosing interval $(\tau) = 6\,\text{h}$
elimination rate constant $(K) = 0.1386\,\text{h}^{-1}$
systemic clearance
$\quad \text{Cl}_s = KV = 9494.1\,\text{mL\,h}^{-1}\ (9.4941\,\text{L\,h}^{-1})$

$$(\text{AUC})_0^\infty = \frac{\text{Dose}}{VK} = \frac{400\,000\,\mu\text{g}}{9494\,\text{mL\,h}^{-1}}$$

$$= 42.23\,\mu\text{g\,mL}^{-1}\text{h}$$

Substituting for the term AUC in the equation will permit us to determine

$$(\bar{C}_p)_{ss}$$

for the dosage regimen:

$$(\bar{C}_p)_{ss} = \frac{(\text{AUC})_0^\infty}{\tau} = \frac{42.23\,\mu\text{g\,mL}^{-1}\text{h}}{6\,\text{h}}$$

$$= 7.021\,\mu\text{g\,mL}^{-1}.$$

b. It takes time infinity to reach the true steady-state condition.

c.
$$\frac{D_L}{D_m} = \frac{1}{1 - e^{-K\tau}}$$

$$D_L = D_m\left(\frac{1}{1 - e^{-K\tau}}\right)$$

$$D_L = 400\,000\,\mu\text{g}\left(\frac{1}{1 - e^{-(0.1386)(6)}}\right)$$

$$= \left(\frac{400\,000\,\mu\text{g}}{1 - 0.4353}\right) = \left(\frac{400\,000\,\mu\text{g}}{0.5647}\right)$$

$$= 708\,340\,\mu\text{g} = 708\,\text{mg}.$$

Question 4 answer

a. Following any extravascular administration of a drug:

$$R = \left(\frac{1}{1 - e^{-K\tau}}\right)\left(\frac{1}{1 - e^{-K_a\tau}}\right)$$

dosing interval $(\tau) = 24\,\text{h}$
elimination rate constant $(K) = 0.1155\,\text{days}^{-1}$

$$R = \left(\frac{1}{1 - e^{-(0.1155)(1)}}\right)\left(\frac{1}{1 - e^{-(1.40)(24)}}\right)$$

$$= \left(\frac{1}{1 - 0.8909}\right)\left(\frac{1}{1 - 0.00000025}\right)$$

$$= \left(\frac{1}{0.1091}\right)\left(\frac{1}{1}\right) = 9.16$$

Please note that elimination half life of this drug is 6 days (i.e. 144 h) and the dose is administered every 24 h $(N = 0.166$ half life). The more frequent the administration of the dose, greater is the drug accumulation.

Question 5 answer

a.
$$\text{MTC} = \frac{600\,\text{mg}}{14\,\text{L}} = 42.85\,\text{mg\,L}^{-1}$$

The desired 'average' steady-state plasma concentration, $(\bar{C}_p)_{ss}$, must be between the MTC $(42.85\,\text{mg\,L}^{-1})$ and the MEC $(10\,\text{mg\,L}^{-1})$. Therefore,

$$\text{Target }(\bar{C}_p)_{ss} = \frac{42 + 10}{2} = 26\,\text{mg\,L}^{-1}.$$

$$(\bar{C}_p)_{ss} = \frac{F\text{Dose}}{VK\tau} = \frac{FX_0}{VK\tau}$$

$$\text{Dose} = \frac{26\,\text{mg L}^{-1} \times 14\,\text{L} \times 0.18\,\text{h}^{-1} \times 4\,\text{h}}{F(=1)}$$

$$= 262.1\,\text{mg}.$$

This is the maintenance dose administered every 4 h. Since tablets are available in 125 mg and 250 mg strengths, it is recommended that one 250 mg tablet is taken every 4 h.

$$(\bar{C}_p)_{ss} = \frac{(1)(250\,\text{mg})}{(14\,\text{L})(0.18\,\text{h}^{-1})(4\,\text{h})} = 24.80\,\text{mg L}^{-1}$$

The dosage regimen of 250 mg every 4 h will provide an 'average' steady-state plasma concentration of 24.80 mg L^{-1}, which is quite close to 26 mg L^{-1}.

Question 6 answer

a. Weight of the patient $= 88\,\text{lb} = 40\,\text{kg}$.

administered dose $= 8$ tablespoonfuls $= 120\,\text{mL}$
administered daily dose $= 640\,\text{mg}$ theophylline
absolute bioavailability $(F) = 1.00$
   Elimination rate constant $(K) = 0.100\,\text{h}^{-1}$
$V = 0.50\,\text{L kg} = 20\,\text{L}$
dosing interval $(\tau) = 24\,\text{h}$.

$$(\bar{C}_p)_{ss} = \frac{F\text{Dose}}{VK\tau} = \frac{FX_0}{VK\tau}$$

$$(\bar{C}_p)_{ss} = \frac{1 \times 640\,000\,\mu\text{g}}{(20\,000\,\text{mL})(0.100\,\text{h}^{-1})(24\,\text{h})}$$

$$= \frac{640\,000\,\mu\text{g}}{48\,000\,\text{mL}} = 13.33\,\mu\text{g mL}^{-1}.$$

b. Solution contains 20 mL alcohol in 100 mL of solution. Therefore, 120 mL (8 tablespoonfuls) contains 24 mL of alcohol.

$$\frac{(120\,\text{mL})(20\,\text{mL})}{(100\,\text{mL})} = 24\,\text{mL of ethanol}.$$

This patient will consume 24 mL of alcohol daily.

Question 7 answer

a. For oral or extravascularly administered drug,

dosing interval $(\tau) =$ every 24 h
administered dose $= 20\,\text{mg}$ daily

$$(\bar{C}_p)_{ss} = \frac{F\text{Dose}}{VK\tau} = \frac{F(X)_0}{VK\tau}$$

$$(\bar{C}_p)_{ss} = \frac{0.30 \times 20\,000\,\mu\text{g}}{(8\,352\,\text{mL h}^{-1})(24\,\text{h})}$$

$$= \frac{6000\,\mu\text{g}}{200\,448\,\text{mL}} = 0.0299\,\mu\text{g mL}^{-1}.$$

The 20 mg per day dosing of lisinopril will provide an 'average' plasma concentration within the therapeutic range of the drug.

Alternatively, for extravascularly administered dose of a drug:

$$(\text{AUC})_0^\infty = \frac{FX_0}{VK} = \frac{FX_0}{\text{Cl}_s}$$

$$(\text{AUC})_0^\infty = \frac{0.30 \times 20\,000\,\mu\text{g}}{8\,352\,\text{mL h}^{-1}}$$

$$= 0.71839\,\mu\text{g mL}^{-1}\,\text{h}.$$

$$(\bar{C}_p)_{ss} = \frac{(\text{AUC})_0^\infty}{\tau} = \frac{0.71839\,\mu\text{g mL}^{-1}\,\text{h}}{24\,\text{h}}$$

$$= 0.0299\,\mu\text{g mL}^{-1}.$$

Question 8 answer

a. Initial plasma concentration $(C_p)_0 = \text{Dose}/V$

$$(C_p)_0 = 4500\,\mu\text{g kg}^{-1}/470\,\text{mL kg}^{-1}$$
$$= 9.574\,\text{mg mL}^{-1}.$$

$$(C_{p\infty})_{\text{max}} = \frac{(C_p)_0}{1 - e^{-K\tau}}$$

$$(C_{p\infty})_{\text{max}} = \frac{9.574\,\mu\text{g mL}^{-1}}{1 - e^{-0.1155 \times 6}}$$

$$= \frac{9.574\,\mu\text{g mL}^{-1}}{1 - 0.500}$$

$$= \frac{9.574\,\mu\text{g mL}^{-1}}{0.500}$$

$$= 19.148\,\mu\text{g mL}^{-1}.$$

$$(C_{p\infty})_{min} = \frac{(C_p)_0}{1 - e^{-K\tau}} \times e^{-K\tau}$$

$$(C_{p\infty})_{min} = \frac{9.574\,\mu g\,mL^{-1}}{1 - e^{-0.1154(6)}} \times e^{-0.1154(6)}$$

$$= \frac{9.574\,\mu g\,mL^{-1}}{1 - 0.500} \times 0.500$$

$$= 9.574\,\mu g\,mL^{-1}.$$

Alternatively, as the elimination rate constant (K) is $0.1155\,h^{-1}$

$$(C_{p\infty})_{min} = (C_{p\infty})_{max} \times e^{-Kt}$$
$$(C_{p\infty})_{min} = 19.148\,\mu g\,mL^{-1} \times e^{-0.1154 \times 6}.$$
$$(C_{p\infty})_{min} = 9.574\,\mu g\,mL^{-1}.$$

For an intravenous bolus administration:

$$(\bar{C}_p)_{ss} = \frac{F Dose}{V K\tau} = \frac{F X_0}{V K\tau}$$

$$(\bar{C}_p)_{ss} = \frac{4\,500\,\mu g\,kg^{-1}}{(470\,mL\,kg^{-1})(0.1154\,h^{-1})(6\,h)}$$

$$= 13.82\,\mu g\,mL^{-1}.$$

or

$$(\bar{C}_p)_{ss} = \frac{(AUC)_0^\infty}{\tau}$$

$$(\bar{C}_p)_{ss} = \frac{(AUC)_0^\infty}{\tau} = \frac{82.895\,\mu g\,mL\,h}{6\,h}$$

$$= 13.82\,\mu g\,mL^{-1}.$$

These calculations show that this dosage regimen will provide peak, trough and 'average' plasma vancomycin concentrations within the therapeutic range of the drug.

b. Drug accumulation factor (R) of a drug can be determined by employing several approaches:

$$R = \frac{1}{1 - e^{-K\tau}}$$

$$R = \frac{1}{1 - e^{-(0.1155)(6)}} = \frac{1}{1 - e^{-0.693}}$$

$$= \frac{1}{0.5} = 2.00$$

When the dosing interval is equal to one half life of a drug, the drug accumulation factor is always equal to 2.0.
   Alternatively,

$$R = \frac{(C_{p\infty})_{max}}{(C_{p1})_{max}} = \frac{19.148\,\mu g\,mL^{-1}}{9.574\,\mu g\,mL^{-1}} = 2.00$$

$(C_{p1})_{max}$ is also equal to initial plasma concentration, $(C_p)_0$, when the drug is administered intravenously.
   Alternatively,

$$R = \frac{(C_{p\infty})_{min}}{(C_{p1})_{min}} = \frac{9.574\,\mu g\,mL^{-1}}{4.787\,\mu g\,mL^{-1}} = 2.00$$

$(C_{p1})_{min}$ is the minimum plasma concentration following the intravenous administration of the first dose of a drug, and it can be obtained as follows:

$$(C_{p1})_{min} = (C_p)_0 e^{-K\tau}$$
$$(C_{p1})_{min} = 9.574\,\mu g\,mL^{-1} \times e^{-0.1155 \times 6}$$
$$(C_{p1})_{min} = 9.574\,\mu g\,mL^{-1} \times 0.500$$
$$(C_{p1})_{min} = 4.787\,\mu g\,mL^{-1}.$$

Question 9 answer

Further data:

- elimination rate constant (K) = $0.2475\,h^{-1}$
- absorption rate constant (K_a) = $1.205\,h^{-1}$

$$I = 44\,ng\,mL^{-1} = \frac{K_a F X_0}{V(K_a - K)}$$

a. $$t_{max} = \frac{\ln(K_a/K)}{K_a - K} = \frac{\ln(1.205\,h^{-1}/0.2475\,h^{-1})}{1.205\,h^{-1} - 0.2475\,h^{-1}}$$

$$= \frac{1.5828}{0.9575\,h^{-1}} = 1.654\,h.$$

b. $$t'_{max} = \frac{2.303}{K_a - K} \log\left(\frac{(K_a)(1 - e^{-K\tau})}{(K)(1 - e^{-K_a\tau})}\right)$$

$$t'_{max} = \frac{2.303}{1.205 - 0.247} \log\left(\frac{(1.205)(1 - e^{-(0.247)(8)})}{(0.247)(1 - e^{-(1.205)(8)})}\right)$$

$$t'_{max} = \frac{2.303}{0.958} \log\left(\frac{(1.205)(1 - 0.1386)}{(0.247)(1 - 0.0000)}\right)$$

$$= 2.404 \log \frac{1.038}{0.247} = 1.498\,h$$

c. Dosage regimen of 10 mg every 4 h oral or extravascularly administered drug:

$$(\bar{C}_p)_{ss} = \frac{F\text{Dose}}{VK\tau} = \frac{FX_0}{VK\tau}$$

$$(\text{AUC})_0^\infty = \frac{F(X)_0}{VK}$$

$$(\text{AUC})_0^\infty = I\left(\frac{1}{K} - \frac{1}{K_a}\right)$$

$$(\text{AUC})_0^\infty = (22 \text{ ng mL}^{-1})$$
$$\times\left(\frac{1}{0.247 \text{ h}^{-1}} - \frac{1}{1.205 \text{ h}^{-1}}\right)$$

$$= (22 \text{ ng mL}^{-1})(4.0485 \text{ h} - 0.8299 \text{ h})$$

$$(\text{AUC})_0^\infty = 22 \text{ ng mL}^{-1} [3.21863 \text{ h}] = 70.809 \text{ ng mL}^{-1}\text{h}.$$

$$(\bar{C}_p)_{ss} = \frac{(\text{AUC})_0^\infty}{\tau} = \frac{70.809 \text{ ng mL}^{-1}\text{h}}{4 \text{ h}}$$

$$= 17.70 \text{ ng mL}^{-1}$$

For the dosage regimen of 20 mg every 8 h:
$(\text{AUC})_0^\infty = 141.622 \text{ ng mL}^{-1}\text{h}$. Similarly,

$$(\bar{C}_p)_{ss} = (\text{AUC})_0^\infty/\tau$$
$$= 141.622 \text{ ng mL}^{-1} \text{ h}/8 \text{ h}$$

$$(\bar{C}_p)_{ss} = 17.70 \text{ ng mL}^{-1}.$$

d. For 10 mg every 6 h,

$$R = \left(\frac{1}{1 - e^{-K\tau}}\right)\left(\frac{1}{1 - e^{-K_a\tau}}\right)$$

$$= \left(\frac{1}{1 - e^{-(0.247)(6)}}\right)\left(\frac{1}{1 - e^{-(1.205)(6)}}\right)$$

$$= (1.294)(1.0007) = 1.295$$

For 20 mg every 6 h, the calculation is independent of dose and yields the exact same answer: R = 1.295

e. For 20 mg every 4 h,

$$R = \left(\frac{1}{1 - e^{-(0.247)(4)}}\right)\left(\frac{1}{1 - e^{-(1.205)(4)}}\right)$$

$$= (1.593)(1.008) = 1.606$$

This shows that more frequent dosing gives rise to a larger value for the accumulation factor, R.

13

Two-compartment model

Objectives

Upon completion of this chapter, you will have the ability to:

- explain why pharmacokinetics of some drugs can be best described by employing a two-compartment model
- calculate plasma drug concentration at any time t after the administration of an intravenous bolus dose of a drug exhibiting two-compartment model
- calculate the distribution rate constant (α), and the post-distribution rate constant (β) from plasma drug concentration versus time data
- calculate and distinguish between the three volumes of distribution (V_C, V_b and V_{ss}) associated with a drug that exhibits two-compartment model characteristics
- calculate and distinguish between the rate constants (α, β, K_{10}, K_{12} and K_{21}) associated with a drug that exhibits two-compartment model characteristics.

13.1 Introduction

At the outset of this chapter, it is strongly recommended that you review the section on the compartmental concept in Ch. 1.

Most drugs entering the systemic circulation require a finite time to distribute completely throughout the body. This is particularly obvious upon rapid intravenous administration of drugs. During this distributive phase, the drug concentration in plasma will decrease more rapidly than in the post-distributive phase. Whether or not such a distributive phase is apparent will depend on the frequency with which blood samples are collected. A distributive phase may last for few minutes, for hours or, very rarely, even for days.

If drug distribution is related to blood flow, highly perfused organs such as the liver and kidneys should, generally, be in rapid distribution equilibrium with blood. The blood and all other readily accessible fluids and tissues, therefore, may often be treated kinetically as a common homogeneous unit, which is referred to as the central compartment. The kinetic homogeneity, please note, does not necessarily mean that drug distribution to all tissues of the central compartment at any given time is the same. However, it does assume that any change which occurs in plasma concentration of drug putatively reflects a change that occurs in all central compartment tissue concentrations. Consequently, following intravenous administration of a drug that exhibits multi-compartment pharmacokinetics, the

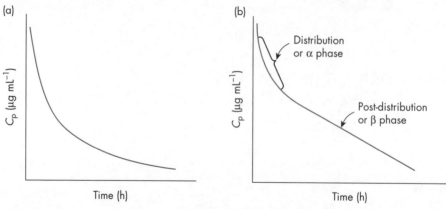

Figure 13.1   Typical plasma concentration (C_p) versus time profiles for a drug that obeys a two-compartment model following intravenous bolus administration. (a) rectilinear plot; (b) semilogarithmic plot.

concentrations of drug in all tissues and fluids associated with the central compartment (analogous to plasma and serum drug concentrations) should decline more rapidly during the distributive phase than during the post-distributive phase (Fig. 13.1).

However, drug concentrations in poorly perfused tissues (generally, muscle, lean tissues and fat) will first increase, reach a maximum and then begin to decline during the post-distributive phase (Fig. 13.2).

At some point in time, a pseudo-distribution equilibrium is attained between the tissues and fluid of the central compartment and the poorly perfused or less-readily accessible tissues (peripheral compartment). Once such a pseudo-distribution equilibrium has been established, loss of drug from plasma can be described by a mono-exponential process, indicating kinetic homogeneity with respect to drug concentrations in all fluids and tissues of the body. The access of drug to various perfused tissues may occur at different rates. However, frequently, for a given drug these rates will appear to be very similar and, therefore, cannot be differentiated based solely on plasma concentration data. Therefore, all poorly perfused tissues are often "lumped" into a single peripheral (or tissue) compartment, as illustrated in Fig. 13.3.

Figure 13.4 shows that, after an intravenous bolus injection, the central compartment fills up with drug virtually instantaneously; while the peripheral (tissue) compartment fills up with drug slowly, reaching an equilibrium with the amount of drug in the central compartment after a period of time.

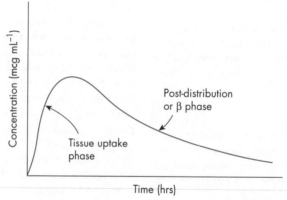

Figure 13.2   A typical concentration versus time profile for a drug in the peripheral compartment (also called the tissue compartment or compartment 2) and that obeys a two-compartment model following intravenous bolus administration.

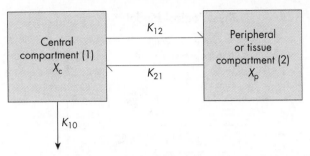

Figure 13.3 A schematic representation of a two-compartment model. K_{12}, K_{21}, transfer rate constants; K_{10}, elimination rate constant; X, mass of drug in a compartment.

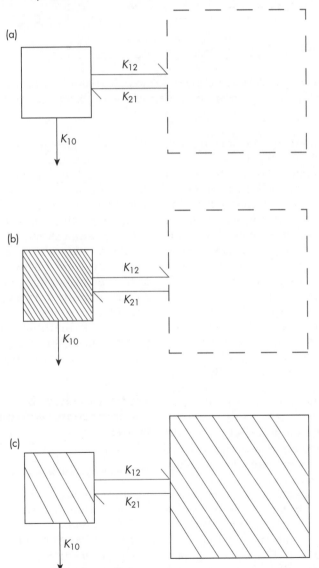

Figure 13.4 A two-compartment model prior to the administration of a drug (a), immediately after the administration of the drug (b) and after the attainment of distribution equilibrium (c). K_{12}, K_{21}, transfer rate constants; K_{10}, elimination rate constant.

Physiological Model

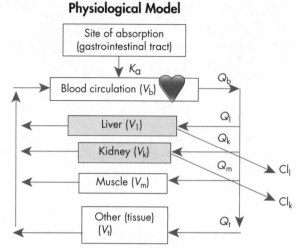

Figure 13.5 Scheme illustrating the distribution of a drug in the central compartment and various body tissues and fluid. V_b, volume of blood; Q, blood flow; l, liver; k, kidney; m, muscle; t, other tissues; b, blood; Cl, clearance.

It must be kept in mind that the time course of drug concentrations in the hypothetical peripheral compartment, as inferred or construed from the mathematical analysis of plasma concentration data, may not exactly correspond to the actual time course of drug concentrations in any real tissue or organ. The peripheral compartments of pharmacokinetic models are, at best, hybrids of several functional physiological units. Theoretically, one can assign a compartment for each organ, as illustrated in Fig. 13.5.

However, justification of such an approach is difficult, mathematically as well as practically, unless the differences in the drug behavior in each organ are dramatically and significantly different. Frequently, for a given drug, the differences in the drug behavior in each organ would appear not to be significantly different and, therefore, cannot be differentiated based solely on plasma concentration data. As a result, all poorly perfused tissues are often grouped into a single peripheral or tissue or compartment 2, as illustrated in Figs 13.3 13.6 and 13.7.

The particular compartment (i.e. central or peripheral) with which certain tissues or part of tissues or organs may be associated often depends on the properties of the particular drug being studied. For instance, the brain is a highly perfused organ; however, it is clearly separated from the blood by an apparent lipophilic barrier. Therefore, for lipid-soluble drugs, the brain would probably be in the central compartment, while for more polar drugs, the brain would probably be considered as a part of the peripheral compartment.

Although there are three possible types of two-compartment model based on the site(s) of elimination (as seen in Fig. 13.6), the most useful and common two-compartment model (called the mammillary model) has drug elimination occurring from the central compartment (Fig. 13.7).

Figure 13.8 and Table 13.1 compare and contrast the kinetics of drugs conferring one or two-compartment characteristics on the body.

13.2 Intravenous bolus administration: two-compartment model

The following assumptions are made.

1. Distribution, disposition and/or elimination of a drug follow the first-order process and passive diffusion.
2. The drug is being monitored in blood.
3. The organ responsible for removal of the drug is in the central compartment.

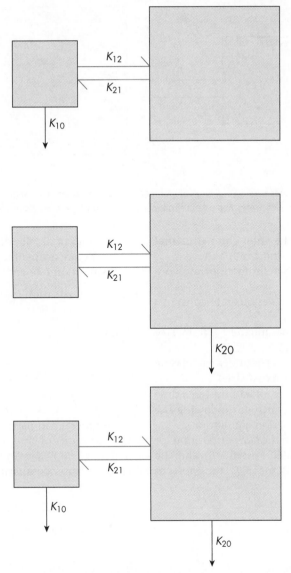

Figure 13.6   A schematic representation of three types of two-compartment models consisting of a central and a peripheral compartment. Please note the difference in each type is reflected in the placement of an organ responsible for the elimination of the drug from the body. K_{12}, K_{21}, transfer rate constants; K_{10}, K_{20}, elimination rate constants.

Useful equations and pharmacokinetic parameters

1. Equation for predicting plasma concentration during distribution and post- distribution phases.

2. Determination of post-distribution (or slow disposition, or terminal) half life $(t_{1/2})_\beta$ and its corresponding rate constant (β).

3. Determination of the distribution half life $(t_{1/2})_\alpha$ and distribution rate constant (α).

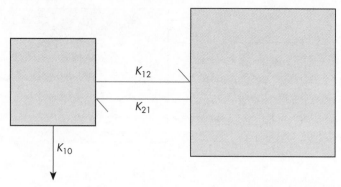

Figure 13.7   A schematic representation of a two-compartment model most commonly employed to describe the kinetics of drugs that are slowly distributed following their administration. K_{12}, K_{21}, transfer rate constants; K_{10}, elimination rate constant.

4. Determination of the inter-compartmental (or transfer) rate constants (K_{21} and K_{12})
5. Determination of the elimination rate constant (K_{10}).
6. Relationship between various rate constants (α, β, K_{12}, K_{21} and K_{10}).
7. Determination of the apparent volumes of drug distribution (V_C, V_b, and V_{ss}).
8. Determination of the area under the plasma concentration time curve, $(AUC)_0^\infty$.
9. Fraction, or percentage, of administered dose present in each compartment following the attainment of distribution equilibrium.
10. Relationship between the slow disposition (or post-distribution) rate constant (β) and the elimination rate constant (K_{10}), the apparent

volumes of distribution (V_C and V_b), and the inter-compartmental rate constant (K_{21}) and distribution rate constant (α).

Differential equation for the set up and scheme:

$$\frac{dX_C}{dt} = K_{21}X_p - K_{12}X_C - K_{10}X_C \qquad (13.1)$$

where dX_C/dt is the the rate of change in the mass (amount) of drug in the central compartment (e.g. $\mathrm{mg\,h^{-1}}$); X_p is the mass (amount) of drug in the peripheral compartment (e.g. mg); X_C is the mass (amount) of drug in the central compartment (e.g. mg); K_{21} and K_{12} are the apparent first-order inter-compartmental distribution, or

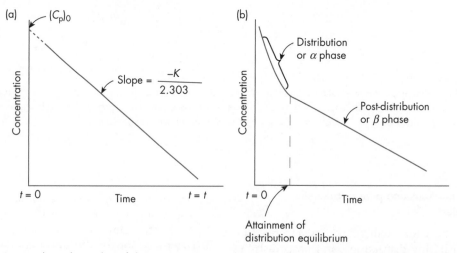

Figure 13.8   Semilogarithmic plots of drug concentration in the plasma for a one-compartment drug (a) and for a two-compartment drug (b).

Table 13.1 The kinetics of drugs conferring one- or two-compartment characteristics on the body

Body as One Compartment	Body as Two Compartments
Rapid or prompt equilibrium is attained.	Distribution equilibrium is slow (takes finite time).
There is a single disposition phase, i.e. the separation of distribution and elimination is neither desired nor possible.	Distribution and post-distribution are two distinct phases.
Equal rates into and out of tissues occur immediately.	Equal rates occur at a finite time.

transfer, rate constants (e.g. $\min^{-1}$); and K_{10} is the apparent first-order elimination rate constant (e.g. $\min^{-1}$) from the central compartment.

It should be noted that, in Eq. 13.1, the term $K_{21}X_p$ represents the rate of transfer of drug from compartment 2 (i.e. tissue or peripheral) to compartment 1 (i.e. central), the term $K_{12}X_C$ represents the rate of transfer from compartment 1 (i.e. central) to compartment 2 (i.e. peripheral or tissue), and the term $K_{10}X_C$ represents the rate of transfer of drug from compartment 1 (i.e. central) to outside the body (i.e. the elimination rate). Also, only one of the rates shows a positive sign. (Why?)

When distribution equilibrium is attained at a finite time (from a few minutes to a few hours), build up of drug in the tissue compartment stops and the body begins to behave as a single homogeneous compartment, with drug in both the central and peripheral compartments declining exponentially with the same rate constant β.

Using Laplace transforms and matrix algebra to solve the resulting simultaneous equations, Equation 13.1 becomes:

$$X_C = \frac{X_0(\alpha - K_{21})}{\alpha - \beta}e^{-\alpha t} + \frac{X_0(K_{21} - \beta)}{\alpha - \beta}e^{-\beta t}$$

$$(13.2)$$

where X_0 is the the administered dose (e.g. mg); α is the the distribution rate constant, which is associated with the distributive or α phase; (e.g. h^{-1}); β is the the slow disposition, or post-distribution, rate constant, which is associated with the slow disposition phase (β phase or terminal linear phase) (e.g. h^{-1}).

However, since

$$X_C = V_C C_p \qquad (13.3)$$

where V_C is the apparent volume of distribution for the central compartment (e.g. mL) and C_p is the plasma concentration (e.g. $\mu g\,mL^{-1}$), Eq. 13.2 can be written in concentration terms as follows:

$$C_p = \frac{X_0(\alpha - K_{21})}{V_C(\alpha - \beta)}e^{-\alpha t} + \frac{X_0(K_{21} - \beta)}{V_C(\alpha - \beta)}e^{-\beta t}$$

$$(13.4)$$

Equation 13.4 can be rearranged to solve for the dose that would produce a given C_p at time t:

$$X_0 = \frac{C_p V_c(\alpha - \beta)}{(\alpha - K_{21})e^{-\alpha t} + (K_{21} - \beta)e^{-\beta t}} \qquad (13.5)$$

Equation 13.4 can be written as:

$$C_p = Ae^{-\alpha t} + Be^{-\beta t} \qquad (13.6)$$

A semilogarithmic plot of plasma concentration versus time will yield a biexponential curve (Fig. 13.9).

In Eq. 13.6, A is an empirical constant (intercept on y-axis) with units of concentration (e.g. $\mu g\,mL^{-1}$).

$$A = \frac{X_0(\alpha - K_{21})}{V_C(\alpha - \beta)} \qquad (13.7)$$

B is also an empirical constant (intercept on y-axis) with units of concentration (e.g. $\mu g\,mL^{-1}$).

$$B = \frac{X_0(K_{21} - \beta)}{V_C(\alpha - \beta)} \qquad (13.8)$$

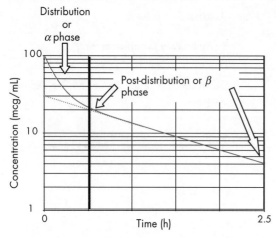

Figure 13.9 A typical plasma concentration (C_p) versus time profile for a drug that obeys a two-compartment model following intravenous bolus administration (semilogarithmic plot).

Please note the values of A and B are directly proportional to the dose administered since the empirical constants A and B have concentration units and the drug is assumed to follow the first-order process (i.e. concentration-independent kinetics) and passive diffusion. All the rate constants involved in a two-compartment model, therefore, will have units consistent with the first-order process.

For ordinary pharmacokinetics, the distribution rate constant (α) is greater than the slow disposition, or post-distribution rate constant (β)

and, hence, at some time, t (generally at a time following the attainment of distribution equilibrium), the term $Ae^{-\alpha t}$ of Eq. 13.6 will approach zero while the term $Be^{-\beta t}$ will still have a finite value. At some finite time, therefore, Eq. 13.6 will collapse to:

$$C_p = Be^{-\beta t} \tag{13.9}$$

which, in common logarithmic form, becomes:

$$\log(C_p)_t = \log B - \frac{\beta t}{2.303} \tag{13.10}$$

13.3 Determination of the post-distribution rate constant (β) and the coefficient (B)

The slow disposition, or post-distribution, rate constant (β) and the empirical constant B may be obtained graphically by plotting plasma concentration (C_p) versus time data on semilogarithmic paper.

The following procedure is used.

1. Determine $(t_{1/2})_\beta$ from the graph by using the method employed in previous chapters.
2. $\beta = 0.693/(t_{1/2})_\beta$; or $(slope) \times 2.303 = -\beta\,h^{-1}$; please note that slope will be negative and, hence, β will be positive.
3. The y-axis intercept of the extrapolated line is B (e.g. $\mu g\,mL^{-1}$).

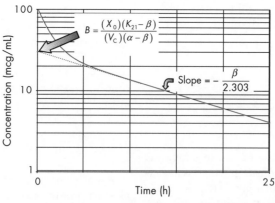

Figure 13.10 A plasma concentration (C_p) versus time profile for a drug that obeys a two-compartment model following intravenous bolus administration plotted on semilogarithmic paper. β, slow disposition, or post-distribution, rate constant; B, empirical constant; V_c, apparent volume of distribution for the central compartment; K_{21}, transfer rate constant; X_0, administered dose; α, distribution rate constant.

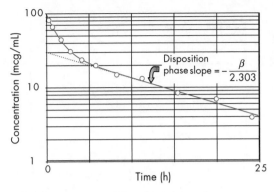

Solid curve = curve of best fit to data points
Dotted line = extrapolation of terminal linear segment
of curve

Figure 13.11 A plasma concentration (C_p) versus time profile for a drug that obeys a two-compartment model following intravenous bolus administration (semilogarithmic plot). β, slow disposition, or post-distribution, rate constant.

13.4 Determination of the distribution rate constant (α) and the coefficient (A)

The method of residuals is a commonly employed technique for resolving a curve into various exponential terms. This method is also known as feathering or curve stripping (see p.102). The curve from the observed data and that for the extrapolated line are depicted in Fig. 13.11. Table 13.2 gives the headings for the data that can be extracted from the figure.

The difference between plasma concentrations measured and those obtained by extrapolation $(C_p)_{diff}$ (values from column 4) versus time (values from column 1) are then plotted on the same or separate semilogarithmic paper (Fig. 13.12).

The following procedure is used.

1. Determine $(t_{1/2})_\alpha$ phase.
2. $\alpha = 0.693/(t_{1/2})_\alpha$ or (slope) $\times 2.303 = -\alpha\,h^{-1}$; again, note that slope will be negative and the distribution rate constant (α) will be positive. The distribution rate constant (α) is greater than the slow disposition rate constant (β).
3. The y-axis intercept is A (e.g. $\mu g\,mL^{-1}$).

When an administered drug exhibits the characteristics of a two-compartment model, the difference between the distribution rate constant (α) and the slow (post-) distribution rate constant (β) plays a critical role. The greater the difference between these, the more conspicuous is the existence of a two-compartment model and, therefore, the greater is the need to apply all the equations for a two-compartment model. Failure to do so will, undoubtedly, result in inaccurate clinical predictions. If, however, the difference between the distribution and the slow post-distribution rate constant is small and will not cause any significant difference in the clinical predictions, regardless of the model chosen to describe the pharmacokinetics of a drug, then it may be prudent to follow the principle of

Table 13.2 Method of residuals to calculate the difference between the extrapolated and observed plasma concentrations values

Time (h)	$(C_p)_{obs}$ $(\mu g\,mL^{-1})$	$(C_p)_{extrap}$ $(\mu g\,mL^{-1})$	$(C_p)_{diff}$ $(\mu g\,mL^{-1})$
0.25			
0.50			
0.75			
1.0			

$(C_p)_{extrap}$, extrapolated plasma concentrations; $(C_p)_{obs}$, observed plasma concentrations; $(C_p)_{diff}$, difference between extrapolated and observed values for each time in the absorption phase.

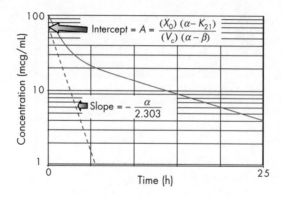

Solid curve = curve of best fit curve to observed plasma drug
levels
Dashed line = residual line, $(C_p)_{diff}$, related to rate of distribution
of drug

Figure 13.12 A semilogarithmic plot of the difference between plasma concentrations measured and those obtained by extrapolation $[(C_p)_{diff}]$ for a drug that obeys a two-compartment model following intravenous bolus administration. β, slow disposition, or post-distribution, rate constant; A, empirical constant; V_c, apparent volume of distribution for the central compartment; K_{21}, transfer rate constant; X_0, administered dose; α, distribution rate constant.

parsimony when selecting the compartment model by choosing the simpler of the two available models (e.g. the one-compartment model) to describe the pharmacokinetics of that drug.

Questions

1. Is it possible to have the slow disposition rate constant greater than the fast disposition rate constant? The answer to this is "No". The slower rate constant (having the smaller value) is always associated with the terminal slope of the curve.
2. Is it possible for the rate constant associated with elimination to have a greater value than that for the distribution rate constant? The answer to this is "Yes." This type of flip-flop kinetics occurs for the aminoglycoside antibiotic gentamicin. In the case of gentamicin, the terminal (β) portion of the curve, which represents the slower process, corresponds to distribution; while the steep feathered line, whose slope is $-\alpha/2.303$, corresponds to the faster process (the elimination process in this case). Ordinarily, for most drugs, this is not the case, and we can refer to α as the distribution rate constant and to β as the post-distribution rate constant.
3. Is it possible that a two-compartment model will need to be employed for a drug when it

is administered intravenously and a one-compartment model when the same drug is administered by an extravascular route? In other words, can the inflection of the curve indicative of two-compartment kinetics be hidden under the peak that occurs in the graph of the plasma concentration for extravascularly administered drug? (Answer is "Yes".)

13.5 Determination of micro rate constants: the inter-compartmental rate constants (K_{21} and K_{12}) and the pure elimination rate constant (K_{10})

Once the values of distribution rate constant and the post-distribution rate constant, as well as the values of the two empirical constants A and B (the two y-axis intercepts) are obtained by the methods described above, or are taken to be the values reported in the literature, the micro rate constants for elimination and inter-compartmental transfer can be generated using Equation 13.6:

$$C_p = Ae^{-\alpha t} + Be^{-\beta t}$$

where X_0 is the administered dose of drug, and A and B are the dose-dependent empirical constants (the y-axis intercepts on the concentration versus time plot).

Alternatively, the volume of distribution of the central compartment may also be obtained as follows:

$$V_C = \frac{X_0}{K_{10}\int_0^\infty C_p dt} = \frac{X_0}{K_{10}(\text{AUC})_0^\infty} \tag{13.20}$$

where $(\text{AUC})_\infty^0$ is the area under the plasma concentration–time curve from $t = 0$ to $t = \infty$ and K_{10} is the elimination rate constant.

Determination of apparent volume of distribution of drug in the body

We define:

$$f_C^* = \frac{X_C^*}{X^*} \tag{13.21}$$

where f_C^* is the is the the fraction, or percentage, of the administered dose in the central compartment after the attainment of distribution equilibrium; X_C^* is the mass or amount of drug remaining in the central compartment at a time after the occurrence of distribution equilibrium; and X^* is the total amount of drug remaining in the body after distribution equilibrium $(X_p^* + X_C^*)$.

Rearrangement of Eq. 13.21 yields:

$$X^\star = X_C^*/f_C^* \tag{13.22}$$

However,

$$X_C = V_C C_p \text{ and } X_C^* = V_C C_p^* \tag{13.23}$$

and $\quad f_C^* = \beta/K_{10} \tag{13.24}$

Substituting for X_C^* and f_C^* in Eq. 13.22 with Eq. 13.23 and 13.24, yields:

$$X^* = \frac{V_C C_p^*}{\beta/K_{10}} \tag{13.25}$$

or

$$\frac{X^*}{C_p^*} = \frac{V_C K_{10}}{\beta} \tag{13.26}$$

In the post-distribution phase,

$$\frac{X}{C_p} = \frac{X^*}{C_p^*}$$

which equals the apparent volume of distribution of drug in the body (V_b). Thus,

$$V_b = \frac{V_C K_{10}}{\beta} \tag{13.27}$$

This equation shows that the apparent volume of distribution of drug in the body is dependent on both elimination and distribution characteristics of the drug. The parameter, V_b, will relate the amount of drug remaining in the body at any given time to the plasma concentration at that time, providing that distribution equilibrium has been established.

Alternatively, the apparent volume of distribution of drug in the body may be obtained as follows:

$$V_b = \frac{X_0}{\beta(\text{AUC})_0^\infty} \tag{13.28}$$

From Eqs 13.20 and 13.28, it should become apparent that knowledge of the AUC is essential for determining the volumes of drug distribution.

Determination of volume of distribution at steady state

The following two equations may be used to calculate the volume of distribution at steady state, depending on the information at hand.

Volume of distribution at steady state can be expressed in terms of the volume of distribution in the central compartment:

$$V_{ss} = V_C \frac{K_{12} + K_{21}}{K_{21}} \tag{13.29}$$

It may also be expressed in terms of apparent volume of distribution of drug in the body:

$$V_{ss} = V_b \frac{K_{12} + K_{21}}{\alpha} \qquad (13.30)$$

In Eq. 13.30, evaluation of the expression $(K_{12} + K_{21})/\alpha$ results in a number less than 1. Thus, volume of distribution at steady state is less than the apparent volume of distribution of drug in the body ($V_{ss} < V_b$). This means that the volume of distribution at steady state (after elimination equilibrium has been established) has actually contracted in size when compared with the apparent volume of distribution of drug in the body, a volume of distribution calculated at an earlier time: when distribution equilibrium had been reached.

13.7 How to obtain the area under the plasma concentration–time curve from time zero to time *t* and time ∞

The trapezoidal rule

Chapter 4 should be reviewed for the trapezoidal rule, which employs a rectilinear plot of plasma drug concentration against time. The AUC is calculated for all data points (i.e. from $t = 0$ to t*), where t* is the time at which the last plasma concentration was measured.

$$(AUC)_0^{t^*} = \int_0^{t^*} C_p dt = \text{sum of all trapezoids}$$

$$(AUC)_{t^*}^{\infty} = C_p^* / \beta \qquad (13.31)$$

$$AUC = (AUC)_0^{t^*} + (AUC)_{t^*}^{\infty} \qquad (13.32)$$

Please note that in Eq. 13.31 the last observed plasma concentration is divided by the post-distribution rate constant (β) because of the presence of a two-compartment model. Compare Eq. 13.31 with Eq. 4.26 (p. 66) and Eq. 7.15 (p. 134), which were employed when the administered drug exhibited the characteristics of a one-compartment model.

Another approach to obtain AUC or $\int_0^{\infty} C_p dt$ is to use Eq. 13.6: $C_p = Ae^{-\alpha t} + Be^{-\beta t}$. Upon integration of this equation from $t = 0$ to $t = \infty$, the following equation is obtained:

$$\int_0^{\infty} C_p dt = (AUC)_0^{\infty} = A \int_0^{\infty} e^{-\alpha t} dt + B \int_0^{\infty} e^{-\beta t} dt$$

$$= \frac{A}{\alpha} + \frac{B}{\beta} \qquad (13.33)$$

A and B are the two empirical constants (i.e. y-axis intercepts) of the plasma concentration versus time plot, and α and β are the two rate constants associated with the two phases of the concentration versus time plot.

13.8 General comments

1. The distribution (α) and post-distribution (β) rate constants are complex constants that serve to define other constants which unequivocally characterize distribution or elimination processes.

2. Using Laplace transforms and the general solution for the quadratic equation, it has been proven that:

$$\beta = \frac{1}{2} \Big[(K_{12} + K_{21} + K_{10})$$

$$- \sqrt{(K_{12} + K_{21} + K_{10})^2 - 4K_{21}K_{10}} \Big]$$

and

$$\alpha = \frac{1}{2} \Big[(K_{12} + K_{21} + K_{10})$$

$$+ \sqrt{(K_{12} + K_{21} + K_{10})^2 - 4K_{21}K_{10}} \Big]$$

Since both the α and β rate constants depend on the pure distribution rate constants (K_{12} and K_{21}) and on the pure elimination rate constant (K_{10}), they are termed "hybrid" rate constants.

3. A clear distinction must be made between the elimination rate constant (K_{10}) and the slow disposition or post-distribution rate constant (β). The constant K_{10} is the elimination rate constant from the central compartment at any time; while the disposition or post-distribution

rate constant (β) reflects the drug elimination from the body in the "post-distributive phase." Although there is a clear distinction between K_{10} and β, these two rate constants may be related to each other as follows, Eq. 13.15:

$$\alpha\beta = K_{10}K_{21}$$

and Eq. 13.16

$$\alpha + \beta = K_{12} + K_{21} + K_{10}$$

Equation 13.16 may be rearranged:

$$\alpha = K_{12} + K_{21} + K_{10} - \beta \qquad (13.34)$$

Substitute for α (Eq. 13.34) in Eq. 13.15:

$$(K_{12} + K_{21} + K_{10} - \beta)\beta = K_{10}K_{21} \qquad (13.35)$$

Simplification of Eq. 13.35 yields:

$$(K_{12} + K_{21} - \beta)\beta = K_{10}K_{21} - K_{10}\beta$$

which is equivalent to:

$$(K_{12} + K_{21} - \beta)\beta = K_{10}(K_{21} - \beta)$$

Therefore,

$$\beta = \frac{K_{10}(K_{21} - \beta)}{(K_{12} + K_{21} - \beta)} \qquad (13.36)$$

In general, the fraction drug in the central compartment, f_C is equal to:

$$\frac{X_C}{X_C + X_p}$$

After distribution equilibrium has been attained, this fraction, now called f_C^*, can be shown to be:

$$f_C^* = \frac{\beta}{K_{10}} = \frac{(K_{21} - \beta)}{(K_{12} + K_{21} - \beta)} \qquad (13.37)$$

where f_C^* is the fraction of the drug in the central compartment in the post-distributive phase. Therefore,

$$\beta = K_{10}f_C^* \qquad (13.38)$$

If, after the attainment of distribution equilibrium, the fraction of drug in the central compartment is equal to 1, then, from Eq. 13.38, $\beta = K_{10}$. That is, the slow disposition rate constant would be equal to the elimination rate constant. What does this mean?

13.9 Example

Compound HI-6 has been shown to be very effective in the treatment of laboratory animals poisoned with the organophosphate anticholinesterase chemical Soman (GD, or O-pinacolyl methylphosphonofluoridate). The pharmacokinetics of HI-6 have been studied by Simons and Briggs (1983) following intravenous administration to beagle dogs (9.04 kg is the average weight of the group of seven dogs used). After administration of a 20 mg kg^{-1} intravenous dose to each dog (solution concentration of 250 mg mL^{-1}), the mean plasma concentrations of HI-6 were as given in Table 13.3.

Table 13.3   Plasma concentration versus time data for the example

Time (min)	Mean concentration (μg mL^{-1} [$\pm$SD])
2.0	93.08 $\pm$ 10.82
7.0	69.11 $\pm$ 4.80
10.0	63.82 $\pm$ 4.14
15.0	54.79 $\pm$ 2.02
20.0	48.73 $\pm$ 3.68
30.0	38.63 $\pm$ 3.40
45.0	27.85 $\pm$ 4.04
60.0	24.29 $\pm$ 5.43
75.0	19.12 $\pm$ 2.61
90.0	13.62 $\pm$ 2.89
105.0	11.95 $\pm$ 1.93
120.0	8.74 $\pm$ 2.41

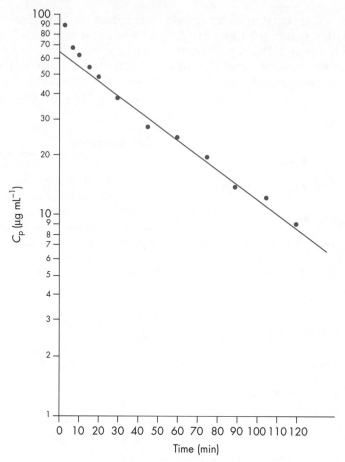

Figure 13.13   Plasma concentration (C_p) versus time plot for the example in text using data in Table 13.3 (semilogarithmic plot).

Determination of the slow disposition rate constant and the empirical constant B

Figure 13.13 is the plasma concentration versus time plot from which the slow disposition rate constant and the empirical constant B can be obtained.

1. $(t_{1/2})_\beta = 40$ min (from the resulting graph not shown).
2. $\beta = 0.693/(t_{1/2})_\beta = 0.693/40\,\mathrm{min} = 0.0173\,\mathrm{min}^{-1}$; or it can be calculated from slope $\times 2.303 = -\beta$.
3. The y-axis intercept of the extrapolated line for the β phase (or terminal linear phase) of a semilogarithmic plot of plasma concentration versus time provides the empirical constant B: $B = 64\,\mu\mathrm{g\,mL}^{-1}$.

Determination of the distribution rate constant and the empirical constant A

Table 13.4 gives data for the difference between the observed and the extrapolated plasma concentrations $(C_p)_{\mathrm{diff}}$ at various times, from which the distribution rate constant (α) and the empirical constant A can be obtained.

A plot of $(C_p)_{\mathrm{diff}}$ (values from column 4 in Table 13.4) against time on a semilogarithmic paper allows the following to be derived.

1. $(t_{1/2})_\alpha = 5.0$ min (from the resulting graph not shown)
2. $\alpha = 0.693/(t_{1/2})_\alpha = 0.693/5.0\,\mathrm{min} = 0.138\,\mathrm{min}^{-1}$; or it can be calculated from (slope) $\times 2.303 = -\alpha$.

Table 13.4 Differences between the observed and the extrapolated plasma concentration data at various times for the example

Time (min)	$(C_p)_{obs}$ (µg mL^{-1})	$(C_p)_{extrap}$ (µg mL^{-1})	$(C_p)_{diff}$ (µg mL^{-1})
2.0	93.08	62.0	31.08
7.0	69.11	57.0	12.11
10.0	63.82	54.0	9.82
15.0	54.79	50.0	4.79
20.0	48.73	45.0	3.73

$(C_p)_{extrap}$, extrapolated plasma concentrations; $(C_p)_{obs}$, observed plasma concentrations; $(C_p)_{diff}$, difference between extrapolated and observed values for each time in the absorption phase.

3. The y-intercept of the "feathered" or residual line is the empirical constant A: $A = 41.0\,\mu g\,mL^{-1}$.

Determination of the inter-compartmental (K_{21} and K_{12}) rate constants and the elimination rate constant (K_{10})

Determination of K_{21}

From Equation 13.14:

$$\frac{A\beta + B\alpha}{(A + B)} = K_{21}$$

$A = 41\,\mu g\,mL^{-1}$, $B = 64\,\mu g\,mL^{-1}$, $\alpha = 0.138$ min^{-1} and $\beta = 0.0173$ min^{-1}. So,

$$\frac{(41\mu g\,mL^{-1})(0.0173\,min^{-1}) + (64\,\mu g\,mL^{-1})(0.138\,min^{-1})}{41\,\mu g\,mL^{-1} + 64\,\mu g\,mL^{-1}} = K_{21}$$

$$\frac{0.7093\,\mu g\,mL^{-1}\,min^{-1} + 8.832\,\mu g\,mL^{-1}\,min^{-1}}{105\,\mu g\,mL^{-1}} = K_{21}$$

$$\frac{9.5413\,\mu g\,mL^{-1}\,min^{-1}}{105\,\mu g\,mL^{-1}} = K_{21}$$

$$K_{21} = 0.09086\ min^{-1}.$$

Determination of K_{10}

From Eq. 13.15:
$$\alpha\beta = K_{10}K_{21}$$

So,

$$\alpha\beta / K_{21} = K_{10}$$

$$\frac{(0.138\ min^{-1})(0.0173\ min^{-1})}{0.09086\ min^{-1}} = K_{10}$$

$$K_{10} = 0.02627\ min^{-1}$$

Determination of K_{12}

From Eq. 13.18:

$$\alpha + \beta = K_{12} + K_{21} + K_{10}$$

$$K_{12} = \alpha + \beta - (K_{21} + K_{10})$$

$\alpha = 0.138$ min^{-1}, $\beta = 0.0173$ min^{-1}, $K_{21} = 0.09086$ min^{-1}, $K_{10} = 0.02627$ min^{-1}.
So,

$$K_{12} = 0.138\ min^{-1} + 0.0173\ min^{-1}$$
$$- (0.09086\ min^{-1} + 0.02627\ min^{-1})$$

$$K_{12} = 0.03817\ min^{-1}.$$

Determination of the volumes of distribution

There are three volumes of distribution: distribution in the central compartment (V_C), distribution in the body (V_b) and distribution at steady state (V_{ss}).

Volume of distribution of central compartment

$$V_C = X_0 / (C_p)_0$$

$$X_0 = \text{dose} = 180.80\ mg\ \text{or}\ 180\,800\ \mu g$$

$$(C_p)_0 = A + B = 105\ \mu g\,mL^{-1}$$

$$V_C = 180\,800\ \mu g / 105\ \mu g\,mL^{-1}$$
$$= 1721.9\ mL = 1.72\ L.$$

Alternatively, V_C can be calculated from $V_C = X_0/K_{10}(AUC)_\infty^0$

$$K_{10} = 0.0263 \text{ min}^{-1}$$

$$(AUC)_0^\infty = (A/\alpha) + (B/\beta)$$
$$= (41 \,\mu\text{g ml}^{-1}/0.138 \text{ min}^{-1})$$
$$+ (64 \,\mu\text{g mL}^{-1}/0.0173 \text{ min}^{-1})$$
$$(AUC)_0^\infty = 297.1 \,\mu\text{g min mL}^{-1}$$
$$+ 3699.42 \,\mu\text{g min mL}^{-1}$$

$$(AUC)_0^\infty = 3996.52 \,\mu\text{g mL}^{-1} \text{ min}$$

Then,

$$V_C = \frac{180\,800 \,\mu\text{g}}{(0.0263 \text{ min}^{-1})(3996.52 \,\mu\text{g mL}^{-1} \text{ min})}$$

$$V_C = 180\,800/105.10 \text{ mL}^{-1}$$

$$= 1720.26 \text{ mL or } 1.72 \text{ L}.$$

Volume of distribution in the body

$$V_b = V_C K_{10}/\beta$$
$$V_C = 1721.9 \text{ mL}$$
$$K_{10} = 0.0263 \text{ min}^{-1}$$
$$\beta = 0.0173 \text{ min}^{-1}$$
$$V_b = \frac{(1729.9 \text{ mL})(0.0263 \text{ min}^{-1})}{0.0173 \text{ min}^{-1}} = \frac{45.0286 \text{ mL}}{0.0173}$$
$$V_b = 2617.68 \text{ mL or } 2.617 \text{ L}$$

Alternatively, V_b can be caluculated from $V_b = X_0/\beta(AUC)_\infty^0$

$$V_b = \frac{180\,800 \,\mu\text{g}}{(0.0173 \text{ min}^{-1})(3996.52 \,\mu\text{g mL}^{-1} \text{ min})}$$
$$V_b = 180\,800 \,\mu\text{g}/69.1398 \,\mu\text{g mL}^{-1}$$

$$= 2614 \text{ mL} = 2.61 \text{ L}.$$

13.10 Futher calculations to perform and determine the answers

The following calculations should be carried out for this example and the answers determined.

1. Ratio of volume of distribution of drug in the central compartment (V_C) over the volume of distribution of drug in the body (V_b).
2. Ratio of the disposition or post-distribution rate constant (β) over the elimination rate constant.
3. Ratio of the inter-compartmental transfer rate constant associated with the transfer of drug from the peripheral compartment to the central compartment over the distribution rate constant.
4. Determination of the fraction of drug in the central compartment following the attainment of distribution equilibrium (by employing Eq. 13.37).
5. Determination of the fraction of drug in the peripheral, or tissue, compartment following the attainment of distribution equilibrium.
6. Attempt to determine the systemic clearance of the drug in as many ways as possible from the available information.

Since we have more than one volume of drug distribution and more the one rate constant, unlike the case for the one-compartment model, should we have more than one systemic clearance for a drug that manifests the characteristics of a two-compartment model? (The answer is "No", but be prepared to explain why.)

Problem set 6

Problems for Chapter 13

Question 1

Foord (1976) reported on human pharmacokinetics of cefuroxime, a parenteral cephalosporin. Following an intravenous bolus administration of 1.0 g cefuroxime to three subjects, the following mean serum concentrations shown in Table P6.1 were reported.

Plot the data and, using the plot, determine the following.

a. The disposition half life, $(t_{1/2})_\beta$.
b. The disposition rate constant (β) and the intercept of the elimination phase (terminal linear segment of the curve) (B).
c. The distribution half life $(t_{1/2})_\alpha$.
d. The distribution rate constant (α) and the intercept of the extrapolated line (A).

Table P6.1

Time (min)	Serum concentrations ($\mu g\ mL^{-1}$)
3.0	99.2
10.0	75.4
30.0	43.2
60.0	27.2
120.0	11.7
180.0	7.4
240.0	3.6
360.0	1.1
480.0	0.3

e. The intercompartmental transfer rate constants (K_{12} and K_{21}) and the elimination rate constant (K_{10}).
f. The area under the plasma concentration time curve, $(\text{AUC})_0^\infty$, by the trapezoidal method and by the use of an equation.
g. The apparent volumes of distribution volume in the central compartment (V_c) and in the body (V_b).
h. The fraction of drug remaining in the central compartment (f_c^*) following the attainment of distribution equilibrium.

Answers

The following are our answers to the questions and, as discussed in earlier problem sets, your answers may differ slightly from these.

Question 1 answer

From the terminal linear portion of a plot of plasma concentration versus time data on semilogarithmic paper and the intercept of the line on the y-axis, we obtained:

a. $(t_{1/2})_\beta = 70.0\ \text{min}$.
b. Disposition rate constant $\beta = 0.0099\ \text{min}^{-1}$
   $B = 37.0\ \mu g\ mL^{-1}$.
   From the feathered line and the intercept of the feathered line in a plot of $(C_p)_{\text{diff}}$ against time on semilogarithmic paper, the following were determined:
c. Distribution half life $(t_{1/2})_\alpha = 13.00\ \text{min}$.
d. Distribution rate constant $\alpha = 0.0533\ \text{min}^{-1}$
   $A = 74.0\ \mu g\ mL^{-1}$.

Please note that the distribution rate constant α is greater than the disposition rate constant β.

e. $K_{21} = 0.0242 \, \text{min}^{-1}$
$K_{12} = 0.0171 \, \text{min}^{-1}$
$K_{10} = 0.0216 \, \text{min}^{-1}$.

The answers obtained can be used to verify the following relationship between the 'hybrid' rate constant and the micro rate constants:

$$\alpha + \beta = K_{10} + K_{12} + K_{21}.$$

f. trapezoidal method $(AUC)_0^\infty = 5634.70 \, \mu\text{g mL}^{-1} \text{min}$

employing equation, $(AUC)_0^\infty = 5133.59 \, \mu\text{g mL}^{-1} \text{min}$

g. $V_c = 9018.35 \, \text{mL} \, (9.018 \, \text{L})$

$V_b = 19\,677.29 \, \text{mL}$

Please note that V_b is greater than V_c.

h.

$$f_c^* = \frac{\beta}{k_{10}} = \left(\frac{0.0099 \, \text{min}^{-1}}{0.0216 \, \text{min}^{-1}}\right) = 0.458$$

$$f_c^* = \frac{V_c}{V_b} = \left(\frac{9.018 \, \text{L}}{19.677 \, \text{L}}\right) = 0.458$$

14

Multiple intermittent infusions

Objectives

Upon completion of this chapter, you will have the ability to:

- calculate plasma drug concentrations during an intermittent infusion
- determine the dosing regimen (infusion rate [Q] and the duration of infusion [t_{inf}]) that will result in target plasma drug concentrations
- calculate a *loading* infusion rate
- apply theoretical pharmacokinetic principles to real-world intermittent infusion regimens of aminoglycosides and vancomycin
- adjust the method of calculating "peak" (C_{PK}) and trough (C_{TR}) plasma drug concentrations when these concentrations are not collected exactly at their scheduled times.

14.1 Introduction

Drugs administered by constant-rate intravenous infusion are frequently infused *intermittently* rather than continuously. The following example of a particular dosing regimen for the antibiotic vancomycin may be illustrative. In a particular patient, vancomycin was infused at a rate of 800 mg h^{-1} for 1 h, with a period of 12 h elapsing before this process was repeated. While drug was being infused, it was entering the body at a constant rate, namely 800 mg h^{-1} in this example. However, the lapse of 12 h between each 1 h infusion defines this process as an *intermittent* administration of drug.

Figure 14.1 is a graph, on *rectilinear* co-ordinates, of plasma vancomycin concentration for this regimen. In this figure we see the fairly rapid attainment (after approximately 36 h) of steady-state conditions, where successive peak drug concentrations ($C_{PK})_{ss}$ are equal to each other and

successive trough concentrations ($C_{TR})_{ss}$ are equal to each other. We see also that the dosing interval (τ) can be measured either from peak to peak or from trough to trough. Finally, we see that the interval τ comprises the time that the infusion is running (t_{inf}, which is 1 h in this example) plus the time that the infusion is not running (i.e. the time from the end of one infusion to the beginning of the next infusion [$\tau - t_{inf}$]: 11 h in this example.) Therefore, $\tau - t_{inf}$ is also the length of time between the peak and trough times.

Figure 14.2 is the same data plotted on *semilogarithmic* co-ordinates. At time zero, the plasma drug concentration would also equal zero. (A value of zero cannot be shown on the logarithmic *y*-axis of this graph; therefore, we have to imagine the plasma drug concentration coming up from zero for an infinitely long distance along the *y*-axis.) This figure also shows that the declining blood concentrations after

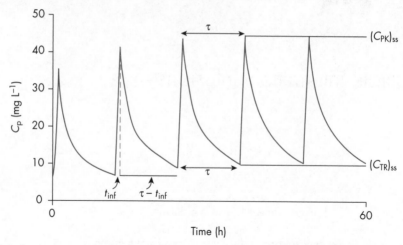

Figure 14.1 Multiple intermittent infusions shown in a rectilinear plot. C_p, plasma drug concentration; $(C_{PK})_{ss}$, peak drug concentration at steady state; $(C_{TR})_{ss}$, trough drug concentration at steady state; τ, dosing interval; t_{inf}, time infusion is running.

each short infusion exhibit a terminal linear segment. This occurs when distribution of drug to tissues has reached equilibrium. Finally, there is an extension of the terminal linear segment for 1 h beyond the commencement of the next short infusion. This is equal to $(C_{TR})_{ss}(e^{-Kt_{inf}})$, an expression which is found in the equation for calculation of the volume of distribution:

$$V = \frac{(S)(Q)(1 - e^{-Kt_{inf}})}{(K)((C_{PK})_{ss} - (C_{TR})_{ss}e^{-Kt_{inf}})} \tag{14.1}$$

Once steady state has been attained, the following equation can be used to calculate drug concentration at any time, t, from the time of peak concentration up to the time of trough

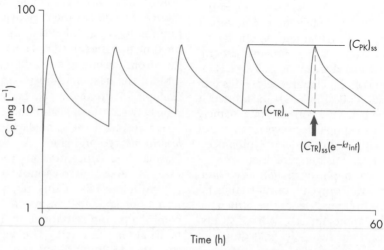

Figure 14.2 Multiple intermittent infusion shown in a semilogarithmic plot. Abbreviations as in Fig. 14.1.

Table 14.1   Peak, trough and other points with respect to Equation 14.2

Point described	$t=$	$t - t_{inf}=$
Peak (the highest point; it occurs immediately before the infusion is stopped)	$=t_{inf}$ (e.g. $t=1$ h)	$=t_{inf} - t_{inf} = 0$ (so $t - t_{inf}$ always equals 0 at time of peak)
Points between peak and trough	$\tau > t > t_{inf}$ (e.g. t is between 1 and 8 h)	$7 > t - t_{inf} > 0$ (i.e. $t - t_{inf}$ will range between 0 and 7 h for this example)
Trough (the lowest point; it occurs immediately before the next infusion is started)	$=\tau$ (e.g. $t=8$ h)	$=\tau - t_{inf}$ (e.g. $t - t_{inf} = 7$ h)
Trough extends for 1 h into the *next* interval (serves as a baseline under the next peak)	$=\tau + t_{inf}$ (e.g. $t=9$ h)	$=\tau$ (e.g. $t - t_{inf} = 8$ h)

τ, dosing interval (measured from peak to peak or from trough to trough); t_{inf}, time infusion running; $\tau - t_{inf}$, the time from the end of one infusion to the beginning of the next infusion (also the length of time between the peak and trough times).

concentration (right before the next infusion is begun):

$$C_{ss} = (C_{PK})_{ss}(e^{-K(t - t_{inf})}) \qquad (14.2)$$

Table 14.1 shows what happens when various values are substituted for t in the above equation. The numerical values in the table are based on a dosing interval equal to 8 h and an infusion time equal to 1 h.

14.2 Drug concentration guidelines

Table 14.2 presents target plasma steady-state peak and trough drug concentrations for four aminoglycoside antibiotics. These target values vary depending upon the severity of the patient's infection but give a guideline when calculating the ideal dosing regimen for a particular patient in a particular condition. Below is a worked example of the determination of a multiple intermittent infusion dosing regimen for the aminoglycoside gentamicin.

Table 14.2   Aminoglycoside target plasma levels

	Severity of infection	Gentamicin, tobramycin or netilmicin	Amikacin
Target *peak* concentration (μg mL^{-1})	Less severe	5–8	20–25
	Life-threatening	8–10[a]	25–48
Target *trough* concentration (μg mL^{-1})	Less severe	0.5–1	1–4
	Life-threatening	1–2[a]	4–8

[a] In select patients with life-threatening infections, netilmicin has been used with troughs 2–4 μg mL^{-1} and peaks 12–16 μg mL^{-1}.

14.3 Example: determination of a multiple intermittent infusion dosing regimen for an aminoglycoside antibiotic

The aminoglycoside antibiotics display some two-compartment characteristics, but not as markedly as vancomycin. For a 1 h infusion, the true peak plasma gentamicin concentration (immediately after the infusion is stopped) is often used. The rationale for this is that distribution equilibrium for gentamicin is essentially complete in 1 h. However, for a 30 min infusion, it is common to wait for an additional 30 min after the infusion is stopped and to call this the gentamicin "peak" concentration.

Patient information:

$$
\begin{aligned}
t_{1/2} &= 4.91\,\text{h} \\
V &= 0.25\,\text{L kg}^{-1} \\
\text{height} &= 200\,\text{cm} \\
\text{weight} &= 60\,\text{kg} \\
\text{drug} &= \text{gentamicin sulfate}\left(\text{for which} \right. \\
&\left. \text{the salt value } (S) \approx 1\right).
\end{aligned}
$$

1. An intermittent intravenous infusion dosing regimen needs to be designed that will achieve peak steady-state plasma drug concentrations of $6\,\mu\text{g mL}^{-1}$ and trough steady-state plasma drug concentrations of $1\,\mu\text{g mL}^{-1}$ for an infusion over 1 h.
2. Using convenient, practical values for infusion rate (Q) and dosing interval (τ), what exact peak and trough steady-state plasma drug concentrations will be achieved?
3. Calculate a one-time-only loading infusion rate.

1. First solve for the interval τ, using the following equation:

$$
\tau = \frac{\ln\dfrac{(C_{PK})_{ss}}{(C_{TR})_{ss}}}{K} + t_{inf} \tag{14.3}
$$

$$
\tau = \frac{\ln\left(\dfrac{6\,\text{mg L}^{-1}}{1\,\text{mg L}^{-1}}\right)}{0.693/4.91\,\text{h}} + 1\,\text{h} = 13.7\,\text{h}
$$

A convenient interval $= 12\,\text{h}$.

In order to solve for the infusion rate Q, the following equation is used:

$$
Q = (C_{PK})_{ss}VK\left(\frac{1-e^{-K\tau}}{1-e^{-Kt_{inf}}}\right) \tag{14.4}
$$

$$
\begin{aligned}
Q &= (6\,\text{mg L}^{-1})(0.25\,\text{L kg}^{-1}) \\
&\quad \times (60\,\text{kg})(0.141\,\text{h}^{-1})\left(\frac{1-e^{-(0.141)(12)}}{1-e^{-(0.141)(1)}}\right) \\
&= 78.7\,\text{mg h}^{-1}
\end{aligned}
$$

A round number is $80\,\text{mg h}^{-1}$.

So, the infusion would be of $80\,\text{mg h}^{-1}$ for 1 h. This would be repeated every 12 h.

2. Because of rounding off, the peak will not be exactly $6\,\mu\text{g mL}^{-1}$, nor will the trough be exactly $1\,\mu\text{g mL}^{-1}$.

To calculate the peak value, rearrange Eq. 14.4 as follows:

$$
(C_{PK})_{ss} = \left(\frac{Q}{VK}\right)\left(\frac{1-e^{-Kt_{inf}}}{1-e^{-K\tau}}\right) \tag{14.5}
$$

Then,

$$
\begin{aligned}
(C_{PK})_{ss} &= \left(\frac{80\,\text{mg h}^{-1}}{(15\,\text{L})(0.141\,\text{h}^{-1})}\right) \\
&\quad \times \left(\frac{1-e^{-(0.141)(1)}}{1-e^{-(0.141)(12)}}\right) = 6.10\,\text{mg L}^{-1}
\end{aligned}
$$

To calculate the trough value, use:

$$
(C_{TR})_{ss} = (C_{PK})_{ss}(e^{-K(\tau-t_{inf})}) \tag{14.6}
$$

So,

$$
\begin{aligned}
(C_{TR})_{ss} &= (6.10\,\text{mg L}^{-1})(e^{-(0.141)(12-1)}) \\
&= 1.29\,\text{mg L}^{-1}
\end{aligned}
$$

3. A one-time-only loading infusion rate avoids waiting to achieve a steady state; a single loading infusion rate that, exactly 1 h (when it is discontinued), will provide the desired steady-state peak drug concentration of $6\,\mu\text{g mL}^{-1}$ is calculated by:

$$
Q_L = \frac{(C_{PK})_{desired}(V)(K)}{1-e^{-Kt_{inf}}}
$$

$$Q_L = \frac{(6\,\text{mg L}^{-1})(15\,\text{L})(0.141\,\text{h}^{-1})}{1 - e^{-(0.141)(1)}}$$

$$= 96.5\,\text{mg h}^{-1}$$

$$\approx 100\,\text{mg h}^{-1} \text{ for 1 h only,}$$

given one time only.

Adjusting for the severity of infection

In light of the guidelines (Table 14.2), suppose the patient in the dosing regimen calculation above was categorized as having a less-severe, non-life-threatening infection. In this case, it would be important not to risk possible side effects from the calculated trough steady-state concentration of $1.29\,\text{mg L}^{-1}$. Since the peak concentration is acceptable, the trough concentration can be lowered by judiciously increasing the dosing interval. The calculations can be reworked substituting a dosing interval of 16 h for the original interval of 12 h. First Eq. 14.4 is used to solve for the new infusion rate:

$$Q = (6\,\text{mg L}^{-1})(0.25\,\text{L kg}^{-1})(60\,\text{kg})$$

$$\times (0.141\,\text{h}^{-1})\left(\frac{1 - e^{-(0.141)(16)}}{1 - e^{-(0.141)(1)}}\right)$$

$$= 86.4\,\text{mg h}^{-1}$$

Rounded off to the nearest $10\,\text{mg h}^{-1}$, $Q = 90\,\text{mg h}^{-1}$.

If the infusion rate is $90\,\text{mg h}^{-1}$ and the new dosing interval is 16 h, but the original infusion length of 1 h is unchanged, what changes would be expected in the steady-state peak and trough concentrations?

Using Eq. 14.5, the calculation is:

$$(C_{PK})_{ss} = \left(\frac{90\,\text{mg h}^{-1}}{(15\,\text{L})(0.141\,\text{h}^{-1})}\right)$$

$$\times \left(\frac{1 - e^{-(0.141)(1)}}{1 - e^{-(0.141)(16)}}\right) = 6.25\,\text{mg L}^{-1}$$

which is a modest increase.

Next, using Eq. 14.6, the calculation is:

$$(C_{TR})_{ss} = (6.25\,\text{mg L}^{-1})(e^{-(0.141)(16-1)})$$

$$= 0.754\,\text{mg L}^{-1}$$

Since this falls between 0.5 and $1\,\text{mg L}^{-1}$, the regimen is acceptable.

14.4 Dose to the patient from a multiple intermittent infusion

Table 14.3 shows the dose to the patient from two multiple intermittent infusion regimens which differ in the length of the infusion. This table makes use of the equation:

$$X_0 = Q/t_{inf} \qquad (14.7)$$

Notice in this table that $X_0/t_{inf} = Q$, the infusion rate, which was the same for both regimens in the

Table 14.3 Effect of the time a transfusion is running on dose to the patient and on average steady-state plasma drug concentration

Dosing regimen	Infusion rate (Q) [mg h^{-1}]	Infusion time $(t_{inf}$ [h])	Dosing interval $(\tau$ [h])	Dose (mg)	Dose/τ (proportional to average steady-state drug concentration) (mg h^{-1})
$100\,\text{mg h}^{-1}$ given over 1 h every 12 h	100	1	12	100	$100/12 = 8.333$
$100\,\text{mg h}^{-1}$ given over 0.5 h every 12 h	100	0.5	12	50	$100/12 = 4.167$

example above; whereas X_0/τ was lower for the shorter infusion time regimen. This indicates that $(C_{ave})_{ss}$ will also be lower, since $(C_{ave})_{ss} = \frac{SF}{KV}\left(\frac{X_0}{\tau}\right)$.

14.5 Multiple intermittent infusion of a two-compartment drug: vancomycin "peak" at 1 h post-infusion

In Fig. 14.2, plasma concentrations of vancomycin plotted versus time were plotted using semilogarithmic co-ordinates. Even though this figure was graphed using a logarithmic y-axis, the post-infusion plasma drug concentration shows curvature for a period of time, until finally settling down to a straight line. This initial curvature indicates the presence of a multi-compartment drug. Vancomycin is, in fact, a classical two-compartment drug. In theory, use of a two-compartment equation would exactly characterize the vancomycin plasma concentration versus time curve. However, in practice, it is rare to have enough plasma concentration data on a patient to be able to calculate the two-compartment parameters. So, instead, a usable "peak" plasma vancomycin concentration (on the more nearly linear part of the curve) is drawn, assayed, and recorded at 1 h after the end of the infusion.

Figure 14.3 is a semilogarithmic plot showing the point on the declining plasma drug concentration curves at which sufficient linearity is reached to use simple one-compartment equations. This occurs at approximately 1 h after each short infusion has ended. Curvature of the graph before this time prevents the *true* peak concentration (immediately after the infusion ends) to be used in calculations. The concentration 1 h post-infusion is the useable peak level $(C_{"PK"})_{ss}$. In this figure, lines (with slope proportional to the elimination rate constant) are extended downward from the true peak concentration and from $(C_{"PK"})_{ss}$ to the concentration immediately before the next short infusion. The line originating from the 1 h post-infusion "peak" level is a closer estimate of the actual plasma vancomycin concentration curve. The slope of the line from the useable peak level to the trough value at steady state yields an apparent one-compartment, first-order elimination rate constant, which can be denoted K.

Modification of equations for the time from the end of the infusion to the "peak" (t')

The multiple intermittent infusion equation must be modified to reflect the use of the "peak" concentration for vancomycin, as defined above. The modified equation for steady-state peak plasma drug concentration is as follows:

$$(C_{"PK"})_{ss} = \frac{(Q)(1 - e^{-Kt_{inf}})(e^{-Kt'})}{(V)(K)(1 - e^{-K\tau})} \tag{14.8}$$

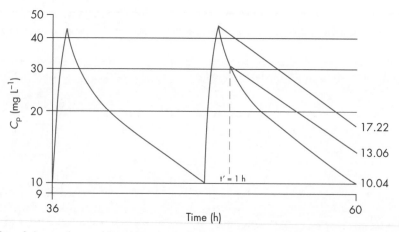

Figure 14.3 Effect of choice of time of "peak" vancomycin concentration on estimate of trough level. C_p, plasma drug concentration.

where t' is the time from the end of the infusion to the "peak" (this is set to equal 1 h for vancomycin in the discussion above); t_{inf} is the duration of the infusion; τ is the interval between short infusion doses.

The trough equation must be modified as well:

$$(C_{TR})_{ss} = (C''_{PK''})_{ss}(e^{-K(\tau - t_{inf} - t')}) \qquad (14.9)$$

The equation for volume of distribution then becomes:

$$V = \frac{(S)(Q)(1 - e^{-Kt_{inf}})(e^{-Kt'})}{(C''_{PK''})_{ss}(K)(1 - e^{-K\tau})}$$
$$= \frac{(S)(Q)(1 - e^{-Kt_{inf}})(e^{-Kt_{wait}})}{(C''_{PK''})_{ss}(K)(1 - e^{-K\tau})} \qquad (14.10)$$

The only difference in these two equations is whether one prefers the notation t' or t_{wait}, both of which terms stand for the same thing.

14.6 Vancomycin dosing regimen problem

Now we are able to solve a vancomycin problem. A patient has a vancomycin elimination half life of 8 h (elimination rate constant, $0.08663\,h^{-1}$) and a volume of distribution of 35 L.

1. Calculate a dosing interval τ to achieve a steady-state plasma drug "peak" concentration (measured 1 h after the end of the infusion) equal to $30\,mg\,L^{-1}$ and a steady-state plasma drug trough concentration equal to $11\,mg\,L^{-1}$. Use a 1 h infusion duration for doses $< 1000\,mg$. and a 2 h infusion duration for doses ≥ 1000 mg. The following equation is used:

$$\tau = \frac{\ln\dfrac{(C''_{PK''})_{ss}}{(C_{TR})_{ss}}}{K} + t_{inf} + t' \qquad (14.11)$$

where t' is the time from the end of the infusion to the "peak" and t_{inf} is the the duration of the infusion.

2. Calculate a multiple intermittent infusion rate, Q, that will deliver a "peak" steady-state plasma vancomycin concentration of $30\,mg\,L^{-1}$,

assuming that the salt form correction factor (S) is 1.0. Equation 14.8 is rearranged to solve for R.

First, Eq. 14.11 is used to solve for τ. Tentatively $t_{inf} = 1\,h$ is used until the magnitude of the dose is known.

$$\tau = \frac{\ln\dfrac{30}{11}}{0.08663} + 1 + 1 = 13.6\,h.$$

For practical purposes, $\tau = 12\,h$ is used.
Second, the multiple intermittent infusion rate is calculate using:

$$Q = \frac{(C''_{PK''})_{ss}(V)(K)(1 - e^{-K\tau})}{(1 - e^{-Kt_{inf}})(e^{-Kt'})}$$
$$= \frac{(30\,mg\,L^{-1})(35\,L)(0.08663\,h^{-1})(1 - e^{-(0.08663)(12)})}{(1 - e^{-(0.08663)(1)})(e^{-(0.08663)(1)})}$$

$Q = 773\,mg\,h^{-1}$.
For practical purposes, an infusion rate of $800\,mg\,h^{-1}$ is used.

Since each dose to the patient will equal 800 mg, there is no need to go back and redo the calculations based on a $t_{inf} = 2\,h$.

Since values for τ and Q were rounded off, the expected values of the steady-state peak and trough concentrations need to be calculated.

This is done using a simple proportion for the "peak" calculation.

$$(C_{PK})_{ss} = (\text{rounded off}\,Q/\text{caculated}\,Q)(\text{target peak})$$
$$= (800/773)(30\,mg\,L^{-1}) = 31.05\,mg\,L^{-1}.$$

This is close to the desired "peak" value.
Equation 14.9 is used to obtain the trough value:

$$(C_{TR})_{ss} = (31.05\,mg\,L^{-1})(e^{-(0.08663)(12-1-1)})$$
$$= 13.06\,mg\,L^{-1}.$$

This predicted trough level is higher than the desired trough of $11\,mg\,L^{-1}$. If it is deemed too high, the dosing interval would need to be increased. For example, increasing the interval to 16 h would produce a trough level equal to $9.23\,mg\,L^{-1}$.

14.7 Adjustment for early or late drug concentrations

In the real world, "peak" and trough blood concentrations after a multiple intravenous infusion at steady state are not always taken exactly at the appropriate time. For example, a delayed "peak" plasma drug concentration will be deceptively low, while an early trough concentration will be falsely high. A mathematical technique is needed to adjust these readings so that judgements can be made on the suitability of the dosing regimen for the patient.

As long as we are in the *post-distribution* phase of the drug concentration–time curve (the part that is linear when the data for the curve are plotted using a logarithmic y-axis), there is a simple way of adjusting the observed drug concentrations to yield the corresponding "peak" and trough concentrations. This method relies on the fact that the drug concentration is declining monoexponentially in the post-distribution phase of the curve. Therefore, for two points on this curve:

$$(C_p)_{LO} = (C_p)_{HI}(e^{-\lambda \Delta t})$$

where $(C_p)_{LO}$ is the lower of the two points; $(C_p)_{HI}$ is the higher of the two points; λ is a general symbol for the first-order rate constant of disappearance of drug from the plasma.

Since we are approximating two-compartment kinetics by employing a one-compartment equation in the terminal (i.e. elimination) phase of the plasma drug concentration versus time curve, the elimination rate constant K can be substituted for λ, to give:

$$(C_p)_{LO} = (C_p)_{HI}(e^{-K \Delta t})$$

Specifically, if a "peak" plasma concentration $(C_p)_{HI}$ is sampled somewhat late (e.g. 1.5 h late), the above equation can be used to adjust $(C_p)_{HI}$ to the (higher) plasma drug concentration that would have been recorded if the concentration had been collected on time. Then,

$$(C_p)_{"PK"} = (C_p)_{HI}/(e^{-K1.5})$$

where $(C_p)_{"PK"}$ is a more accurate estimate of the "peak" concentration than was $(C_p)_{HI}$. This process can be described as *sliding up* the plasma concentration curve from right to left by exactly $t = t_{PKlate} = 1.5\,h$.

Similarly, if a trough plasma concentration $(C_p)_{LO}$ is sampled somewhat early (e.g. 2 h early), this concentration will be falsely high; so the equation can be used to adjust $(C_p)_{LO}$ to the (lower) plasma drug concentration that would have been recorded if the concentration had been collected on time. Then,

$$(C_p)_{TR} = (C_p)_{LO}(e^{-K2})$$

where $(C_p)_{TR}$ is a more accurate estimate of the trough concentration than was $(C_p)_{LO}$. This process can be described as *sliding down* the plasma concentration curve from left to right by exactly $t = t_{TRearly} = 2.0\,h$.

Next, we ought to consider whether any other possibilities exist besides the two cases just described. For example, could a "peak" concentration need adjustment because it was collected too early? In fact, this case would represent a real problem since the drug concentration would have been collected in a part of the curve where distribution is still going on. Adjusting the observed concentration with the monoexponential equation would not be appropriate in this case since it would generate an erroneous estimate of the "peak" concentration.

What about a trough being collected too late? Well.... The right time to collect a trough concentration is immediately before the next infusion is begun. Therefore, collecting a trough too late would imply that it was collected during the next dose (while plasma drug concentration is rising!) Needless to say, this is not done.

This leaves the following four possibilities.

A. Both "peak" and trough concentrations are collected on time according to the guidelines for the particular drug.

B. The trough concentration is sampled too early.

C. The "peak" concentration is sampled late.

D. A combination of scenarios B and C occur, where the trough concentration is sampled

Table 14.4 Adjustment for early and late collection of plasma drug concentrations

Scenario	Adjustment for actual "peak" or trough value	Δt in the equation for K^a	Volume of distribution, $V=$
A: peak and trough levels collected on time	No adjustment: $(C_p)_{HI}=$"peak" and $(C_p)_{LO}=$trough	$=\tau - t_{inf} - t_{wait}$	$\dfrac{Q(1-e^{-Kt_{inf}})(e^{-Kt_{wait}})}{C_{"PK"}(K)(1-e^{-K\tau})}$
B: observed trough level [$(C_p)_{LO}$] sampled too early	Trough is $(C_p)_{LO}(e^{-(K)(t_{TRearly})})$	$=\tau - t_{inf} - t_{wait} - t_{TRearly}$	$\dfrac{Q(1-e^{-Kt_{inf}})(e^{-Kt_{wait}})}{C_{"PK"}(K)(1-e^{-K\tau})}$
C: observed "peak" level [$(C_p)_{HI}$] sampled late	"Peak" is $(C_p)_{HI}/(e^{-(K)(t_{PKlate})})$	$=\tau - t_{inf} - t_{wait} - t_{PKlate}$	$\dfrac{Q(1-e^{-Kt_{inf}})(e^{-K(t_{wait}+t_{PKlate})})}{(C_p)_{HI}(K)(1-e^{-K\tau})}$
D: trough sampled too early *and* "peak" sampled late	Trough is $(C_p)_{LO}(e^{-(K)(t_{TRearly})})$; "Peak" is $(C_p)_{HI}/(e^{-(K)(t_{PKlate})})$	$=\tau - t_{inf} - t_{wait} - t_{TRearly} - t_{PKlate}$	$\dfrac{Q(1-e^{-Kt_{inf}})(e^{-K(t_{wait}+t_{pklate})})}{(C_p)_{HI}(K)(1-e^{-K\tau})}$

$^a K = [\ln(C_p)_{HI}/\ln(C_p)_{LO}]/\Delta t$

Δt, time between high concentration sample $(C_p)_{HI}$ and low concentration sample $(C_p)_{LO}$; tr, actual trough concentration; "PK", actual "peak"; τ, interval between infusions; Q, infusion rate; t_{inf}, length of infusion; t_{wait}, recommended time after infusion is stopped to wait until sampling (0.5 h for gentamicin and 1.0 h for vancomycin); $t_{TRearly}$, how much earlier than the recommended time the trough concentration was actually collected; $t_{PK\ late}$, how much later than the recommended time the "peak" concentration was actually collected.

too early *and* the "peak" concentration is sampled late.

As shown above, early/late sampling will require the use of equations to adjust observed high and low concentrations to achieve more accurate estimates of the "peak" and trough concentrations. Early/late sampling will also have ramifications for the equations used to for solve for the apparent volume of distribution and the elimination rate constant by using two steady-state plasma drug concentrations sampled after a multiple intravenous infusion. Table 14.4 summarizes these equations.

Example problem: adjustment for early or late drug concentrations

In the vancomycin problem discussed in this chapter, what would be the effect of collecting the trough concentration 2.5 h before the end of the infusion (i.e. 2.5 h too early). The concentration recorded at that time was $16.2\,\mathrm{mg\,L^{-1}}$. This would be called $(C_p)_{LO}$. The following questions need to be answered.

1. What is a more accurate estimate of the trough plasma vancomycin concentration in this patient?
2. Based on the measured $(C_p)_{LO}$ value and the $C_{"PK"}$ value of $31.05\,\mathrm{mg\,L^{-1}}$, what is this patient's elimination rate constant?
3. What is an estimate of the patient's volume of distribution?

Figure 14.4 will help to visualize the situation in this problem.

First, from Table 14.4, we obtain:

$$(C_p)_{TR} = (C_p)_{LO}(e^{-K(t_{TRearly})})$$
$$(C_p)_{TR} = 16.2\,\mathrm{mg\,L^{-1}}(e^{-0.08663 \times 2.5})$$
$$= 13.05\,\mathrm{mg\,L^{-1}}.$$

Notice that this agrees with the earlier estimate of $(C_p)_{TR}$.

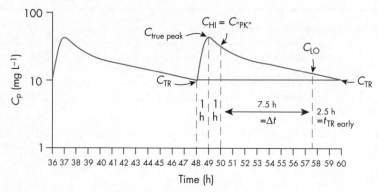

Figure 14.4 Visualization of "trough" vancomycin level collected too early. C_p, plasma drug concentration; $C_{"PK"}$, apparent peak drug concentration; C_{HI}, highest drug concentration measured; C_{LO}, lowest drug concentration measured; C_{TR}, trough drug concentration.

In order to calculate K, Δt must be calculated first; this is the time between the $(C_p)_{"PK"}$ value and the $(C_p)_{LO}$ value. Therefore,

$$\Delta t = \tau - t_{inf} - t_{wait} - t_{TRearly} = 12 - 1 - 1 - 2.5 = 7.5\ \text{h}.$$

Then,

$$K = \frac{\ln\frac{C_{HI}}{C_{LO}}}{\Delta t} = \frac{\ln\frac{C_{"PK"}}{C_{LO}}}{\Delta t} = \frac{\ln\frac{31.05}{16.2}}{7.5} = 0.0867\ \text{h},$$

which is also in good agreement with the earlier estimate.

Finally volume of distribution can be calculate from scenario B of Table 14.4.

$$V = \frac{(S)(Q)(1 - e^{-Kt_{inf}})(e^{-Kt_{wait}})}{(C_{"PK"})_{ss}(K)(1 - e^{-K\tau})}$$

$$= \frac{(1)(800\ \text{mg h}^{-1})(1 - e^{-K(1)})(e^{-K(1)})}{(31.05\ \text{mg/L})(0.0867\ \text{h}^{-1})(1 - e^{-(0.0867)(12)})}$$

$$= 35.0\ \text{L}.$$

Problem set 7

Problems for Chapter 14

Question 1

At the end of a 1 h loading infusion of 12 mg tobramycin, a plasma drug concentration of $6.5\ \mu g\ mL^{-1}$ was recorded in a 30-year-old white female with *Pseudomonas* sp. infection. At 3 h post-infusion, the plasma drug concentration had declined to $5.0\ \mu g\ mL^{-1}$, and by 7 h post-infusion to $3.5\ \mu g\ mL^{-1}$. Linear regression of the log of plasma concentration (C_p) versus time yielded a elimination rate constant (K) of $0.088\ h^{-1}$.

a. Calculate the volume of distribution (V) for this patient.
b. Predict the steady-state peak, $(C_{PK})_{ss}$, and trough, $(C_{TR})_{ss}$, concentrations if a maintenance infusion of 70 mg over 1 h every 12 h is administered.
c. Will this keep the patient at the same peak concentration as the loading infusion?
d. If the loading infusion were allowed to *continue indefinitely* (a grave error), what theoretical steady-state tobramycin concentration would be predicted (assuming that the patient was still alive)?
e. If the loading infusion were *repeated intermittently* (another error) as a 1 h infusion every 12 h, what steady-state peak concentration would ensue?
f. What steady-state *average* concentration would occur from the regimen in part (e)?
g. What steady-state *trough* concentration would occur from the regimen in part (e)?
h. What *continuous* infusion rate (Q) would yield a final plasma concentration, $(C_p)_\infty$ of $6.5\ mg\ L$?

Answers

Question 1 answer

a. $$V = \frac{Q_L}{C_p K}(1 - e^{-Kt'})$$

Specifically,

$$V = \frac{Q_L}{(C_p)_{PK} K}(1 - e^{-Kt_{PK}})$$

$$V = \frac{125\ mg\ h^{-1}}{(6.5\ mg\ L^{-1})(0.088\ h^{-1})}$$

$$\times (1 - e^{-(0.088\ h^{-1})(1\ h)}) = 18.4\ L.$$

b. With the maintenance infusion;

$$(C_{PK})_{ss} = \left(\frac{Q}{VK}\right)\frac{1 - e^{-Kt_{inf}}}{1 - e^{-K\tau}}$$

$$= \left(\frac{70\ mg\ h^{-1}}{(18.4\ L)(0.088\ h^{-1})}\right)\frac{1 - e^{-(0.088)(1)}}{1 - e^{-(0.088)(12)}}$$

$$= 5.6\ mg\ L^{-1}$$

$$(C_{TR})_{ss} = (C_{PK})_{ss}(e^{-K(\tau - t_{inf})})$$
$$= 5.6\ mg\ L^{-1}(e^{-(0.088)(12-1)})$$
$$= 2.1\ mg\ L^{-1}$$

c. The C_{PK} from the loading infusion is $6.5\ mg\ L$, which is *not* equal to that at steady state, $(C_{PK})_{ss}$, $5.6\ mg\ L^{-1}$

d. Continuing the loading dose:

$$(C_p)_\infty = \frac{Q_L}{VK} = \frac{125\ mg\ h^{-1}}{(18.4\ L)(0.088\ h^{-1})}$$

$$= 77.2\ mg\ L^{-1}, \text{ a massively toxic level.}$$

e. Repeating the loading infusion intermittently:

$$(C_{PK})_{ss} = \left(\frac{Q}{VK}\right)\frac{1 - e^{-Kt_{inf}}}{1 - e^{-K\tau}}$$

$$= \left(\frac{125\ mg\ h^{-1}}{(18.4\ L)(0.088\ h^{-1})}\right)\frac{1 - e^{-(0.088)(1)}}{1 - e^{-(0.088)(12)}}$$

$$= 9.97\ mg\ L^{-1}.$$

This is also too high.

f. The loading infusion repeated intermittently as a 1 h infusion every 12 h would give:

$$(C_{ave})_{ss} = \frac{FX_0}{\tau KV}$$

$$= \frac{(1)(125\ mg)}{(12\ h)(0.088\ h^{-1})(18.4\ L)}$$

$$= 6.43\ mg\ L^{-1}.$$

This is too high.

g. The loading infusion repeated intermittently as a 1 h infusion every 12 h would give:

$$(C_{TR})_{ss} = (C_{PK})_{ss}(e^{-K(\tau - t_{inf})})$$

$$= 9.97\ mg\ L^{-1}(e^{-(0.088)(12-1)})$$

$$= 3.79\ mg\ L^{-1}.$$

This is also too high.

h. For a continuous infusion,

$$Q = VK(C_p)_{\infty}$$

$$= (18.4\ L)(0.088\ h^{-1})(6.5\ mg\ L^{-1})$$

$$= 10.5\ mg\ h^{-1}.$$

15

Non-linear pharmacokinetics

Objectives

Upon completion of this chapter, you will have the ability to:

- perform pharmacokinetic calculations for drugs that have partially saturated their metabolic sites (capacity-limited metabolism)
- obtain values of the Michaelis–Menten elimination parameters from plasma drug concentration data, either graphically or by equation
- estimate the daily dosing rate necessary to attain a target steady-state plasma drug concentration
- calculate the steady-state plasma drug concentration that will be attained from a given daily dosing rate
- estimate the time necessary to reach 90% of steady-state plasma drug concentrations
- calculate target phenytoin concentrations for a patient with hypoalbuminemia.

15.1 Introduction

Pharmacokinetic parameters, such as elimination half life ($t_{1/2}$), the elimination rate constant (K), the apparent volume of distribution (V) and the systemic clearance (Cl) of most drugs are not expected to change when different doses are administered and/or when the drug is administered via different routes as a single or multiple doses. The kinetics of these drugs is described as linear, or dose-independent, pharmacokinetics and is characterized by the first-order process. The term linear simply means that plasma concentration at a given time at steady state and the area under the plasma concentration versus time curve (AUC) will both be directly proportional to the dose administered, as illustrated in Fig. 15.1.

For some drugs, however, the above situation may not apply. For example, when the daily dose of phenytoin is increased by 50% in a patient from 300 mg to 450 mg, the average steady-state plasma concentration [$(C_p)_{ss}$] may increase by as much as 10-fold. This dramatic increase in the concentration (greater than directly proportional) is attributed to the non-linear kinetics of phenytoin.

For drugs that exhibit non-linear or dose dependent kinetics, the fundamental pharmacokinetic parameters such as clearance, the apparent volume of distribution and the elimination half life may vary depending on the administered dose. This is because one or more of the kinetic processes (absorption, distribution and/or elimination) of the drug may be occurring via a mechanism other than simple first-order kinetics. For these drugs, therefore, the relationship between the AUC or the plasma concentration at a given time at steady state and the administered dose is not linear (Fig. 15.2).

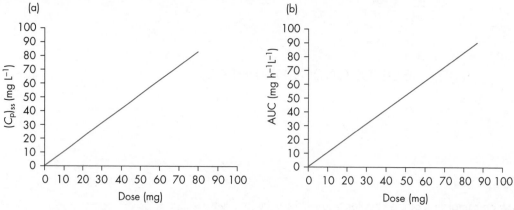

Figure 15.1   Relationship between the plasma concentration (C_p) at a time at steady state (a) and the area under the plasma concentration versus time (AUC) curve (b) against the administered dose for a drug that exhibits *dose-independent* pharmacokinetics.

Furthermore, administration of different doses of these drugs may not result in parallel plasma concentration versus time profiles expected for drugs with linear pharmacokinetics (Fig. 15.3).

For drugs with non-linear metabolism, the initial rate of decline in the plasma concentrations of high doses of drug may be less than proportional to the decline in plasma concentration; by comparison, after the administration of lower doses, the decline will be proportional to plasma concentration and the proportionality constant will be K (Fig. 15.4).

This means that the rate of elimination is not directly proportional to the plasma concentration for these drugs. The reason for this non-linearity is explained as follows:

Non-linearity may arise at at any one of the various pharmacokinetic steps, such as absorption, distribution and/or elimination. For example, the extent of absorption of amoxicillin decreases with an increase in dose. For distribution, plasma protein binding of disopyramide is saturable at the therapeutic concentration, resulting in an increase in the volume of distribution

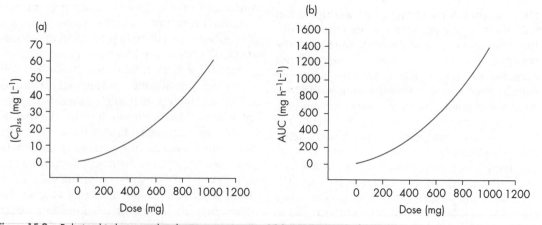

Figure 15.2   Relationship between the plasma concentration (C_p) at a time at steady state (a) and the area under the plasma concentration versus time (AUC) curve (b) against the administered dose for a drug that exhibits *dose-dependent* pharmacokinetics.

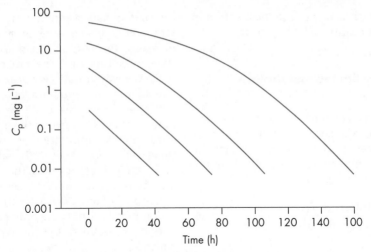

Figure 15.3 The relationship between plasma concentration (C_p) and time following the administration of different doses of a drug that exhibits dose-dependent elimination pharmacokinetics.

with an increase in dose of the drug. As for non-linearity in renal excretion, it has been shown that the antibacterial agent dicloxacillin has saturable active secretion in the kidneys, resulting in a decrease in renal clearance as dose is increased.

Both phenytoin and ethanol have saturable metabolism, which means an increase in dose results in a decrease in hepatic clearance and a more than proportional increase in AUC. In the remainder of this chapter, non-linearity in

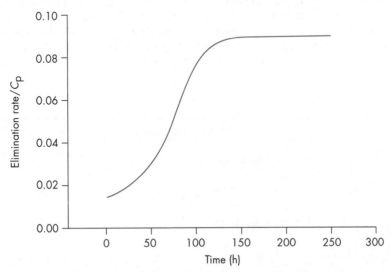

Figure 15.4 Plot of elimination rate (dC_p/dt) normalized for plasma drug concentration (C_p) versus time. Early after a dose of drug, when drug levels are high, dose-dependent elimination kinetics may apply. In this case, the elimination rate is less than proportional to plasma drug concentration. When plasma drug levels have declined sufficiently (after about 100h in this figure), the elimination rate is directly proportional to C_p, with proportionality constant K (horizontal section).

metabolism, which is one of the most common sources of non-linearity, will be discussed.

15.2 Capacity-limited metabolism

Capacity-limited metabolism is also called saturable metabolism, Michaelis–Menten kinetics or mixed-order kinetics. The process of enzymatic metabolism of drugs may be explained by the relationship depicted below

$$\text{Enzyme} + \text{Substrate(drug)} \rightarrow \text{Enzyme–drug}$$
$$\text{complex} \rightarrow \text{Enzyme} + \text{Metabolite}$$

First the drug interacts with the enzyme to produce a drug–enzyme intermediate. Then the intermediate complex is further processed to produce a metabolite, with release of the enzyme. The released enzyme is recycled back to react with more drug molecules.

According to the principles of Michaelis–Menten kinetics, the rate of drug metabolism changes as a function of drug concentration, as illustrated in Fig. 15.5.

Based on this relationship, at very low drug concentration, the concentration of available enzymes is much greater than the number of drug molecules or the drug concentration. Therefore, when the concentration of drug is increased, going from left to right in Fig. 15.5, the rate of metabolism is also increased proportionally

(linear elimination kinetics). However, after a certain point, as the drug plasma concentration increases, the rate of metabolism increases less than proportionally. The other extreme occurs when the concentration of drug is very high relative to the concentration of available enzyme molecules. Under this condition, all of the enzyme molecules are saturated with the drug molecules and, when concentration is increased further, there will be no change in the rate of metabolism of the drug. In other words, the maximum rate of metabolism (V_{max}) has been achieved.

The rate of metabolism, or the rate of elimination if metabolism is the only pathway of elimination, is defined by the Michaelis–Menten equation:

$$\text{Metabolism rate} = \frac{V_{max}C}{K_m + C} \qquad (15.1)$$

where V_{max} is the maximum rate ($\mathrm{mg\,h^{-1}}$) of metabolism; K_m is the Michaelis–Menten constant ($\mathrm{mg\,L^{-1}}$) and C is the drug concentration ($\mathrm{mg\,L^{-1}}$).

The maximum rate of metabolism (i.e. V_{max}) is dependent on the amount or concentration of enzyme available for metabolism of the drug; K_m is the concentration of the drug that results in a metabolic rate equal to one half of V_{max} ($V_{max}/2$). In addition, K_m is inversely related to the affinity of the drug for the metabolizing enzymes (the higher the affinity, the lower the K_m value).

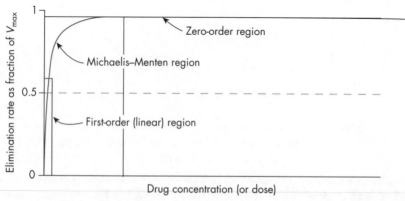

Figure 15.5 Relationship between elimination rate and the plasma concentration of a drug that exhibits dose-dependent pharmacokinetics. At high drug concentrations, where saturation occurs, the elimination rate approaches its maximum, V_{max}.

The unit for the maximum rate of metabolism is the unit of elimination rate and is normally expressed as amount per unit time (e.g. $mg\,h^{-1}$). However, in some instances, it may be expressed as concentration per unit time (e.g. $mg\,L^{-1}h^{-1}$).

Equation 15.1 describes the relationship between the metabolism (or elimination) rate and the concentration over the entire range of concentrations. However, different regions of the Michaelis–Menten curve (Fig. 15.5) can be examined with regard to drug concentrations. At one extreme, the drug concentration may be much smaller than K_m. In this case, the concentration term may be deleted from the denominator of Eq. 15.1, yielding:

$$\text{Metabolism rate} = \frac{V_{max}C}{K_m} \qquad (15.2)$$

Because both V_{max} and K_m are constants, the metabolism rate is proportional to the drug concentration and a constant (i.e. first-order process) in this region:

$$\text{Metabolism rate} = KC \qquad (15.3)$$

$$K = \frac{V_{max}}{K_m}$$

where units of K are $\frac{mg\,L^{-1}\,h^{-1}}{mg\,L^{-1}} = h^{-1}$

Equation 15.3 is analogous to the classical first-order rate equation ($-dX/dt = KX$).

At the other extreme, the drug concentrations are much higher than K_m; therefore, the term K_m may be deleted from the denominator of Eq. 15.1:

$$\text{Metabolism rate} = \frac{V_{max}C}{C} = V_{max} \qquad (15.4)$$

Equation 15.4 is analogous to the zero-order equation ($-dX/dt = K_0$). Equation 15.4 shows that, when the drug concentration is much higher than K_m, the rate of metabolism is a constant (V_{max}), regardless of drug concentration. This situation is similar to zero-order kinetics; at drug concentrations around the K_m, a mixed order is observed, which is defined by the Michaelis–Menten equation (Eq. 15.1).

15.3 Estimation of Michaelis–Menten parameters (V_{max} and K_m)

Estimation of Michaelis–Menten parameters from administration of a single dose

Following the administration of a drug as an intravenous solution, drug plasma concentration is measured at various times. This gives a set of concentration versus time data (Fig. 15.6).

Use concentration versus time data and follow the following steps to obtain the information necessary to determine V_{max} and K_m.

Determine dC_p/dt (rate; units of $mg\,L^{-1}h^{-1}$): for example,

$$\frac{(C_p)_0 - (C_p)_1}{t_1 - t_0} = \frac{\Delta C_p}{\Delta t}$$

Determine the midpoint concentration (i.e. average concentration; units of $mg\,L^{-1}$):

$$\frac{(C_p)_0 + (C_p)_1}{2}$$

The practical expression of Michaelis–Menten equation becomes:

$$\left(\frac{\Delta C_p}{\Delta t}\right)_{\bar{t}} = \frac{V_{max}(\overline{C}_p)_{\bar{t}}}{K_m + (\overline{C}_p)_{\bar{t}}} \qquad (15.5)$$

There are two ways to linearize Eq. 15.5, which will then enable determination of V_{max} and K_m.

Lineweaver–Burke plot

Take the reciprocal of Eq. 15.5

$$\frac{1}{\left(\frac{\Delta C_p}{\Delta t}\right)_{\bar{t}}} = \left(\frac{K_m}{V_{max}} \cdot \frac{1}{(C_p)_{\bar{t}}}\right) + \frac{1}{V_{max}} \qquad (15.6)$$

The plot of $\dfrac{1}{\left(\frac{\Delta C_p}{\Delta t}\right)_{\bar{t}}}$ against $\dfrac{1}{(C_p)_{\bar{t}}}$ yields a straight line (Fig. 15.7).

On this plot, the intercept is $1/V_{max}$.
So $V_{max} = 1/\text{intercept}$.
The slope of the plot is given by K_m/V_{max}.

(a)

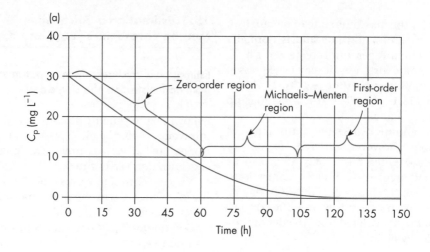

(b)

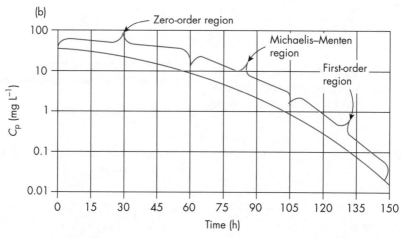

Figure 15.6   Plasma concentration (C_p) versus time profile following the administration of an intravenous bolus dose of a drug that exhibits the characteristics of dose-dependent pharmacokinetics. (a) Rectilinear plot; (b) semilogarithmic plot.

So using two corresponding sets of values on the line for x and y, the slope will equal $(Y_2 - Y_1)/(X_2 - X_1)$ and will have units of $(\text{h L mg}^{-1})/(\text{L mg}^{-1}) = \text{h}$ (i.e. units of time).

The calculated slope then equals K_m/V_{max}.

Slope (h) $\times V_{max}$ (mg L^{-1} h^{-1}) $= K_m$ (mg L^{-1}).

A second way of linearizing equation 15.6

$$\frac{1}{\left(\frac{\Delta C_p}{\Delta t}\right)_{\bar{t}}} = \left(\frac{K_m}{V_{max}} \cdot \frac{1}{(\bar{C}_p)_{\bar{t}}}\right) + \frac{1}{V_{max}}$$

Each side of Eq. 15.6 is multiplied by $(\bar{C}_p)_{\bar{t}}$

$$\frac{(\bar{C}_p)_{\bar{t}}}{\left(\frac{\Delta C_p}{\Delta t}\right)_{\bar{t}}} = \frac{K_m}{V_{max}} + \frac{(\bar{C}_p)_{\bar{t}}}{V_{max}} \qquad (15.7)$$

The plot of $\dfrac{(\bar{C}_p)_{\bar{t}}}{\left(\frac{\Delta C_p}{\Delta t}\right)_{\bar{t}}}$ versus $(\bar{C}_p)_{\bar{t}}$ will yield a straight line (Fig. 15.8).

The slope of this line is found as before, $(Y_2 - Y_1)/(X_2 - X_1)$, and will have units of $(\text{h})/(\text{mg L}^{-1}) = \text{h L mg}^{-1}$. The slope is $1/V_{max}$. So $V_{max} = 1/\text{slope}$ (units of mg L^{-1} h^{-1}).

The intercept is K_m/V_{max}.

Intercept (h) $\times V_{max}$ (mg L^{-1} h^{-1}) $= K_m$ (mg L^{-1}).

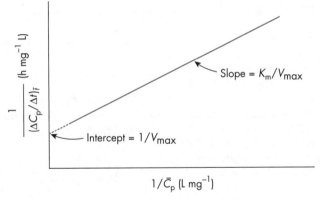

Figure 15.7 Lineweaver–Burke plot to estimate the fundamental pharmacokinetic parameters of a drug that exhibits non-linear kinetics. Km, Michaelis–Menten constant; V_{max}, maximum velocity.

Estimation of Michaelis–Menten parameters following administration of multiple doses

If the drug is administered on a multiple-dosing basis, then the rate of metabolism (or elimination) at steady state will be a function of the steady-state plasma concentration [i.e. $(C_p)_{ss}$]:

Elimination rate or metabolism rate $= -\dfrac{dX}{dt}$

$$= \frac{V_{max}(C_p)_{ss}}{K_m + (C_p)_{ss}}$$

Please note that at steady state, *the rate of elimination is equal to the drug dosing rate (R)*:

$$R = \frac{V_{max}(C_p)_{ss}}{K_m + (C_p)_{ss}} \tag{15.8}$$

In order to estimate V_{max} and K_m, Eq. 15.8 must first be linearized. The following approach may be used. Equation 15.8 is rearranged as follows.

$$R[K_m + (C_p)_{ss}] = V_{max}(C_p)_{ss}$$

$$RK_m + R(C_p)_{ss} = V_{max}(C_p)_{ss}$$

$$R(C_p)_{ss} = V_{max}(C_p)_{ss} - RK_m$$

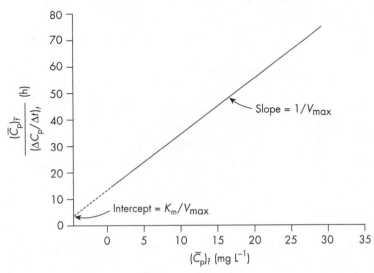

Figure 15.8 Wolf's plot to estimate the fundamental pharmacokinetic parameters of a drug that exhibits non-linear kinetics. Abbreviations as in Fig. 15.7.

$$R = [V_{\max}(C_p)_{ss} - RK_m]/(C_p)_{ss}$$

$$R = V_{\max} - [K_m \times R/(C_p)_{ss}] \tag{15.9}$$

Equation 15.9 indicates that a plot of R versus $R/(C_p)_{ss}$ will be linear, with a slope of $-K_m$ and a y-axis intercept of $V_{\max}$.

To construct such a plot and estimate the values of Michaelis–Menten parameters (i.e. $V_{\max}$ and K_m), one needs at least two sets (three or four is ideal) of doses along with their corresponding steady state plasma concentration values.

Calculation of K_m from two steady-state drug concentrations arising from two infusion rates

The equation derived above (Eq. 15.9) can be used to derive two steady-state drug concentrations (e.g. for a drug such as phenytoin, which undergoes capacity-limited metabolism) arising from two infusion rates:

$$R = V_{\max} - [K_m \times R/(C_p)_{ss}]$$

This equation forms the basis for the linear plot of R versus $R/(C_p)_{ss}$, as seen in Fig. 15.9, with a slope of $-K_m$ and a y-axis intercept of $V_{\max}$. In practice, two pairs of infusion-rate, steady-state drug concentration data will suffice to define the straight line of this plot and evaluate $V_{\max}$

in a patient. The two rates will be

$$R_1 = V_{\max} - [K_m \times R_1/(C_{p1})_{ss}] \tag{15.10}$$

$$R_2 = V_{\max} - [K_m \times R_2/(C_{p2})_{ss}] \tag{15.11}$$

Now, the slope of the line connecting the points $[R_1, R_1/(C_{p1})_{ss}]$ and $[R_2, R_2/(C_{p2})_{ss}]$ will equal $\Delta Y/\Delta X$, or

$$\frac{R_1 - R_2}{\dfrac{R_1}{(C_{p1})_{ss}} - \dfrac{R_2}{(C_{p2})_{ss}}}$$

Substituting the values of R_1 and R_2 from Eqs 15.10 and 15.11 into the numerator of the above expression yields:

$$\frac{V_{\max} - K_m \dfrac{R_1}{(C_{p1})_{ss}} - V_{\max} + K_m \dfrac{R_2}{(C_{p2})_{ss}}}{\dfrac{R_1}{(C_{p1})_{ss}} - \dfrac{R_2}{(C_{p2})_{ss}}}$$

$$= \frac{-K_m \dfrac{R_1}{(C_{p1})_{ss}} + K_m \dfrac{R_2}{(C_{p2})_{ss}}}{\dfrac{R_1}{(C_{p1})_{ss}} - \dfrac{R_2}{(C_{p2})_{ss}}}$$

Upon simplification, this equals:

$$\frac{K_m \left(\dfrac{R_2}{(C_{p2})_{ss}} - \dfrac{R_1}{(C_{p1})_{ss}} \right)}{\dfrac{R_1}{(C_{p1})_{ss}} - \dfrac{R_2}{(C_{p2})_{ss}}} = -K_m$$

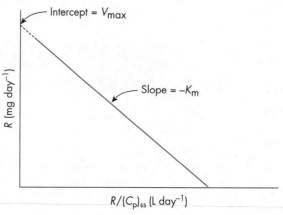

Figure 15.9   The use of dosing rate (R) and the corresponding steady-state plasma concentrations to obtain the pharmacokinetic parameters for a drug that exhibits non-linear kinetics. Abbreviations as in Fig. 15.7.

Once we have the value of K_m, we can obtain the patient's V_{max} by rearrangement of Eq. 15.8, as follows:

$$V_{max} = \frac{R[K_m + (C_p)_{ss}]}{(C_p)_{ss}}$$

Example: estimation of dosing rate (R) and steady-state plasma concentration (C_p)_ss for phenytoin from Michaelis–Menten parameters

If the Michaelis–Menten parameters are known in a patient or are reported in the literature, the dosing rate necessary to obtain a desired steady-state plasma concentration can be estimated.

For example, for phenytoin, the estimated value of K_m and V_{max} are $6.5\,mg\,L^{-1}$ and $548\,mg\,day^{-1}$, respectively. It is desired to obtain a steady-state plasma concentration of $15\,mg\,L^{-1}$. The dosing rate can be determined from Eq. 15.8:

$$R = \frac{V_{max} \times (C_p)_{ss}}{K_m + (C_p)_{ss}}$$

$$R = \frac{548\,mg\,day^{-1} \times 15\,mg\,L^{-1}}{6.5\,mg\,L^{-1} + 15\,mg\,L^{-1}}$$
$$= 382\,mg\,day^{-1}$$

Alternately, if the Michaelis–Menten parameters and the administered dosing rate are known, the steady-state plasma concentration can be predicted. Equation 15.8 may be rearranged to solve for $(C_p)_{ss}$:

$$(C_p)_{ss} = \frac{K_m \times R}{V_{max} - R} \qquad (15.12)$$

In the earlier example, if a dose of $400\,mg\,day^{-1}$ is administered,

$$(C_p)_{ss} = \frac{6.5\,mg\,L^{-1} \times 400\,mg\,day^{-1}}{548\,mg\,day^{-1} - 400\,mg\,day^{-1}}$$
$$(C_p)_{ss} = 17.56\,mg\,L^{-1}.$$

Using Eq. 15.12 and administered daily doses of phenytoin of 100, 200, 300 and 450 mg, the steady-state plasma concentration can be calculated for each dose.

For 100 mg dose:

$$(C_p)_{ss} = \frac{6.5\,mg\,L^{-1} \times 100\,mg\,day^{-1}}{548\,mg\,day^{-1} - 100\,mg\,day^{-1}}$$
$$(C_p)_{ss} = 1.45\,mg\,L^{-1}.$$

For 200 mg dose:

$$(C_p)_{ss} = \frac{6.5\,mg\,L^{-1} \times 200\,mg\,day^{-1}}{548\,mg\,day^{-1} - 200\,mg\,day^{-1}}$$
$$(C_p)_{ss} = 3.73\,mg\,L^{-1}.$$

For 300 mg dose:

$$(C_p)_{ss} = \frac{6.5\,mg\,L^{-1} \times 300\,mg\,day^{-1}}{548\,mg\,day^{-1} - 300\,mg\,day^{-1}}$$
$$(C_p)_{ss} = 7.86\,mg\,L^{-1}.$$

For 450 mg dose:

$$(C_p)_{ss} = \frac{6.5\,mg\,L^{-1} \times 4540\,mg\,day^{-1}}{548\,mg\,day^{-1} - 450\,mg\,day^{-1}}$$
$$(C_p)_{ss} = 29.84\,mg\,L^{-1}.$$

1. What $(C_p)_{ss}$ would be achieved by a 548 $mg\,day^{-1}$ dose?
2. Construct a plot of $(C_p)_{ss}$ versus administered dose.

15.4 Relationship between the area under the plasma concentration versus time curve and the administered dose

For a single intravenous bolus eliminated by a first-order process:

$$(AUC)_0^\infty = \int_0^\infty C_p\,dt = \frac{(Dose)}{VK} \qquad (15.13)$$

Whereas for non-linear kinetics, capacity-limited kinetics or Michaelis–Menten kinetics:

$$(\text{AUC})_0^\infty = \int_0^\infty C_p dt$$

$$= \frac{(C_p)_0}{V_{\max}} \left[\frac{(C_p)_0}{2} + K_m \right] \quad (15.14)$$

High doses

At high doses or when $(C_p)_0 \gg K_m$, the value of K_m in Eq. 15.14 is negligible.

$$(\text{AUC})_0^\infty = \int_0^\infty C_p dt = \frac{(C_p)_0^2}{2(V_{\max})}$$

$$= \frac{(X_0)^2}{2(V_{\max})(V)^2} \quad (15.15)$$

where V is the apparent volume of distribution and X_0 is the dose administered.

Equation 15.15 shows that, for a single, relatively high dose of phenytoin, if you double the dose, the AUC will increase by four times; while tripling the dose will increase plasma concentration nine times. In other words, $(\text{AUC})_0^\infty$ is proportional to the square of the dose. Therefore, a relatively modest increase in the dose may produce a dramatic increase in the total AUC. The effect of increasing the size of doses of phenytoin that will be given in a multiple-dosing regimen can have even more dramatic effects. As mentioned in the introduction to this chapter, increasing the daily dose of phenytoin to a size that is large (compared with $V_{\max}$) can cause steady-state phenytoin concentrations to skyrocket. In fact, daily doses equal to or greater than a patient's maximum rate of metabolism ($V_{\max}$) will cause phenytoin concentrations to increase without an upper limit! These assertions can be validated by use of Eq. 15.12.

Low doses

At low doses: When $(C_p)_0 \ll K_m$, or $(C_p)_0/2 \ll K_m$, the value of $(C_p)_0/2$ in Eq. 15.14 is

ignored because it is much smaller than the value of K_m.

$$(\text{AUC})_0^\infty = \int_0^\infty C_p dt = \frac{(C_p)_0 \times K_m}{V_{\max}}$$

Moreover, $V_{\max}/K_m = K$. Therefore, $K_m/V_{\max} = 1/K$ and $(C_p)_0 = \text{Dose}/V$, which yields Eq. 15.13:

$$(\text{AUC})_0^\infty = \frac{\text{Dose}}{VK}$$

For example, for phenytoin, the reported values of the apparent volume of distribution and $V_{\max}$ are 50 L and 548 mg day^{-1}, respectively. Determine the $(\text{AUC})_0^\infty$ following the daily administration of 100, 200, 300 and 450 mg doses of phenytoin. Remember that, for phenytoin, the literature average $K_m = 6.5$ mg L^{-1}. The apparent volume of distribution for phenytoin is 50 L.

$$V_{\max} = 548 \text{ mg day}^{-1}/50 \text{ L}$$
$$= 10.96 \text{ mg L}^{-1} \text{ day}^{-1}.$$

This situation does not qualify for use of the high dose equation (Eq. 15.15). Neither are the plasma drug concentrations obtained small enough to warrant use of the low dose (linear kinetic) equation (Eq. 15.13). This leaves the requirement to use the general equation for Michaelis–Menten elimination kinetics (Eq. 15.14):

$$(\text{AUC})_0^\infty = \int_0^\infty C_p dt = \frac{(C_p)_0}{V_{\max}} \left[\frac{(C_p)_0}{2} + K_m \right]$$

For 100 mg dose:

$$(C_p)_0 = \text{Dose}/V = 100 \text{ mg}/50 \text{ L} = 2 \text{ mg L}^{-1}$$

$$(\text{AUC})_0^\infty = \int_0^\infty C_p dt = \frac{2 \text{ mg L}^{-1}}{10.96 \text{ mg L}^{-1} \text{ day}^{-1}}$$

$$\times \left[\frac{2 \text{ mg L}^{-1}}{2} + 6.5 \text{ mg L}^{-1} \right]$$

$$= 1.37 \text{ mg L}^{-1} \text{ day}$$

For 200 mg dose:

$$(C_p)_0 = \text{Dose}/V = 200\,\text{mg}/50\,\text{L} = 4\,\text{mg}\,\text{L}^{-1}$$

$$(\text{AUC})_0^\infty = \int_0^\infty C_p dt = \frac{4\,\text{mg}\,\text{L}^{-1}}{10.96\,\text{mg}\,\text{L}^{-1}\,\text{day}^{-1}}$$

$$\times \left[\frac{4\,\text{mg}\,\text{L}^{-1}}{2} + 6.5\,\text{mg}\,\text{L}^{-1}\right]$$

$$= 3.10\,\text{mg}\,\text{L}^{-1}\,\text{day}$$

For 300 mg dose:

$$(C_p)_0 = \text{Dose}/V = 300\,\text{mg}/50\,\text{L} = 6\,\text{mg}\,\text{L}^{-1}$$

$$\text{AUC}_0^\infty = \int_0^\infty C_p dt = \frac{6\,\text{mg}\,\text{L}^{-1}}{10.96\,\text{mg}\,\text{L}^{-1}\,\text{day}^{-1}}$$

$$\times \left[\frac{6\,\text{mg}\,\text{L}^{-1}}{2} + 6.5\,\text{mg}\,\text{L}^{-1}\right]$$

$$= 5.20\,\text{mg}\,\text{L}^{-1}\,\text{day}$$

For 450 mg dose:

$$(C_p)_0 = \text{Dose}/V = 450\,\text{mg}/50\,\text{L} = 9\,\text{mg}\,\text{L}^{-1}$$

$$\text{AUC}_0^\infty = \int_0^\infty C_p dt = \frac{9\,\text{mg}\,\text{L}^{-1}}{10.96\,\text{mg}\,\text{L}^{-1}\,\text{day}^{-1}}$$

$$\times \left[\frac{9\,\text{mg}\,\text{L}^{-1}}{2} + 6.5\,\text{mg}\,\text{L}^{-1}\right]$$

$$= 9.03\,\text{mg}\,\text{L}^{-1}\,\text{day}$$

Using these data, a plot of $(\text{AUC})_0^\infty$ against the administered dose can be constructed. From the plot, make an observation of the relationship.

15.5 Time to reach a given fraction of steady state

In non-linear elimination pharmacokinetics, the time required to reach a given fraction of the steady-state concentration varies with the rate of drug administration and depends upon the values of V_{max} and K_m. For a constant rate of infusion or input, the rate of change of a drug in the body, $V(dC_p/dt)$, is the difference between the rate drug in and the rate drug out.

$$V\frac{dC_p}{dt} = R - \frac{V_{max}C_p}{K_m + C_p} = \frac{RK_m + RC_p - V_{max}C_p}{K_m + C_p}$$

Collecting terms with their appropriate differentials,

$$\frac{K_m + C_p}{RK_m + (R - V_{max})C_p}dC_p = \frac{1}{V}dt$$

Multiplying numerator and denominator of the left side by -1 and splitting terms,

$$\frac{-K_m}{-RK_m + (V_{max} - R)C_p}dC_p$$

$$+ \frac{-C_p}{-RK_m + (V_{max} - R)C_p}dC_p$$

$$= \frac{1}{V}dt$$

Integrating from $(C_p)_0$ to $(C_p)_t$,

$$-K_m \int_{(C_p)_0}^{(C_p)_t} \frac{1}{-RK_m + (V_{max} - R)C_p}dC_p$$

$$+ \int_{(C_p)_0}^{(C_p)_t} \frac{-C_p}{-RK_m + (V_{max} - R)C_p}dC_p$$

$$= \frac{1}{V}\int_0^t dt$$

Performing the integrations (using CRC Selby SM (ed.) (1970). Standard Math Tables, 18th edn. Chemical Rubber Co., Cleveland, OH, p. 397. integrals 27 and 30 to for the first two terms),

$$\frac{-K_m}{V_{max} - R}\ln\frac{-RK_m + (V_{max} - R)(C_p)_t}{-RK_m + (V_{max} - R)(C_p)_0}$$

$$-\left(\frac{(C_p)_t}{V_{max} - R} - \frac{(C_p)_0}{V_{max} - R} - \frac{-RK_m}{(V_{max} - R)^2}\ln\frac{-RK_m + (V_{max} - R)(C_p)_t}{-RK_m + (V_{max} - R)(C_p)_0}\right) = \frac{1}{V}t$$

Multiplying through by $V_{max} - R$,

$$-K_m \ln \frac{-RK_m + (V_{max} - R)(C_p)_t}{-RK_m + (V_{max} - R)(C_p)_0}$$

$$-\left((C_p)_t - (C_p)_0 - \frac{-RK_m}{(V_{max} - R)} \ln \frac{-RK_m + (V_{max} - R)(C_p)_t}{-RK_m + (V_{max} - R)(C_p)_0}\right) = \frac{(V_{max} - R)}{V} t$$

which equals:

$$+K_m \ln \frac{-RK_m + (V_{max} - R)(C_p)_0}{-RK_m + (V_{max} - R)(C_p)_t}$$

$$-\left((C_p)_t - (C_p)_0 - \frac{+RK_m}{(V_{max} - R)} \ln \frac{-RK_m + (V_{max} - R)(C_p)_0}{-RK_m + (V_{max} - R)(C_p)_t}\right) = \frac{(V_{max} - R)}{V} t$$

Multiplying the first term by unity in the form of $(V_{max} - R)/(V_{max} - R)$ and expanding yields:

$$\frac{K_m V_{max}}{V_{max} - R} \ln \frac{-RK_m + (V_{max} - R)(C_p)_0}{-RK_m + (V_{max} - R)(C_p)_t}$$

$$-\frac{K_m R}{V_{max} - R} \ln \frac{-RK_m + (V_{max} - R)(C_p)_0}{-RK_m + (V_{max} - R)(C_p)_t}$$

$$+\left(-(C_p)_t + (C_p)_0 + \frac{+RK_m}{(V_{max} - R)} \ln \frac{-RK_m + (V_{max} - R)(C_p)_0}{-RK_m + (V_{max} - R)(C_p)_t}\right) = \frac{(V_{max} - R)}{V} t$$

Cancellation of terms yields:

$$\frac{K_m V_{max}}{V_{max} - R} \ln \frac{-RK_m + (V_{max} - R)(C_p)_0}{-RK_m + (V_{max} - R)(C_p)_t}$$

$$+ [-(C_p)_t] + (C_p)_0$$

$$= \frac{(V_{max} - R)}{V} t$$

Multiplying both numerator and denominator of the logarithmic expression by -1 yields:

$$\frac{K_m V_{max}}{V_{max} - R} \ln \frac{+RK_m - (V_{max} - R)(C_p)_0}{+RK_m - (V_{max} - R)(C_p)_t}$$

$$+ [-(C_p)_t] + (C_p)_0$$

$$= \frac{(V_{max} - R)}{V} t$$

Rearranging to solve for t, the time to go from $(C_p)_0$ to $(C_p)_t$, yields:

$$\frac{K_m V_{max} V}{(V_{max} - R)^2} \ln \frac{RK_m - (V_{max} - R)(C_p)_0}{RK_m - (V_{max} - R)(C_p)_t} - \frac{V(C_p)_t}{V_{max} - R} + \frac{V(C_p)_0}{V_{max} - R} = t \qquad (15.16)$$

If the starting condition is $(C_p)_0 = 0$, then:

$$\frac{K_m V_{max} V}{(V_{max} - R)^2} \ln \frac{RK_m}{RK_m - (V_{max} - R)(C_p)_t} - \frac{V(C_p)_t}{V_{max} - R} = t$$

(15.17)

If the objective is to determine how much time it will take to reach a given fraction of the drug concentration that will be achieved at steady state (i.e. $(C_p)_t = f_{ss}(C_p)_{ss}$), then Eq. 15.12 needs to be modified as follows:

$$(C_p)_t = \frac{f_{ss} K_m R}{V_{max} - R}$$

(15.18)

and

$$(V_{max} - R)(C_p)_t = f_{ss} K_m R$$

(15.19)

Now the expression in Eq. 15.18 for $(C_p)_t$ and the expression in Eq. 15.19 for $(V_{max} - R)(C_p)_t$ can both be substituted into Eq. 15.17:

$$\frac{K_m V_{max} V}{(V_{max} - R)^2} \ln \frac{RK_m}{RK_m - f_{ss} RK_m} - \frac{f_{ss} RK_m V}{(V_{max} - R)^2} = t_{f_{ss}}$$

(15.20)

Cancellation yields:

$$\frac{K_m V_{max} V}{(V_{max} - R)^2} \ln \frac{1}{1 - f_{ss}} - \frac{f_{ss} RK_m V}{(V_{max} - R)^2} = t_{f_{ss}}$$

(15.21)

Combining common factors gives the expression for time to go from an initial concentration of zero to the concentration achieved at a particular fraction of steady state:

$$\frac{K_m V}{(V_{max} - R)^2} \times \left(V_{max} \ln \frac{1}{1 - f_{ss}} - f_{ss} R \right) = t_{f_{ss}}$$

(15.22)

For the commonly used $f_{ss} = 0.9$, we obtain:

$$\frac{K_m V}{(V_{max} - R)^2} (V_{max} \ln(10) - 0.9R)$$

$$= \frac{K_m V}{(V_{max} - R)^2} (2.303 V_{max} - 0.9R) = t_{0.9}$$

(15.23)

Dimensional analysis

The dimensions will be:

$$\frac{(mg\,L^{-1})(L)}{(mg\,day^{-1})^2} (2.303[mg\,day^{-1}] - 0.9[mg\,day^{-1}])$$

$$= \frac{mg}{(mg\,day^{-1})} = time(days)$$

It is clear from Eq. 15.23 that the time required to reach 90% of steady state for drugs with non-linear kinetics is affected by the dosing rate (R) as well as the values of V_{max}, K_m and the apparent volume of distribution (V) of the drug. For a given drug, however, the time required to attain a given fraction of the steady-state concentration is determined by the chosen rate of drug administration (R), the other parameters being constant for a particular drug administered to a particular patient.

15.6 Example: calculation of parameters for phenytoin

The time required to attain 90% of the true steady-state plasma concentration for phenytoin

Let us assume that we are interested in determining the time required to attain 90% of the true steady-state plasma concentration for phenytoin, which is administered at different rates, where $V = 50\,L$, $V_{max} = 500\,mg\,day^{-1}$ and $K_m = 4\,\mu g\,mL^{-1}$ ($= 4\,mg\,L^{-1}$). Using Eq. 15.23, the time required to attain 90% of the steady-state concentration can be determined for various daily doses:

For 100 mg dose:

$$\frac{(4\ \text{mg L}^{-1})(50\text{L})}{(400\ \text{mg day}^{-1})^2}(2.303[500\ \text{mg day}^{-1}]$$

$$-\,0.9[100\ \text{mg day}^{-1}]) = 1.33\ \text{days}$$

For 200 mg dose:

$$\frac{(4\ \text{mg L}^{-1})(50\text{L})}{(300\ \text{mg day}^{-1})^2}(2.303[500\ \text{mg day}^{-1}]$$

$$-\,0.9[200\text{mg day}^{-1}]) = 2.16\ \text{days}$$

For 300 mg dose:

$$\frac{(4\ \text{mg L}^{-1})(50\text{L})}{(200\ \text{mg day}^{-1})^2}(2.303[500\ \text{mg day}^{-1}]$$

$$-\,0.9[300\ \text{mg day}^{-1}]) = 4.41\ \text{days}$$

For 400 mg dose:

$$\frac{(4\ \text{mg L}^{-1})(50\text{L})}{(100\ \text{mg day}^{-1})^2}(2.303[500\ \text{mg day}^{-1}]$$

$$-\,0.9[400\ \text{mg day}^{-1}]) = 15.8\ \text{days}$$

What plasma phenytoin concentrations would be achieved at the times and doses above? The answer is that slight modifications of the steady-state phenytoin concentration can be made as follows (using Eq. 15.12):

$$0.9(C_\text{p})_\text{ss} = 0.9K_\text{m}R/(V_\text{max} - R) \qquad (15.24)$$

From this a table can be constructed (Table 15.1).

What if K_m was equal to $5.7\ \text{mg L}^{-1}$ instead of $4\ \text{mg L}^{-1}$? The answer is that, since K_m appears only in the numerator of Eq. 15.23, there is a direct proportion between K_m and the time to reach 90% of the steady-state phenytoin concentration. Similarly, the value $0.9(C_\text{p})_\text{ss}$ is also directly proportional to K_m. Therefore, each of the above values can be multiplied by the factor $(5.7/4.0)$, resulting in the figures given in Table 15.2.

Table 15.1 Time ($t_{0.9}$) to 90% of steady-state plasma concentration (C_p)$_\text{ss}$ level as a function of daily dose (R)

R (mg/day)	$t_{0.9}$ (days)	$0.9(C_\text{p})_\text{ss}$ (mg L^{-1})
100	1.33	0.90
200	2.16	2.40
300	4.41	5.10
400	15.8	14.4

Alternative equation to calculate the time to reach a given fraction of steady state

If V_max is not known, but the desired steady-state drug (e.g. phenytoin) concentration is known, a different equation must be used to calculate the time required to reach a given fraction of steady state. Equation 15.8 can be easily rearranged to the following expression:

$$V_\text{max} = \frac{RK_\text{m}}{(C_\text{p})_\text{ss}} + R \qquad (15.25)$$

Thus,

$$V_\text{max} - R = \frac{RK_\text{m}}{(C_\text{p})_\text{ss}} \qquad (15.26)$$

Table 15.2 Time ($t_{0.9}$) to 90% of steady-state plasma concentration (C_p)$_\text{ss}$ level as a function of daily dose (R) and K_m

R (mg/day)	$t_{0.9}$ (days)	$0.9(C_\text{p})_\text{ss}$ (mg L^{-1})
100	1.90	1.28
200	3.08	3.42
300	6.28	7.27
400	22.5	20.5

Substitution of the above expressions for V_{max} and $(V_{max} - R)$ into Eq. 15.22 results in:

$$t_{f_{ss}} = \frac{V(C_p)_{ss}}{R}\left(\frac{(C_p)_{ss}}{K_m}\left(\ln\frac{1}{1-f_{ss}} - f_{ss}\right)\right.$$

$$\left. + \ln\frac{1}{1-f_{ss}}\right) \qquad (15.27)$$

For $f_{ss} = 0.9$, this equals:

$$t_{0.9} = \frac{V(C_p)_{ss}}{R}\left(1.403\frac{(C_p)_{ss}}{K_m} + 2.303\right)$$

$$(15.28)$$

The time required for plasma phenytoin concentration to decline from an initial value to a particular value

Rate of metabolism, or more generally elimination, is the decrease of plasma drug concentration over time. Therefore, Eq. 15.1 can be rewritten as:

$$-\frac{dC_p}{dt} = \frac{V_{max}C_p}{K_m + C_p}$$

Collecting terms with their appropriate differentials,

$$-\frac{dC_p}{C_p}(K_m + C_p) = V_{max}dt$$

Expanding,

$$-dC_p - \frac{K_m}{C_p}dC_p = V_{max}dt$$

Taking integrals for $t=0$ to $t=t$,

$$-\int_{(C_p)_t}^{(C_p)_0} dC_p - K_m\int_{(C_p)_t}^{(C_p)_0}\frac{1}{C_p}dC_p$$

$$= V_{max}\int_0^t dt$$

Performing the integration,

$$(C_p)_0 - (C_p)_t + K_m\ln\frac{(C_p)_0}{(C_p)_t} = V_{max}t \qquad (15.29)$$

In this case V_{max} would have units of concentration per unit time. For V_{max} expressed in units of mass per unit time, the equation would be:

$$(C_p)_0 - (C_p)_t + K_m\ln\frac{(C_p)_0}{(C_p)_t} = \frac{V_{max}}{V}t \qquad (15.30)$$

Free and total plasma phenytoin concentrations

Only unbound (free) drug is capable of exerting pharmacological (or toxic) effect. The following example depicts the adjustments required in the case of an atypical free fraction of phenytoin in the blood.

Problem

A patient with hypoalbuminemia has a phenytoin free fraction of 0.22. Calculate a reasonable target total (free + bound) plasma phenytoin concentration in this patient.

Solution

The average percentage phenytoin bound to plasma proteins is 89%, which corresponds to a percentage free equal to $100 - 89 = 11\%$. Expressed as a decimal, the nominal free fraction of phenytoin is 0.11. This is termed the fraction unbound in the plasma (f_{up}).

A reasonable *total* phenytoin concentration at steady state is in the middle of the therapeutic range: $15\,\mu g\,mL^{-1}$. Since unbound drug concentration is equal to the free fraction times the total drug concentration, we define:

$$(C_p)_{free} = f_{up}C_p \qquad (15.31)$$

Therefore, a patient with a nominal free fraction of phenytoin will have a target free phenytoin concentration of $(0.11)\times(15\,\mu g\,mL^{-1}) = 1.65\,\mu g\,mL^{-1}$.

Target total plasma concentrations will be different for different free fractions; however, *the target free plasma phenytoin concentration remains $1.65\,\mu g\,mL^{-1}$.* That is, this value is invariant, regardless of the patient's free phenytoin fraction.

This fact can be used when Eq. 15.31 is rearranged to solve for the target total phenytoin concentration in the patient in this example:

$$
\begin{aligned}
\text{target } (C_p)_{\text{patient}} &= \frac{\text{target } (C_p)_{\text{free}}}{(f_{up})_{\text{patient}}} \\
&= \frac{1.65\,\mu g\ mL^{-1}}{0.22} \\
&= 7.50\,\mu g\ mL^{-1}
\end{aligned}
$$

Notice that, in this problem, the patient's free fraction is twice normal; so, her total plasma phenytoin concentration requirement is exactly one-half of the usual $15\,\mu g\ mL^{-1}$.

Problem set 8

Problems for Chapter 15

Question 1

Patient AB, a 40-year-old female weighing 67 kg presented to the hospital emergency room with epileptiform seizures. A phenytoin assay shows no phenytoin in the plasma. In the absence of individual pharmacokinetic parameters, the literature average values should be used:

- maximum reaction rate $(V_{max}) = 7.5$ mg kg day^{-1}
- Michaelis–Menten constant $(K_m) = 5.7$ mg^{-1} L.
- volume of distribution $(V) = 0.64$ L kg^{-1}
- salt value for sodium phenytoin $= 0.916$
- absolute oral bioavailability $(F_{PO}) = 0.98$.

a. Suggest a loading dose of intravenous sodium phenytoin, $(D_L)_{IV}$, for this patient. Base the desired plasma concentration, $(C_p)_{desired}$, on a maximum concentration $(C_p)_{max}$ of 20 mg L.

b. The patient has been stabilized by a series of short intravenous infusions of sodium phenytoin. For a target average phenytoin concentration of 15 mg L, calculate a daily oral main-tenance dose (D_o) of sodium phenytoin for this patient).

c. If sodium phenytoin capsules are available in 100 mg and 30 mg strengths, what combination of these will closely approximate the daily dose of sodium phenytoin calculated in part (b)?

d. One month later, the patient's regimen is to be reviewed. Steady-state plasma concentrations from two different dosage rates have shown that this patient's V_{max} equals 10 mg kg day^{-1} and her K_m equals 6.0 mg L^{-1}. Calculate a

new daily oral maintenance dose of sodium phenytoin.

e. What intravenous dosing rate in milligrams per day of sodium phenytoin would equal the oral dosing regimen in part (d)?

Question 2

Patient BC, the identical twin of patient AB in question 1, also weighing 67 kg but with a history of hypoalbuminemia, presents to the hospital with epileptiform seizures. A phenytoin assay shows no phenytoin in the plasma. Patient BC is stabilized by a series of short intravenous infusions of sodium phenytoin. Although her seizures have been stabilized, the patient exhibits a plasma total phenytoin concentration of only 7.5 mg L, prompting the determination of a free (unbound) phenytoin concentration. The free phenytoin concentration is 1.65 mg L^{-1}. In the absence of individual pharmacokinetic parameters, employ literature average values:

- maximum reaction rate $(V_{max}) = 7.5$ mg kg day^{-1}
- Michaelis–Menten constant $(K_m) = 5.7$ mg L^{-1}
- volume of distribution $(V) = 0.64$ L kg^{-1}
- salt value for sodium phenytoin $= 0.916$
- absolute bioavailability $(F_{PO}) = 0.98$.

a. What is the free fraction of phenytoin in patient BC?

b. Does the total (bound and free) concentration of 7.5 mg L^{-1} represent a subtherapeutic concentration in this patient?

c. What total phenytoin concentration, $(C_p)_{total}$, would this value of 7.5 mg L^{-1} in patient BC correspond to in a patient with normal serum albumin and a normal free fraction of phenytoin?

d. Calculate a daily oral maintenance dose of sodium phenytoin for patient BC using the literature average values.

Answers

Question 1 answer

a.

$$(D_L)_{IV} = \frac{(0.64\,L\,kg^{-1})(67\,kg)(20\,mg\,L^{-1}-0\,mg\,L^{-1})}{(0.916)(1)}$$

$$= 936\,mg.$$

b. Daily oral maintenance dosage:

$$\frac{D_o}{\tau} = \frac{V_{max}(C_p)_\infty}{[K_m+(C_p)_\infty](SF_{PO})}$$

$$= \frac{(7.5\,mg\,kg^{-1})(67\,kg)(15\,mg\,L^{-1})}{(5.7\,mg\,L^{-1}+15\,mg\,L^{-1})(0.916)(0.98)}$$

$$= 406\,mg.$$

$D_o = 406$ mg sodium phenytoin daily.

c. Four capsules of 100 mg.

d. Revised daily oral maintenance dose:

$$\left(\frac{D_o}{\tau}\right)_{PO} = \frac{(10\,mg\,kg^{-1})(67\,kg)(15\,mg\,L^{-1})}{(6\,mg\,L^{-1}+15\,mg\,L^{-1})(0.916)(0.98)}$$

$$= 533\,mg.$$

$D_o = 533$ mg sodium phenytoin daily.

e. Daily intravenous dose equivalent to oral dose of 533 mg:

$$\left(\frac{D_o}{\tau}\right)_{IV} = (533\,mg)(0.98) = 522\,mg.$$

$D_{IV} = 522$ mg sodium phenytoin daily.

Question 2 answer

a. The free fraction is given by:

$$\frac{(C_p)_{free}}{(C_p)_{total}} = \frac{1.65\,mg\,L^{-1}}{7.5\,mg\,L^{-1}} = 0.22$$

b. In fact a free phenytoin concentration of $1.65\,mg\,L^{-1}$ is in the midrange of the therapeutic window for phenytoin and, as such, represents a useful target.

c. Since the normal free fraction of phenytoin is 0.11, the total phenytoin concentration in a normal person would be:

$$(Cp)_{total} \times 0.11 = 0.22 \times 7.5\,mg\,L^{-1}$$

$$= 15\,mg\,L^{-1}.$$

d. To calculate a daily dose using the Michaelis–Menten equation, the target $(C_p)_{total}$ of 7.5 mg L is not used. Instead, the value used is the $(C_p)_{total}$ to which the observed concentration of 7.5 mg L would correspond if this patient had a normal free fraction. The adjusted total phenytoin concentration, calculated above in (c), equals $15\,mg\,L^{-1}$. This adjusted value is used in the Michaelis–Menten equation. This reflects the fact that more phenytoin is available for elimination when the free fraction is higher than normal. In patient BC, a dose based on a target total phenytoin concentration of 15 mg L should achieve a steady-state,

$$(C_p)_{total} = \left(\frac{0.11}{0.22}\right)(15\,mg\,L^{-1})$$

$$= 7.5\,mg\,L^{-1}$$

and a therapeutic *free* phenytoin concentration,

$$(C_p)_{free} = 0.22 \times 7.5\,mg\,L = 1.65\,mg\,L^{-1}.$$

Now, we can calculate the daily oral dose:

$$\frac{X_o}{\tau} = \frac{V_{max}(C_{p\infty})_{adjusted}}{[K_m+(C_p)_\infty](SF_{PO})}$$

$$= \frac{(7.5\,mg\,kg^{-1})(67\,kg)(15\,mg\,L^{-1})}{(5.7\,mg\,L^{-1}+15\,mg\,L^{-1})(0.916)(0.98)}$$

$$= 406\,mg.$$

Notice that this is the same daily dose as used in patient AB above, the identical twin with normal serum albumin and a normal phenytoin free fraction of 0.11.

We expect that 400 mg day of oral sodium phenytoin will produce a $(C_{p\infty})_{total}$ of 7.5 mg L^{-1} and a $(C_{p\infty})_{free}$ of 1.65 mg L^{-1} in patient BC.

16

Drug interactions

Objectives

Upon completion of this chapter, you will have the ability to:

- predict the effect of a change in hepatic blood flow or intrinsic clearance on hepatic drug clearance
- calculate the change in unbound and total plasma drug concentration after a plasma protein binding displacement interaction
- characterize cytochrome P450-based drug interactions and predict their likely clinical significance
- characterize drug interactions mediated by transporters.

16.1 Introduction

A large fraction of clinically significant drug interactions are mediated by one of the following:

- a change in the intrinsic clearance of free (unbound) drug (Cl'_{int})
- a change in the free fraction of drug in plasma (f_{up})
- change in blood flow to the liver (Q_H).

The bottom line on any drug interaction is whether we expect the effect of the drug to increase, decrease or remain the same after an interaction with another drug. The effect of a drug which has reached steady-state equilibrium is directly (but not linearly) related to the concentration of unbound (free) drug at steady state, $(C_u)_{ss}$.

The concentration of unbound drug at steady state is calculated from:

$$(C_u)_{ss} = (f_{up})(C_{ss}) \qquad (16.1)$$

where C_{ss} is the total drug concentration at steady state.

The term C_{ss} is given by a different formula depending on whether the drug is administered orally or intravenously.

Orally:

$$C_{ss} = (f_{GIT})(\text{Dose}/\tau)/(f_{up})(Cl'_{int}) \qquad (16.2)$$

Intravenously:

$$C_{ss} = (\text{Dose}/\tau)/Cl_H \qquad (16.3)$$

In these equations, f_{GIT} is the fraction of drug traversing the gastrointestinal tract membrane and reaching the portal vein; τ is the dosing interval; f_{up} is the free fraction of drug in plasma; Cl'_{int} is the intrinsic clearance of free drug; and Cl_H is hepatic clearance of drug.

For orally administered drug, the total drug concentration at steady state is seen to be inversely related to the free fraction of drug in plasma and the the intrinsic clearance of free drug and to be unrelated to changes in hepatic clearance of drug. For intravenously administered drug, Eq. 16.3 shows that the total drug concentration at steady state is inversely related to hepatic clearance of drug.

From Chapter 4 (Eq. 4.12) we know that hepatic clearance of drug may be defined as:

$$Cl_H = (Q_H)\frac{Cl_{int}}{Q_H + Cl_{int}} \qquad (16.4)$$

where Cl_H is hepatic clearance from plasma; Q_H is blood flow to the liver; and Cl_{int} is intrinsic plasma clearance of total drug.

Also, from Ch. 4, since Eq. 4.11 states that $Cl'_{int} = (Cl_{int})/f_{up}$, then Eq. 16.5 is formed by substituting $f_{up}Cl'_{int}$ for Cl_{int} in Eq. 16.4:

$$Cl_H = (Q_H)\frac{f_{up}Cl'_{int}}{Q_H + f_{up}Cl'_{int}} \qquad (16.5)$$

This is one step away from having all the tools to predict what will happen in a given drug interaction. Specifically, we need to show what happens to the equation for Cl_H for intravenously administered drug under two situations:

- when $Q_H > f_{up}Cl'_{int}$, which occurs for a drug with a low hepatic extraction ratio (E)
- when $Q_H < f_{up}Cl'_{int}$, which occurs for a drug with a high hepatic extraction ratio.

Recall that for intravenously administered drug, total drug concentration at steady state is inversely related to hepatic clearance.

Moreover, the two equations for Cl_H are:

$$Cl_H(\text{low } E) \sim f_{up}Cl'_{int} \qquad (16.6)$$

$$Cl_H(\text{high } E) \sim Q_H \qquad (16.7)$$

Finally, we have the requisite equations to construct tables of expected outcomes of drug interactions from changes in intrinsic free clearance or in hepatic blood flow (Table 16.1 and Table 16.2.)

16.2 The effect of protein-binding interactions

Drugs may bind, to a greater or lesser extent, to macromolecules found in the blood. The resulting drug–macromolecule complex is too large for the drug to be able to occupy its receptor and exert a pharmacological response. Therefore, unbound (free) drug molecules are responsible for a drug's therapeutic activity. In other words, it is the free, not the total, drug concentration that correlates with effect.

The major drug-binding protein is albumin, a 65 kDa (kilodalton) protein that is present in the blood, normally at a concentration of approximately 4.5%. Albumin binds both anionic (acidic) and cationic (basic) drugs. A drug-binding protein responsible for the binding of many cationic drugs is α_1-acid glycoprotein. Other macromolecules that may play a role in binding of drugs include lipoprotein (for some lipophilic drugs) and globulin (for corticosteroids).

The most significant drug interaction involving protein binding in the blood is where a highly bound (> 90% bound) drug is partially displaced from binding sites by another drug or chemical. A large increase in the free concentration of drug can ensue, with a resulting increase in therapeutic or toxic effect. This effect is more pronounced in the case of highly bound drugs. For example, a decrease in the percentage drug bound from 95% to 90% represents a doubling of the amount of free drug (that is, the free fraction goes from 5 to 10%). Depending on the characteristics of the drug being displaced (size of the volume of distribution, magnitude of the hepatic extraction ratio and whether the drug has been administered orally or intravenously), different changes in various pharmacokinetic parameters and in the concentration of unbound drug may occur. This is illustrated in the example below, where a protein-binding displacement interaction causes a drug's free fraction to double from 0.5% to 1.0%. (Table 16.5, left side).

Changes in volume of distribution

The general equation that expresses the apparent volume of distribution at steady state (V_{ss}) as a function of its contributing parameters is:

$$V_{ss} = 7.5 + 7.5(f_{up}) + V_{incell}\left(\frac{f_{up}}{f_{ut}}\right) \qquad (16.8)$$

where f_{up} is the fraction drug unbound in the plasma; f_{ut} is fraction drug unbound in the

Table 16.1 Consequences of a decrease in intrinsic free clearance $(Cl'_{int})^a$ on parameters and pharmacological effect of a drug currently being administered

Parameters	Oral drug		Intravenous drug	
	Low E	High E	Low E	High E
Cl_H	↓	↔	↓	↔
C_{ss}	↑	↑	↑	↔
$(C_u)_{ss}$	↑	↑	↑	↔
Effect at steady state	↑	↑	↑	↔

E, hepatic extraction ratio; Cl_H, hepatic clearance from plasma; C_{ss}, total drug concentration at steady state; $(C_u)_{ss}$, concentration of unbound (free) drug at steady state; ↓, reduction; ↑, increase; ↔, no change.
[a] Possible causes include development of cirrhosis or addition to a therapeutic regimen of a drug causing inhibition of metabolizing enzymes in the liver.

tissues; and V_{incell} is the intracellular fluid volume available for drug distribution (approximately 27 L for a 70 kg subject).

From this equation, we can see that the degree to which an increase in the fraction of drug unbound in the plasma will tend to increase a drug's apparent volume of distribution is dependent on the size of the ratio of the fraction of drug unbound in the plasma to the fraction unbound in the tissues (f_{up}/f_{ut}). For the case of a drug with a small volume of distribution, this ratio is small,

resulting in little drug distributing into intracellular fluids. In this case, the equation approximates:

$$V_{ss} = 7.5 + 7.5f_{up} \qquad (16.9)$$

for which changes in fraction of drug unbound in the plasma (f_{up}) will have minimal effect on the apparent volume of distribution at steady state. For larger volume of distribution drugs, the full equation (Eq. 16.8) must be used. In this case, changes in fraction drug unbound in the plasma

Table 16.2 Consequences of a decrease in hepatic blood flow $(Q_H)^a$ on parameters and pharmacological effect of a drug currently being administered

Parameters	Oral drug		Intravenous drug	
	Low E	High E	Low E	High E
Cl_H	↔	↑	↔	↓
C_{ss}	↔	↔	↔	↑
$(C_u)_{ss}$	↔	↔	↔	↑
Effect at steady state	↔	↔	↔	↑

E, hepatic extraction ratio; Cl_H, hepatic clearance from plasma; C_{ss}, total drug concentration at steady state; $(C_u)_{ss}$, concentration of unbound (free) drug at steady state; ↓, reduction; ↑, increase; ↔, no change.
[a] Possible causes include development of cirrhosis or addition of a beta-blocker to a therapeutic regimen.

can cause significant changes in the apparent volume of distribution at steady state.

Table 16.3 illustrates a numerical example of the free fraction increasing from 0.005 to 0.010 for both a drug with a low volume of distribution ($f_{ut} = 1$) and one with a large volume of distribution ($f_{ut} = 0.001$):

A change in the fraction of drug unbound in the plasma produces minimal change for the drug with a small volume of distribution drug. (For drugs with a small apparent volume of distribution at steady state and a larger fraction of drug unbound in the plasma than the values in this example, a somewhat larger increase in the apparent volume of distribution can occur.)

For the drug with a large volume of distribution, there is an almost proportional relationship between the fraction of drug unbound in the plasma and the apparent volume of distribution for the drug.

Changes in hepatic clearance

The general equation expressing hepatic clearance as a function of its contributing parameters is Eq. 16.5:

$$Cl_H = \frac{Q_H f_{up} Cl'_{int}}{Q_H + f_{up} Cl'_{int}}$$

where Cl_H is hepatic clearance from plasma; Q_H is plasma flow to the liver; f_{up} is the fraction drug unbound in the plasma; and Cl'_{int} is intrinsic plasma clearance of unbound drug. The product $f_{up}Cl'_{int}$ equals Cl_{int}, the intrinsic clearance of bound plus free drug, as in Ch. 4 Eq. 4.11.

Since it is really blood, not plasma, flowing to the liver (at a nominal rate of $1.35\,L\,min^{-1}$), plasma flow to the liver must be calculated on a case by case basis. For a drug that is known to have no association with the formed elements of blood, the plasma flow to the liver can be calculated from the patient's hematocrit (Hct), in the following manner:

$$Q_H \equiv (Q_H)_{plasma}$$
$$= (Q_H)_{blood}(1 - Hct)$$
$$= (1.35\,L\,min^{-1})(1 - Hct) \quad (16.10)$$

For drugs such as lithium or certain tricyclic antidepressants, which bind to erythrocytes or other formed elements, the ratio of drug concentration in plasma to that in blood (C_{plasma}/C_{blood}) needs to be measured experimentally. Then we can calculate:

$$Cl_H \equiv (Cl_H)_{plasma} = (Cl_H)_{blood}(C_{blood}/C_{plasma})$$

and

$$Q_H \equiv (Q_H)_{plasma}$$
$$= (Q_H)_{blood}(C_{blood}/C_{plasma}) \quad (16.11)$$

Going back to Eq. 16.5, it can be seen that hepatic clearance is determined by three variables: plasma flow to the liver, the fraction of drug unbound in the plasma and the intrinsic plasma clearance of unbound drug (Q_H, f_{up} and Cl'_{int}, respectively). The contribution of these variables to the value of hepatic clearance depends on the relative size of Q_H compared with the product $f_{up}Cl'_{int}$. The numerical example in Table 16.4 shows the effect of changing f_{up} on hepatic clearance for a drug with $f_{up}Cl'_{int} > Q_H$ (left side) and for a drug where $f_{up}Cl'_{int} < Q_H$ (right side). In this example plasma flow to the liver is considered to be constant at $0.8\,mL\,min^{-1}$.

For scenario A (columns 2 and 3) of Table 16.4, where $f_{up}Cl'_{int} \gg Q_H$, doubling the free fraction has a minimal effect on hepatic clearance. Furthermore, hepatic clearance has a value very close to Q_H. In this situation clearance is determined by plasma flow to the liver and cannot exceed this value.

For scenario B (columns 4 and 5) of Table 16.4, where $Q_H \gg f_{up}Cl'_{int}$, doubling the free fraction produces an almost proportional increase in hepatic clearance. Moreover, hepatic clearance has a value very close to $f_{up}Cl'_{int}$. In this situation, clearance is determined by $f_{up}Cl'_{int}$ and cannot exceed this value.

Changes in average total and free drug concentrations at steady state for an intravenously administered drug

Next, we will look at the effect of a change in free fraction on average total and free plasma drug

Table 16.3   Effect of increase in the free fraction on volume of distribution at steady state for a drug with a small volume of distribution ($f_{ut} = 1$) and one with a large volume of distribution ($f_{ut} = 0.001$)

	Drug with small V_{ss}		Drug with large V_{ss}	
	$f_{up} = 0.005$	$f_{up} = 0.010$	$f_{up} = 0.005$	$f_{up} = 0.010$
V_{ss} (L)	7.54	7.58	143	278

f_{up}, fraction drug unbound in plasma; f_{ut}, fraction drug unbound in tissues; V_{ss}, apparent volume of distribution at steady state.

concentrations at steady state. First we will consider drugs administered intravenously and then we will look at drugs administered orally.

The appropriate equation (see also Eq. 11.17 and Eq. 12.19) for average total (bound plus free) plasma drug concentration at steady state is:

$$(\overline{C}_p)_\infty = \frac{X_0}{VK\tau} \qquad (16.12)$$

Therefore,

$$(\overline{C}_p)_\infty = \frac{X_0/\tau}{Cl} \qquad (16.13)$$

For clearance that is exclusively by the liver, this equation becomes:

$$(\overline{C}_p)_\infty = \frac{X_0/\tau}{Cl_H} \qquad (16.14)$$

The appropriate equation for average free (unbound) plasma drug concentration at steady state is:

$$(\overline{C}_u)_\infty = f_{up} \left(\frac{X_0/\tau}{Cl_H} \right) \qquad (16.15)$$

Using an intravenous dosing rate of $1\,mg\,min^{-1}$ and the free fractions and hepatic clearances from Table 16.4, the values in Table 16.5 can be calculated.

In scenario A (columns 2 and 3) of Table 16.5, where (as shown above) clearance is limited by hepatic plasma flow, a doubling of the fraction of drug unbound in the plasma has minimal effect on total steady-state drug concentration but results in a near doubling of free steady-state drug concentration. This increased free concentration will likely increase therapeutic or toxic effect and would require a downward adjustment in dose.

Table 16.4   The effect of changing the fraction of drug unbound in the plasma on hepatic clearance for two drugs, one where the term $f_{up}Cl'_{int}$ is greater than Q_H and one where it is lower than Q_H

	Cl'_{int} 10 000 L min^{-1}		Cl'_{int} 10 L min^{-1}	
f_{up}	0.005	0.01	0.005	0.01
$f_{up}Cl'_{int}$ (L min^{-1})	50	100	0.05	0.10
Q_H (L min^{-1})	0.8	0.8	0.8	0.8
Cl_H (L min^{-1})	0.787	0.794	0.0471	0.089

f_{up}, fraction drug unbound in plasma; Cl'_{int}, intrinsic plasma clearance of unbound drug; $f_{up}Cl'_{int}$, equal to the intrinsic clearance of bound plus free drug; Q_H, plasma flow to the liver; Cl_H, hepatic clearance of drug.

Conversely, in scenario B (columns 4 and 5) Table 16.5, where clearance was limited by $f_{up}Cl'_{int}$, a doubling of the fraction of drug unbound in the plasma results in an almost perfectly inversely proportional change in total steady-state drug concentration but has minimal effect on free steady-state drug concentration. There would be virtually no potential for increased drug effect in this case; however, a clinician monitoring the total drug concentration could be alarmed by its decrease and order an inappropriate increase in the dose in order to increase the total drug concentration.

Changes in average total and free drug concentrations at steady state for an orally administered drug

For an orally administered drug,

$$(\overline{C}_p)_\infty = \frac{F_{po}X_0/\tau}{Cl_H} = \frac{f_{GIT}(1-E)(X_0/\tau)}{Cl_H}$$

$$= \frac{f_{GIT}X_0/\tau}{f_{up}Cl'_{int}} \qquad (16.16)$$

and

$$(\overline{C}_u)_\infty = \frac{f_{up}f_{GIT}X_0/\tau}{f_{up}Cl'_{int}} = \frac{f_{GIT}X_0/\tau}{Cl'_{int}} \qquad (16.17)$$

If, for example, the fraction of drug traversing the gastrointestinal tract membrane and reaching the portal vein (f_{GIT}) is 0.9, then the data in Tables 16.4 and 16.5 can be extended (Table 16.6).

We observe that an increase in free fraction of drug causes an inversely proportional decrease in average total steady-state drug concentration but no change in the corresponding free concentration. These changes are independent of the relative sizes of plasma flow to the liver and the volume of distribution of drug in the body.

Changes in elimination half life

Table 16.7 shows the effects of doubling the fraction of drug unbound in the plasma on the elimination half life of a drug. These effects occur irrespective of whether an oral or an intravenous

dosage form is employed. Half life is directly proportional to the apparent volume of distribution at steady state and inversely proportional to total clearance (and to hepatic clearance for a drug that is exclusively eliminated by metabolism). The magnitude of the change in elimination half life will differ depending on whether a drug has a small or a large volume of distribution and on the relative size of the plasma flow to the liver (Q_H) compared with the term $f_{up}Cl'_{int}$.

In scenario A (columns 2–5) of Table 16.7, where $f_{up}Cl'_{int} \gg Q_H$, a doubling of free fraction causes an almost proportional increase in elimination half life in the case of drugs with a large volume of distribution and minimal change in the half life of drugs with a smaller volume of distribution. In scenario B (columns 6–9) of Table 16.7, where $Q_H \gg f_{up}Cl'_{int}$, a doubling of free fraction causes an almost proportional *decrease* in elimination half life for drugs with a small volume of distribution and minimal change in the half life of drugs with a large volume of distribution.

Transient changes in free drug concentration

Up to this point, the discussion about the effect of a change in free fraction on free and total drug concentrations has been restricted to steady-state concentrations. However, there is the possibility that a drug, immediately after being displaced from a binding protein and before elimination equilibrium has been achieved, will have a transient change in its total or free concentration.

Table 16.8 presents transient effects on free drug concentrations after a protein binding displacement interaction resulting in an increase in free fraction. These transient effects can either differ from, or be the same as, the sustained effects at steady state. The immediate effect of an increase of free fraction is to increase the unbound concentration of drug for those drugs with small volumes of distribution. For drugs with large volumes of distribution, most displaced drug is quickly diluted throughout the volume of distribution and, thus, has less transient effect on concentration of unbound drug in the plasma. Effects are shown for both orally and intravenously administered drugs.

Table 16.5 The effect of a change in free fraction on average total and free plasma drug concentrations at steady state for intravenous administration of the drugs in Table 16.4

f_{up}	Cl'_{int} 10 000 L min^{-1}		Cl'_{int} 10 L min^{-1}	
	0.005	0.01	0.005	0.01
$(\overline{C}_p)_\infty$ (mg L^{-1}) (IV dose)	1.27	1.26	21.23	11.24
$(\overline{C}_u)_\infty$ (mg L^{-1}) (IV dose)	0.00635	0.0126	0.1062	0.1124

V_{ss}, apparent volume of distribution at steady state; f_{up}, fraction drug unbound in plasma; $(\overline{C}_u)_\infty$, average free (unbound) plasma drug concentration at steady state; $(\overline{C}_p)_\infty$, average total (bound plus free) plasma drug concentration at steady state.

Table 16.6 The effect of a change in the free fraction on average total and free plasma drug concentrations at steady state for orally administered drug ($f_{git} = 0.9$)

f_{up}	Cl'_{int} 10 000 L min^{-1}		Cl'_{int} 10 L min^{-1}	
	0.005	0.01	0.005	0.01
$(\overline{C}_p)_\infty$ (mg L^{-1}) (oral dose)	0.018	0.009	18	9
$(\overline{C}_u)_\infty$ (mg L^{-1}) (oral dose)	0.00009	0.00009	0.09	0.09

V_{ss}, apparent volume of distribution at steady state; f_{up}, fraction drug unbound in plasma; $(\overline{C}_u)_\infty$, average free (unbound) plasma drug concentration at steady state; $(\overline{C}_p)_\infty$, average total (bound plus free) plasma drug concentration at steady state.

Table 16.7 The effects of doubling the fraction of drug unbound in the plasma on the elimination half life of a drug

f_{up}	$f_{up}Cl'_{int} \gg Q_H$				$Q_H \gg f_{up}Cl'_{int}$			
	0.005	0.01	0.005	0.01	0.005	0.01	0.005	0.01
V_{ss} (L)	7.54	7.58[a]	143	278	7.54	7.58[a]	143	278
Cl_H (L min^{-1})	0.787	0.794	0.787	0.794	0.0471	0.089	0.0471	0.089
$t_{1/2}$ (min)	6.64	6.62[a]	126	243	111	59.0	2104	2165
$t_{1/2}$ (h)	0.111	0.110	2.10	4.04	1.85	0.98	35.1	36.1[a]

f_{up}, fraction drug unbound in plasma; V_{ss}, apparent volume of distribution at steady state; Cl_H, hepatic clearance of drug; $t_{1/2}$, elimination half life; $f_{up}Cl'_{int}$, equal to the intrinsic clearance of bound plus free drug.
[a] Changes in these parameters can be larger for drugs with high free fractions.

Table 16.8 Transient effects on free drug concentrations after a protein-binding displacement interaction results in an increase in free fraction

	Intravenous drug				Oral drug			
	$f_{up}Cl'_{int} \gg Q_H$		$Q_H \gg f_{up}Cl'_{int}$		$f_{up}Cl'_{int} \gg Q_H$		$Q_H \gg f_{up}Cl'_{int}$	
V_β	Small	Large	Small	Large	Small	Large	Small	Large
Immediate effect on C_u	↑ (S)	→ (T)	↑ (T)	→ (S)	↑ (T)	→ (S)	↑ (T)	→ (S)
Effect on $(C_u)_\infty$	↑	↑	→	→	→	→	→	→

S, immediate effect on C_u is *sustained* through steady state; T, immediate effect on C_u is *transient*; V_β, volume of distribution during the terminal phase.

If we relied only on a table of steady-state effects, the three examples of transient increases in the unbound (free) drug shown in Table 16.8 would be missed. These so-called "transient" changes can be in effect until steady-state equilibrium is achieved (a period of time equal to several half lives of a drug). During this time, a large increase in free concentration of the displaced drug may cause significant or even dangerous increases in therapeutic or toxic effect.

Example: calculation of changes in pharmacokinetic parameters after a plasma protein-binding displacement interaction

Drug X is eliminated exclusively by hepatic metabolism. Initially, in a 70 kg male patient, pharmacokinetic parameters are as follows: $V_{ss} = 0.1553$ L kg^{-1}, hepatic extraction ratio $= 0.2$, $f_{up} = 0.005$, and $f_{ut} = 0.0405$. Drug Y is added to the regimen, causing some displacement of drug X from plasma protein (new $f_{up} = 0.01$). Assume $Q_H = 0.8$ L min^{-1}, $V_{incell} = 0.386$ L kg^{-1} and that the transfer of an oral dose of drug X is complete ($f_{GIT} = 1.0$). Also assume one-compartment distribution and linear elimination kinetics.

1. What new V_{ss} can be predicted for drug X?
2. What was the intrinsic clearance (Cl$_{int}$, which is the product of $f_{up}Cl'_{int}$) before the displacement interaction?
3. Find the value of the intrinsic free clearance (Cl$'_{int}$). Will this be the same before and after the interaction?

4. Find the intrinsic clearance after the interaction.
5. Find the new value for the hepatic extraction ratio (E).
6. Before the interaction, what was the fraction of drug X (F') escaping the first-pass effect? What is this fraction after the interaction?
7. Find the pre-interaction value for the total clearance of drug from the plasma (Cl).
8. Find the new, post-interaction value for the total clearance.
9. Find the pre-interaction elimination half life.
10. Find the post-interaction elimination half life.
11. If drug X is administered as an intravenous infusion at a constant rate of 50 mg h^{-1}, find the following values: old $(\overline{C}_p)_\infty$, old $(\overline{C}_u)_\infty$, new $(\overline{C}_p)_\infty$ and new $(\overline{C}_u)_\infty$. If the old $(\overline{C}_u)_\infty$ represents the desired steady-state concentration of unbound drug X, does the new post-interaction $(\overline{C}_u)_\infty$ indicate the necessity of changing the dose of drug X?
12. For an oral drug X dose of 200 mg every 4 h, find values of old $(\overline{C}_p)_\infty$, old $(\overline{C}_u)_\infty$, new $(\overline{C}_p)_\infty$ and new $(\overline{C}_u)_\infty$. Compare old and new values of $(\overline{C}_u)_\infty$.
13. Are any transient changes in the free plasma concentration of drug X expected when it is given by intravenous infusion? Are any expected with an oral dose? What are the ramifications for dosing drug X?

Calculations to obtain answers

1. $V_{ss} = 7.5 + 7.5f_{up} + V_{incell}(f_{up}/f_{ut})$.

   New $V_{ss} = 7.5 + 7.5(0.01) + (0.386\,L\,kg^{-1})$
   $(70\,kg)(0.01/0.0405) = 14.24\,L$.

   Old $V_{ss} = 7.5 + 7.5(0.005) + (0.386\,L\,kg^{-1})$
   $(70\,kg)(0.005/0.0405) = 10.87\,L$.

   Comparing old and new: the volume has increased by approximately 31%.

2. Old $Cl_{int} = Q_H E/(1-E) = [(0.8\,L\,min^{-1})(0.2)]/$
   $(1-0.2) = 0.20\,L\,min^{-1}$.

3. Old $Cl'_{int} = Cl_{int}/f_{up} = 0.20\,L\,min^{-1}/0.005 =$
   $40\,L\,min^{-1}$.

   This also equals the new Cl'_{int}.

4. New $Cl_{int} = (40\,L\,min^{-1})$
   $(0.010) = 0.40\,L\,min^{-1}$.

5. New $E = Cl_{int}/(Q_H + Cl_{int}) = 0.40/$
   $(0.80 + 0.40) = 0.33$.

6. Old $F' = 1 - 0.2 = 0.8$. New $F' = 1 - 0.33 =$
   0.67.

7. Old $Cl =$ old $Cl_H = Q_H E_{old} = (0.80\,L\,min^{-1})$
   $(0.2) = 0.16\,L\,min^{-1}$.

8. New $Cl =$ new $Cl_H = Q_H E_{new} = (0.80\,L\,min^{-1})$
   $(0.33) = 0.264\,L\,min^{-1}$.

   This is a 65% increase in clearance.

9. Old $t_{1/2} = 0.693(V_{ss})_{old}/Cl_{old} = [(0.693)$
   $(10.87\,L)]/0.16\,L\,min^{-1} = 47.1\,min$.

10. New $t_{1/2} = 0.693(V_{ss})_{new}/Cl_{new} = [(0.693)$
    $(14.24\,L)]/0.264\,L\,min^{-1} = 37.4\,min$

    This is a 21% decrease in elimination half life.

11. The total and unbound drug concentrations for the intravenous infusion are given in Table 16.9. $(\overline{C}_p)_\infty$ shows a 40% decrease and $(\overline{C}_u)_\infty$ shows a 22% increase. See answer 13 below for comments on the significance of this.

12. The total and unbound drug concentrations for oral dosing are given in Table 16.10. $(\overline{C}_p)_\infty$ shows a 50% decrease and $(\overline{C}_u)_\infty$ shows no change from the old value.

13. Because of the relatively small volume of distribution of drug X, there will be an immediate increase in its unbound concentration C_u. This increase can be substantial and will occur whether drug X is dosed intravenously or orally. This immediate effect will be transient for an orally administered drug but will persist to some degree (22% higher $(\overline{C}_u)_\infty$ in this example) for intravenously administered drug. What are the ramifications of this? If the displacing drug can be avoided, this should be done. If the displacing drug must be given, the dose of drug X can be lowered or a dose of drug X could possibly be skipped to allow equilibrium to occur.

16.3 The effect of tissue-binding interactions

Up to this point, the discussion has centered on the changes caused by binding of drug by proteins in the plasma. That is, changes in pharmacokinetic parameters caused by a change in the fraction drug unbound in the plasma have been discussed.

Using the equations generated above, changes in pharmacokinetic parameters occasioned by a changes in the fraction unbound in the tissues can be examined.

The apparent volume of distribution at steady state is given by the general equation, Eq. 16.8:

$$V_{ss} = 7.5 + 7.5(f_{up}) + V_{incell}\left(\frac{f_{up}}{f_{ut}}\right)$$

In the case of drugs with a large volume of distribution, the ratio of the fraction of drug unbound in the plasma to the fraction unbound in the tissues (f_{up}/f_{ut}) is large and the full equation (Eq. 16.8) must be used, in which case an increase in the fraction unbound in tissue will cause an almost proportional decrease in the volume of distribution at steady state.

In the case of drugs with a small volume of distribution, the ratio f_{up}/f_{ut} is small, with the result that a change in the fraction unbound in tissue will have minimal effect on the volume of distribution at steady state.

Equation 16.5 describes hepatic clearance:

$$Cl_H = \frac{Q_H f_{up} Cl'_{int}}{Q_H + f_{up} Cl'_{int}}$$

Table 16.9 The total and unbound drug concentrations for the intravenous infusion in the example problem

	$(\overline{C}_p)_\infty$	$(\overline{C}_u)_\infty = f_{up}(\overline{C}_p)_\infty$
Old concentration	$\dfrac{(50\ \text{mg h}^{-1})}{(0.16\ \text{L min}^{-1})(60\ \text{min h}^{-1})} = 5.21\ \text{mg L}^{-1}$	$f_{up}^{old}(5.21\ \text{mg L}^{-1}) = (0.005)(5.21) = 0.026\ \text{mg L}^{-1}$
New concentration	$\dfrac{(50\ \text{mg h}^{-1})}{(0.264\ \text{L min}^{-1})(60\ \text{mg h}^{-1})} = 3.15\ \text{mg L}^{-1}$	$f_{up}^{new}(3.15\ \text{mg L}^{-1}) = (0.01)(3.15) = 0.0315\ \text{mg L}^{-1}$
	This is a 40% decrease.	This is a 22% increase.

See text for abbreviations.

This equation does not contain the expression f_{ut} and, therefore, hepatic clearance is independent of changes in tissue binding of drug.

From Chapter 4 (Eq. 4.14) we know that the elimination half life for a drug that is eliminated by metabolism can be described by:

$$t_{1/2} = \frac{0.693(V_{ss})}{Cl_H} \qquad (16.18)$$

This indicates that the half life is inversely proportional to hepatic clearance (which is unaffected by changes in tissue binding) and directly proportional to the apparent volume of distribution at steady state, which is inversely proportional to the fraction of drug unbound in tissues for drugs with large volumes of distribution.

Therefore, for such drugs, an increase in fraction unbound in the tissues will cause a nearly proportional decrease in the half life.

Since the factor f_{ut} is not present in any of the four equations in Table 16.11, we expect no change in average steady-state free or total drug concentrations in response to a change in tissue binding. This is true irrespective of the mode of administration of drug:

16.4 Cytochrome P450-based drug interactions

Drug–drug interactions involving the induction or inhibition of the metabolism of one drug by a

Table 16.10 The total and unbound drug concentrations for oral dosing in the example problem

	$(\overline{C}_p)_\infty = \dfrac{f_{GIT}F'D_0/\tau}{Cl_H}$	$(\overline{C}_u)_\infty = f_{up}(\overline{C}_p)_\infty$
Old concentration	$\dfrac{f_{GIT}(\text{old }F')(200\ \text{mg}/4\ \text{h})}{Cl_{old}}$	$\dfrac{f_{up}^{old}(f_{GIT})(\text{old }F')(200\ \text{mg}/4\ \text{h})}{Cl_{old}}$
	$= (1.0)(0.8)(5.21\ \text{mg L}^{-1})$	$= (0.005)(1.0)(0.8)(5.21\ \text{mg L}^{-1}) = 0.021\ \text{mg L}^{-1}$
	$= 4.17\ \text{mg L}^{-1}$	
New concentration	$\dfrac{f_{GIT}(\text{new }F')(200\ \text{mg}/4\ \text{h})}{Cl_{new}}$	$\dfrac{f_{up}^{new}(f_{GIT})(\text{new }F')(200\ \text{mg}/4\ \text{h})}{Cl_{new}}$
	$= (1.0)(0.67)(3.15\ \text{mg L}^{-1}) = 2.1\ \text{mg L}^{-1}$	$= (0.01)(1.0)(0.67)(3.15\ \text{mg L}^{-1}) = 0.021\ \text{mg L}^{-1}$
	(a 50% decrease)	(no change from old value)

See text for abbreviations.

Table 16.11 Equations describing average steady-state total and unbound drug concentrations with oral and intravenous dosing

	$(\overline{C}_p)_\infty$	$(\overline{C}_U)_\infty$
Intravenous	$(\overline{C}_p)_\infty = \dfrac{D_0/\tau}{Cl_H}$	$(\overline{C}_U)_\infty = f_{up}\dfrac{D_0/\tau}{Cl_H}$
Oral	$(\overline{C}_p)_\infty = \dfrac{f_{GIT}D_0/\tau}{f_{up}Cl'_{int}}$	$(\overline{C}_U)_\infty = \dfrac{f_{GIT}D_0/\tau}{Cl'_{int}}$

See text for abbreviations.

second drug administered concomitantly are best understood by examining the specific isozyme of the cytochrome P450 system that is involved in the interaction. If a given drug is a substrate for (i.e. metabolized by) a particular isozyme of cytochrome P450, its metabolism can be speeded up (induced) by a drug that is an inducer of this isozyme. Conversely, this drug will have its metabolism slowed (inhibited) by a drug that is an inhibitor of this isozyme. Induction is usually a relatively slow process (1 to 2 weeks) requiring the production of new protein, while inhibition can occur quite rapidly. It must be borne in mind that prescription pharmaceuticals are not the only substances that can cause these drug–drug interactions. Over-the-counter medications, herbal remedies, nutraceuticals and even some foods can act as inducers or inhibitors of certain drugs.

Table 16.12 presents a number of the clinically relevant substrates, inducers and inhibitors of various cytochrome P450 (CYP) isozymes. Of particular note is the large number of drugs metabolized by the CYP3A4, CYP3A5 and CYP3A6 isoforms. It has been estimated that CYP3A4 is involved in the metabolism of 60% of drugs undergoing oxidative metabolism.

Population differences in the metabolizing efficiency of certain CYP isozymes may have a genetic basis. The incidence, among certain populations, of individuals with poor metabolic activity of isoenzymes CYP2B6, CYP2C19, CYP2C9 and CYP2D6 may be ascribed to genetic polymorphism. CYP3A4 activity may differ among individuals, but the mechanism is not known to be genetic. Knowledge of pharmacogenetics can be used to monitor, and to mitigate, drug interactions caused by genetic polymorphism.

Examples of cytochrome P450-based drug interactions

CYP3A4 interactions

Some inhibitors of CYP3A4 are also inhibitors of P-glycoprotein

These include amiodarone, clarithromycin, diltiazem, erythromycin, itraconazole, ketoconazole, ritonavir, verapamil and grapefruit juice. Enhanced interactions involving these dual inhibitors may occur for drugs that are substrates of both CYP3A4 and P-glycoprotein, namely atorvastatin, cyclosporin, diltiazem, erythromycin, several retroviral protease inhibitors, lidocaine, lovastatin, paclitaxel, propranolol, quinidine, tacrolimus, verapamil and vincristine. Documented interactions of this type include the following.

1. Grapefruit juice and azole antifungal drugs such as ketoconazole can inhibit the elimination of the hydroxymethylglutaryl-coenzyme A (HMG-CoA) reductase inhibitors lovastatin and simvastatin. After oral dosing, these two drugs are normally extracted rapidly by the liver (first-pass effect). Therefore, their bioavailability can be greatly amplified under conditions that inhibit their metabolism in the liver, leading to pronounced physiological effects. As the normal fraction of drug extracted by the liver becomes less, the amplification of bioavailability caused by metabolic inhibition will also become less pronounced.

Table 16.12 Clinically relevant cytochrome P450-based drug interactions

(a) Substrates for CYP isozymes

1A2	2B6	2C8	2C19	2C9	2D6	2E1	3A4,5,7
clozapine cyclobenzaprine imipramine mexiletine naproxen riluzole tacrine theophylline	bupropion cyclophosphamide efavirenz ifosfamide methadone		**Proton Pump Inhibitors:** omeprazole lansoprazole pantoprazole rabeprazole **Anti-epileptics:** diazepam phenytoin phenobarbital **Other drugs:** amitriptyline clomipramine cyclophosphamide progesterone	**NSAIDs:** celecoxib diclofenac ibuprofen naproxen piroxicam **Oral Hypoglycemic Agents:** tolbutamide glipizide **Angiotensin II Blockers:** NOT candesartan irbesartan losartan NOT valsartan **Other drugs:** fluvastatin phenytoin sulfamethoxazole tamoxifen torsemide warfarin	**Beta-blockers:** S-metoprolol propafenone timolol **Antidepressants:** amitriptyline clomipramine desipramine imipramine paroxetine **Antipsychotics:** haloperidol risperidone thioridazine **Other drugs:** aripiprazole codeine dextromethorphan duloxetine flecainide mexiletine ondansetron tamoxifen tramadol venlafaxine	acetaminophen [paracetamol] chlorzoxazone ethanol	**Macrolide Antibiotics:** clarithromycin erythromycin NOT azithromycin telithromycin **Anti-arrhythmics:** quinidine **Benzodiazepines:** alprazolam diazepam midazolam triazolam **Immune Modulators:** cyclosporine tacrolimus (FK506) **HIV Protease Inhibitors:** indinavir ritonavir saquinavir **Prokinetic:** cisapride **Antihistamines:** astemizole chlorpheniramine

Calcium Channel Blockers:
amlodipine
diltiazem
felodipine
nifedipine
nisoldipine
nitrendipine
verapamil

HMG CoA Reductase Inhibitors:
atorvastatin
cerivastatin
lovastatin
NOT pravastatin
NOT rosuvastatin
simvastatin

Other drugs:
aripiprazole
buspirone
Gleevec
haloperidol (in part)
methadone
pimozide
quinine
sildenafil
tamoxifen
trazodone
vincristine

HIV Protease Inhibitors:
indinavir
nelfinavir
ritonavir

(b) Inhibitors of CYP isozymes

cimetidine	thiotepa	gemfibrozil	fluoxetine	amiodarone	amiodarone	disulfiram
fluoroquinolones	ticlopidine	montelukast	fluvoxamine	fluconazole	bupropion	
fluvoxamine			ketoconazole	isoniazid	chlorpheniramine	
ticlopidine			lansoprazole		cimetidine	

(Continued)

Table 16.12 (Continued)

(b) Inhibitors of CYP isozymes						
		omeprazole ticlopidine		clomipramine duloxetine fluoxetine haloperidol methadone mibefradil paroxetine quinidine ritonavir		**Other drugs:** amiodarone NOT azithromycin cimetidine clarithromycin diltiazem erythromycin fluvoxamine grapefruit juice itraconazole ketoconazole mibefradil nefazodone troleandomycin verapamil
(c) Inducers of CYP isozymes						
tobacco	phenobarbital phenytoin rifampin	N/A	rifampin secobarbital	N/A	ethanol isoniazid	carbamazepine phenobarbital phenytoin rifabutin rifampin St. John's wort troglitazone

Reproduced with permission from David A. Flockhart; Accessed on 21 June 2007 at www.drug-interactions.com.

2. Elimination (via CYP3A4 and P-glycoprotein mechanisms) of the immunosuppressant cyclosporin is inhibited by grapefruit juice, azole antfungal drugs and diltiazem.
3. The human immunodeficiency virus (HIV) protease inhibitor ritonavir is an inhibitor of both CYP3A4 and P-glycoprotein. Substrates of these two elimination pathways are particularly susceptible to interactions with ritonavir.
4. Similarly, the calcium channel blockers verapamil and diltiazem are inhibitors of both CYP3A4 and P-glycoprotein. Substrates of these two pathways, such as statins, may have significant increases in blood concentrations when used with these inhibitors.

Some inducers of CYP3A4 are also inducers of P-glycoprotein

These include dexamethasone, rifampin and St. John's wort. The last two have been implicated in the induction of the metabolism of cyclosporin, certain HMG-CoA reductase inhibitors (statins) and several HIV protease inhibitors, with resulting loss of efficacy of these compounds.

Inhibition of the metabolism of warfarin

Ketoconazole and fluconazole inhibit the metabolism of warfarin. The action of these drugs on CYP3A4, and to a lesser extent on CYP1A2 and CYP2C19, will inhibit the metabolism of the (R)-isomer of warfarin. Additionally, metabolism of the (S)-isomer by CYP2C9 may be inhibited by azole antifungal drugs, including fluconazole. There is a also pronounced inhibition of the metabolism of (R)-warfarin by erythromycin, which may lead to hemorrhage. The mechanism is thought to be mainly by inhibition of the CYP3A3 and CYP3A4 pathways. The macrolide azithromycin may be substituted for erythromycin.

Use of sildenafil, a CYP3A4 substrate

Severe side effects, including systemic vasodilation, can occur when sildenafil is used with a CYP3A4 inhibitor.

Drugs that are inhibitors of CYP3A4

In the presence of CYP3A4 inhibitors such as azole antifungal drugs, erythromycin and grapefruit juice, blood concentrations of the antihistamine terfenadine significantly increase, resulting in cardiotoxicity. Terfenadine has been withdrawn from sale in the US.

Drugs that are inducers of CYP3A isozymes

Barbiturates and phenytoin are potent inducers of substrates metabolized by CYP3A4, CYP3A5 and CYP3A6.

CYP2C9 interactions

Inhibition of the metabolism of warfarin

The effect of warfarin is potentiated by concomitant treatment with sulfonamides, including the combination trimethoprim/sulfamethoxazole. This potentiation is likely a result of inhibition of metabolism of the (S)-isomer of warfarin by this class of strong CYP2C9 inhibitor. The bleeding observed in this interaction may also be partly caused by the antibiotic effect of the sulfonamides, which decrease the intestinal flora responsible for production of the anticoagulant vitamin K. The potentiation of warfarin by amiodarone is likely caused by inhibition of CYP2C9 and CYP3A4, CYP3A5 and CYP3A6 by amiodarone.

Inhibition of the metabolism of phenytoin

CYP2C9 inhibitors, such as amiodarone, azole antifungal drugs and fluvoxamine may inhibit the metabolism of phenytoin. This may cause a particularly dangerous increase in phenytoin steady-state concentrations because of the nonlinear elimination kinetics of this drug.

Inhibition of the metabolism of non-steroidal anti-inflammatory drugs (NSAIDs)

CYP2C9 inhibitors will reduce metabolism of NSAIDs.

Induction of CYP2C9

This isozyme is inducible by rifampin and barbiturates. The activity of substrates of this isozyme may be substantially decreased in the present of these agents.

Genetic polymorphism

Approximately 1% of Caucasians are poor metabolizers for drugs metabolized by this isoform. Between 14 and 37% Caucasians and between 2 and 3% Asians show some degree of loss of activity for CYP2C9. Decreases in dosing may be necessary in patients exhibiting poor metabolizer characteristics.

CYP1A2 interactions

Inhibition of the metabolism of warfarin

The potentiation of warfarin by the fluoroquinolone antibiotics is likely caused by a decrease in vitamin K production along with an inhibition of the metabolism of (R)-warfarin by the CYP1A2 pathway.

Modulation of the metabolism of theophylline

Cimetidine, fluoroquinolone antibiotics such as ciprofloxacin and the selective serotonin-reuptake inhibitor (SSRI) fluvoxamine inhibit the metabolism of theophylline, whereas, the its metabolism can be induced by smoking or by the ingestion of char-broiled meats.

CYP2D6 interactions

CYP2D6 is involved in the biotransformation of 15–20% of drugs undergoing oxidative metabolism. Important inhibitors include cimetidine, fluoxetine, paroxetine, amiodarone, quinidine and ritonavir.

Approximately 8% of Caucasians, 4% of African–Americans and 1% of Asians are poor metabolizers for this isoform. There is even a population possessing duplicate genes for CYP2D6; they are "ultra-rapid" metabolizers of CYP2D6 substrates. Normal dosing regimens will produce subtherapeutic concentrations of drugs metabolized by CYP2D6 in this last group.

Activation of codeine

Codeine has little inherent analgesic activity until it is converted by CYP2D6 to morphine. This conversion will be impaired in the case of poor metabolizers or when the activity of CYP2D6 is inhibited by drugs such as the antifungal terbinafine.

Metabolism of the beta blockers metoprolol and timolol

This is decreased among poor metabolizers or in the case of co-administration of a CYP2D6 inhibitor, such as cimetidine.

Metabolism of tricyclic antidepressants

This is decreased when the drugs are administered concomitantly with either fluoxetine or paroxetine.

CYP2C19 interactions

Between 3 and 5% of Caucasians, 2% of African–Americans and between 15 and 20% of Asians are poor metabolizers by CYP2C19.

Metabolism of diazepam

This may be inhibited by the proton pump inhibitor omeprazole, leading to high concentrations of diazepam in the blood.

CYP2E1 interactions

Ethanol

Ethanol is a CYP2E1 substrate. The CYP2E1 inhibitor disulfiram inhibits further metabolism of a metabolic byproduct of ethanol, acetaldehyde. This chemical is responsible for many of the unpleasant side effects of alcohol consumption, such as nausea. The acetaldehyde build up is meant to act as a deterrent to alcohol consumption and is the reason disulfiram (Antabuse) has been prescribed in alcoholism recovery programs.

Chronic ethanol consumption

CYP2E1 activity is induce by chronic ethanol use. If such individuals then take acetaminophen (paracetamol), induction of the phase I metabolism of this drug will occur, with the production of a reactive metabolite that is hepatotoxic. At the same time, chronic alcohol consumption depletes glutathione, which would normally conjugate and inactivate this reactive metabolite. The result of this process is the build up of the hepatotoxic metabolite with potentially life-threatening consequences.

Table 16.13 P-glycoprotein substrates, inhibitors and and inducers

Substrates

Anti-cancer drugs	Actinomycin D, colchicine, daunorubicin, doxorubicin, etoposide, mitomycin C, paclitaxel,[a] vinblastine, vincristine[a]
Antiemetics	Domperidone, ondansetron
Antimicrobial agents	Erythromycin,[a] fluoroquinolones (nalidixic acid and the "floxacins") ivermectin, rifampin
Cardiac drugs	Amiodarone, atorvastatin,[a] diltiazem,[a] digoxin, disopyramide, lovastatin,[a] nadolol, pravastatin, propranolol, quinidine,[a] timolol, verapamil[a]
HIV protease inhibitors	Indinavir,[a] nelfinavir,[a] ritonavir,[a] saquinavir[a]
Immunosuppressants	Cyclosporin,[a] tacrolimus[a]
Rheumatological drugs	Methotrexate
Miscellaneous	Amitriptyline, cimetidine, fexofenadine, lidocaine,[a] loperamide, quinine,[a] telmisartan, terfenadine

Inhibitors

Antimicrobial agents	Clarithromycin,[b] erythromycin,[b] ivermectin, mefloquine, ofloxacin
Azole antifungal agents	Itraconazole,[b] ketoconazole[b]
Cardiac drugs	Amiodarone,[b] carvedilol, diltiazem,[b] dipyridamole, felodipine, nifedipine, propranolol, propafenone, quinidine, verapamil[b]
HIV protease inhibitors	Ritonavir[b]
Immunosuppressants	Cyclosporin,[b] tacrolimus
Psychotropic drugs	Amitriptyline, chlorpromazine, desipramine, doxepin, fluphenazine, haloperidol, imipramine
Steroid hormones	Progesterone, testosterone
Miscellaneous	Grapefruit juice,[b] orange juice isoflavones, telmisartan
Inducers	Dexamethaxone,[c] rifampin,[c] St. John's wort[c]

[a] Also substrate of CYP3A4.
[b] Also inhibitor of CYP3A4.
[c] Also inducer of CYP3A4.

16.5 Drug interactions linked to transporters

Recent studies have shown that carrier-mediated influx and efflux of drugs into organs by transporters is the mechanism responsible for many drug–drug interactions. In the liver, members of the organic anion transporter polypelptides (OATP) family of transporters cause the influx of certain drugs into hepatocytes; while other transporters (such as P-glycoprotein, the product of the multidrug resistance gene *MDR1*) cause the efflux of drugs from the liver by biliary excretion. In the proximal tubule cells of the kidney, members of another organic anion transporter family (OAT) cause influx from blood, while other transporters (including P-glycoprotein, as well as members of the multidrug resistance-associated protein [MRP] family) cause transfer of drug into the lumen, with subsequent excretion. In the small intestine, P-glycoprotein is an important transporter that pumps drug which has entered the enterocyte back into the lumen, thus decreasing drug absorption. P-glycoprotein is a crucial efflux transporter in the brain, preventing many drugs from crossing the blood–brain barrier.

The membrane transfer of drugs that are substrates for a particular transporter will change when that transporter is subject to another drug that induces or inhibits its activity. For example, the action of P-glycoprotein can be inhibited by quinidine, verapamil, erythromycin, clarithromycin and the statins. Inhibition of this transporter can interfere with its ability to keep loperamide out of the brain, resulting in opioid effects in the central nervous system. Similarly, inhibition of P-glycoprotein can cause a decrease in urinary and biliary excretion of digoxin, while at the same time increasing its bioavailability. These three processes in unison will tend to increase the plasma concentration of digoxin, perhaps to dangerous levels. Rifampin will have the opposite effect on P-glycoprotein, causing a decrease in plasma concentrations of digoxin. Morover, in addition to its effects on P-glycoprotein, rifampin can also induce the metabolism of drugs that are substrates for CYP3A4.

The OAT family of transporters can be inhibited by probenecid. If a substrate of this family of transporters, such as penicillin, is administered concomitantly with probenecid, the drug can have decreased renal secretion, with a resulting increase in the plasma penicillin concentration. Cimetidine is an inhibitor of members of the OAT, organic cation transporter (OCT) and OATP families of transporters This inhibition has been shown to result in a decrease in the renal excretion of substrates such as procainamide and levofloxacin, resulting in increased plasma concentrations of these drugs.

Table 16.13 is a list of the substrates, inhibitors, and inducers of P-glycoprotein.

Genetic polymorphism can occur for P-glycoprotein. One study reported subjects with a (homozygous) genetic variance for this protein at amino acid 3435 having a 9.5% increase in oral bioavailability and a 32% decrease in clearance of digoxin, compared with subjects with no genetic variance. Another study showed subjects with this genetic variance to have a 38% increase in digoxin steady-state plasma concentrations compared with subjects with the normal (wild type) P-glycoprotein.

17

Pharmacokinetic and pharmacodynamic relationships

Objectives

Upon completion of this chapter, you will have the ability to:

- use the proper equations to visualize the relationship between plasma drug concentration and therapeutic effect
- contrast a pharmacokinetic drug interaction and a pharmacodynamic drug interaction.

17.1 Introduction

It has been said that pharmacokinetics describes what the body does to the drug (absorption, distribution and elimination); while pharmacodynamics measures what the drug does to the body (therapeutic and/or toxic effect). The entire science of pharmacokinetics is predicated on the observation that, for most drugs, there is a correlation between drug response and drug concentration in the plasma. This correlation is not, however, a linear one. In fact, for most drugs, a sigmoidal (S-shaped) relationship exists between these two factors.

In Fig. 17.1, the therapeutic effect reaches a plateau, where increase in drug concentration will have no further increase in effect. In contrast, the toxic effects of a drug show no such plateau. Toxic effects start at the minimum toxic concentration and continue to rise, without limit, as drug concentration increases (Fig. 17.2).

Upon consideration, it is clear that the best measure of a drug's activity at any given time would be obtained from a direct and quantitative measurement of the drug's therapeutic effect. This is, in fact, possible for a few drugs. For example, the effect of an antihypertensive drug is best measured by recording the patient's blood pressure. There is no need to determine plasma drug concentrations of these drugs. However, for the large majority of drugs whose effect is not quantifiable, the plasma drug concentration remains the best marker of effect. The science of pharmacokinetics allows us to determine a drug dose and dosing interval to achieve and maintain a plasma drug concentration within the therapeutic range. We can also predict the time course of plasma drug concentration over time, observing fluctuations and deciding when a declining concentration becomes low enough to require the administration of another dose.

For some drugs, we can link the parameters and equations of pharmacokinetics to those of pharmacodynamics, resulting in a PKPD model which can predict pharmacological effect over time. This concept is discussed in more detail later in this chapter. (Equation 17.7 is a typical PKPD equation.) Figure 17.3 depicts the relationship of effect versus time for the drug albuterol (salbutamol) and contrasts this with a superimposed plot of plasma drug concentration versus time.

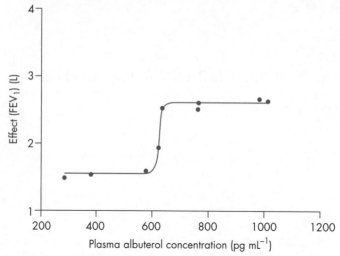

Figure 17.1   Sigmoidal relationship between effect (forced expiratory volume in 1 s [FEV$_1$]) and plasma drug concentration for albuterol.

We can view these plasma drug concentration–effect–time relationships in three-dimensional space, as seen in Fig. 17.4.

The projections of this plot against each co-ordinate plane produces the three plots: plasma drug concentration versus time, drug effect versus time and drug effect versus plasma drug concentration (Fig. 17.5).

17.2 Generation of a pharmacokinetic–pharmacodynamic (PKPD) equation

At any given time, the fraction of a drug's maximum possible pharmacological effect (E/E_{max}) is related to the concentration of drug at the effect

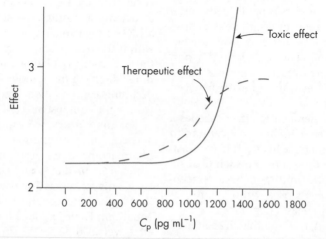

Figure 17.2   While therapeutic effects reach a plateau, toxic effects continue to rise with increasing drug concentration (C_p). Albuterol therapeutic effect is measured by the forced expiratory volume in 1 s (FEV$_1$); while its toxic effects are mainly cardiovascular.

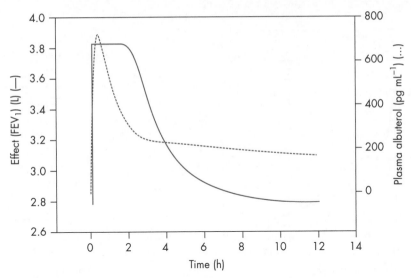

Figure 17.3 Drug effect (solid curve) versus time contrasted with drug concentration (dashed curve) versus time. Albuterol effect is measured by the forced expiratory volume in 1s (FEV_1).

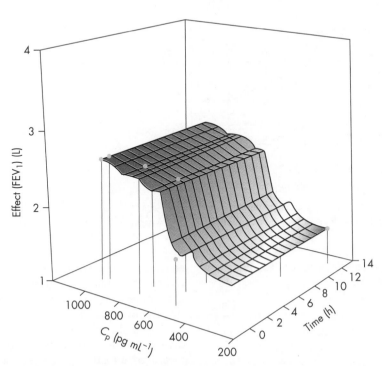

Figure 17.4 Drug concentration and effect over time shown in a three-dimensional plot. Albuterol is administered with a metered dose inhaler to an asthmatic subject and its effect is measured by the forced expiratory volume in 1s (FEV_1).

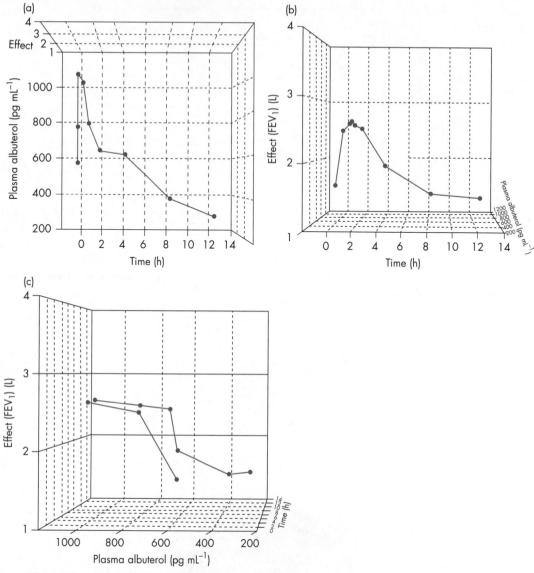

Figure 17.5   Relationship between albuterol plasma concentration, effect (measured by the forced expiratory volume in 1s [FEV$_1$]) and time. (a) Plasma drug concentration versus time; (b) effect versus time; (c) effect versus plasma drug concentration.

site at that same time (C_e), by the following sigmoidal expression:

$$\left(\frac{E}{E_{max}}\right)_t = \frac{(C_e)^n}{[(C_e)_{50}]^n + (C_e)^n} \qquad (17.1)$$

where (C_e)$_{50}$ is the concentration of drug at the effect site that will produce 50% of the maximum

effect (E_{max}) and the exponent n is the sigmoidicity (or shape) factor. Simply stated, the size of n determines how steep the curve corresponding to this equation will be.

Unlike the plasma drug concentration, the drug concentration at the effect site cannot be measured directly. It is, therefore, desirable to replace C_e and (C_e)$_{50}$ in Eq. 17.1 to produce a useable equation.

If an equilibrium exists between drug concentration in plasma and at the effect site (C_p and C_e, respectively) then we can say that $C_e = C_p K_p$ and that $(C_e)_{50} = (C_p)_{50}^{eq} K_p$, where the superscript "eq" represents a condition of equilibrium and K_p is a proportionality constant.

Substituting these values for C_e and $(C_e)_{50}$, respectively, into Eq. 17.1 yields:

$$\left(\frac{E}{E_{max}}\right)_t = \frac{(C_p K_p)^n}{[(C_p)_{50}^{eq} K_p]^n + (C_p K_p)^n} \quad (17.2)$$

where $(C_e)_{50}$ is the plasma drug concentration at equilibrium producing 50% of the maximum effect (E_{max}).

Now numerator and denominator of Eq. 17.2 can be divided by $(K_p)^n$, which generates the following relationship:

$$\left(\frac{E}{E_{max}}\right)_t = \frac{(C_p)^n}{[(C_p)_{50}^{eq}]^n + (C_p)^n} \quad (17.3)$$

For some drugs, equilibrium between C_p and C_e occurs so quickly that we can use the above equation at any time after the administration of drug.

(For drugs at equilibrium and whose effects may be quantified, a PKPD experiment can be conducted in which drug is administered to an experimental subject and the series of plasma drug concentrations and the magnitude of the corresponding effects are recorded. The above equation is then used in a non-linear regression program to estimate the subject's E_{max}, $(C_p)_{50}^{eq}$ and n.)

For other drugs, it takes some time for drug at the effect site to "catch up with" (come into equilibrium with) drug in plasma. The achievement of this equilibrium is a first-order process with a rate constant called $(K_e)_0$. For these drugs, there is a significant time before equilibrium is reached. For example, 95% of this equilibrium will be reached at $(4.32)(0.693)/(K_e)_0$, that is, at a time equal to approximately $3/(K_e)_0$. Before this equilibrium is reached, C_p at any given time is not equal to C_e/K_p and, therefore, a more complex equation involving $(K_e)_0$ is required. In the case of a one-compartment drug administered by intravenous bolus, the equation is:

$$\frac{C_e}{K_p} = \frac{X_0}{V}(e^{-Kt} - e^{-K_{e0}t}) \quad (17.4)$$

Contrast this with the equation for plasma drug concentration of a one-compartment drug administered by intravenous bolus derived in Chapter 3 (Eq. 3.9):

$$C_p = (C_p)_0 e^{-Kt} = \frac{X_0}{V} e^{-Kt}. \quad (17.5)$$

The procedure to obtain a PKPD equation for drugs not in equilibrium begins with division of numerator and denominator of Eq. 17.1 by $(K_p)^n$, producing:

$$\left(\frac{E}{E_{max}}\right)_t = \frac{\left(\frac{C_e}{K_p}\right)^n}{\left(\frac{(C_e)_{50}}{K_p}\right)^n + \left(\frac{C_e}{K_p}\right)^n} \quad (17.6)$$

It has already been determined that, at equilibrium, $(C_e)_{50}^{eq}/K_p = (C_p)_{50}^{eq}$. This is a relation among constants and, therefore, time invariant. Consequently, we are justified in substituting $(C_p)_{50}^{eq}$ for $(C_e)_{50}^{eq}/K_p$ in Eq. 17.6. This results in:

$$\left(\frac{E}{E_{max}}\right)_t = \frac{\left(\frac{C_e}{K_p}\right)^n}{[(C_p)_{50}^{eq}]^n + \left(\frac{C_e}{K_p}\right)^n} \quad (17.7)$$

Finally, (for a one-compartment drug administered by intravenous bolus) the non-equilibrium expression for C_e/K_p in Eq. 17.4 is substituted into Eq. 17.7, obtaining:

$$\left(\frac{E}{E_{max}}\right)_t = \frac{\left(\frac{X_0}{V}(e^{-Kt} - e^{-K_{e0}t})\right)^n}{[(C_p)_{50}^{eq}]^n + \left(\frac{X_0}{V}(e^{-Kt} - e^{-K_{e0}t})\right)^n} \quad (17.8)$$

The above equation predicts fraction of maximal effect at any time for a one-compartment drug given as an intravenous bolus, even when the effect site concentration and the plasma concentration are not at equilibrium.

Once equilibrium is finally achieved, this equation collapses to Eq. 17.3.

Even more complicated equations than Eq. 17.8 are necessary for extravascular or multi-compartment drugs.

17.3 Pharmacokinetic and pharmacodynamic drug interactions

The above considerations help us to discriminate between drug interactions that have a purely pharmacokinetic basis and those that have a pharmacodynamic basis, and from interactions that have both factors at play.

First, a pure pharmacodynamic interaction will be a change in the pharmacological effect resulting from a given plasma drug concentration. This will be evidenced by a change in the value of the

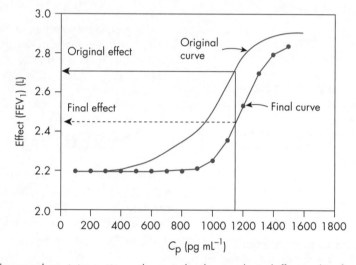

Figure 17.6   Pure pharmacodynamic interaction: a change in the pharmacological effect resulting from a given plasma drug concentration. An increase in $(C_p)_{50}^{eq}$ (plasma concentration at equilibrium that gives a 50% effect) will produce a smaller effect for a given plasma drug concentration.

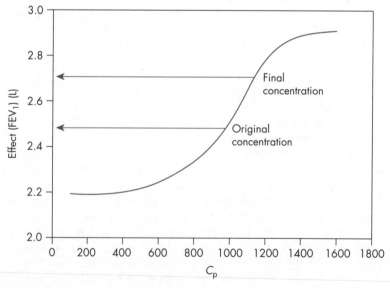

Figure 17.7   Pure pharmacokinetic interaction: increase in C_p (plasma concentration) but no change in $(C_p)_{50}^{eq}$ (plasma concentration at equilibrium that gives a 50% effect).

pharmacodynamic parameter $(C_p)_{50}^{eq}$. For example, an increase in $(C_p)_{50}^{eq}$ will produce a smaller effect for a given plasma drug concentration; that is, the drug will appear to have decreased in potency. On a plot of effect versus drug concentration, this will be seen as a shift of the sigmoidal curve downward and to the right, as seen in Fig. 17.6.

In this figure, this interaction produces a decrease in drug effect, depicted on the y-axis, for the same drug concentration. The converse would be true for a pharmacodynamic interaction producing a decrease in $(C_p)_{50}^{eq}$.

In a pure pharmacokinetic interaction, $(C_p)_{50}^{eq}$ is unchanged. Instead, this interaction results in a change in plasma drug concentration. For example, a pharmacokinetic interaction resulting in an increase in plasma drug concentration can be depicted as a point further up and to the right on the hyperbolic curve. This produces an increase in drug effect (Fig. 17.7).

Combinations of pharmacokinetic and pharmacodynamic interactions are possible. Increases in both plasma drug concentration and $(C_p)_{50}^{eq}$ tend to oppose each other, as do decreases in both these factors. In theory, they could exactly cancel each other, with no resulting change in drug effect.

Changes in plasma drug concentration and $(C_p)_{50}^{eq}$ that are in the opposite direction to each other will reinforce the resulting change in drug effect. For example, an increase in plasma drug concentration and a decrease in $(C_p)_{50}^{eq}$ would potentiate an increase in drug effect, while a decrease in plasma drug concentration along with an increase in $(C_p)_{50}^{eq}$ has the potential to create a large decrease in drug effect.

18

Pharmacokinetics and pharmacodynamics of biotechnology drugs

Objectives

Upon completion of this chapter, you will have the ability to:

- describe the pharmacokinetics and pharmacodynamics of biotechnology drugs, including proteins and peptides, monoclonal antibodies, oligonucleotides, cancer vaccines and other immunotherapeutic agents, and gene therapy agents.

18.1 Introduction

Until very recently the armamentarium of pharmaceuticals almost completely comprised small organic molecules, the vast preponderance of which was synthesized in the laboratory. Steady advances in cellular biology and in biotechnology have allowed scientists to create new therapeutic entities mimicking endogenous bioactive substances. These new products include proteins, peptides, monoclonal antibodies, oligonucleotides, vaccines against microbiological and non-microbiological diseases, and gene therapy treatments. Pharmacists need to understand the pharmacokinetics and pharmacodynamics of these therapeutic products of biotechnology, which will constitute an ever-increasing proportion of the medications that they will be called on to provide to patients.

18.2 Proteins and peptides

Table 18.1 summarizes information about a representative sample of protein and peptide drugs in current use.

Several trends can be discerned from this table.

- Only the smallest peptides in this table are administered orally. This is because large peptides and proteins are subject to degradation and inactivation in the gastrointestinal tract. Systemic bioavailability would be negligible.
- Although one drug (becaplermin) is applied topically (since its site of action is the surface of the skin), the table has no examples of transdermally delivered drugs. This is because the relatively large molecular weights of these compounds interfere with systemic absorption across the skin.
- The majority of these drugs are administered parenterally, either subcutaneously, intramuscularly, or systemically by intravenous injection or infusion. Many of the drugs in this table have very high systemic absorption from subcutaneous and intramuscular dosage forms.
- An example of an inhaled protein is DNase (Pulmozyme). It is an enzyme used to break down thick mucus secretions in the respiratory tracts of patients with cystic fibrosis. An inhaled protein that requires systemic

345

Table 18.1 Protein and peptide drugs in current use

Compound	Molecular mass (kDa)	Volume of distribution (L kg^{-1})	Elimination half life (h)	How administered (systemic availability)	Use
Agalsidase beta; rh-α-galactosidase A (Fabrazyme)	45.4	–	0.75–1.7	IV injection (1.0)	Fabry disease
Aldesleukin; interleukin-2 (Proleukin)	15.3	–	1.42	Intermittent IV infusion (1.0)	Metastatic renal cell carcinoma, metastatic melanoma
Anakinra; interleukin-1 receptor antagonist; IL-1Ra (Kineret)	17.3	–	4–6	SC (0.95)	Rheumatoid arthritis
Antihemophilic factor; factor VIII (Recombinate; Kogenate)	320	–	14.6	IV infusion (1.0)	Hemophilia
Becaplermin; Rh-platelet-derived growth factor (Regranex)	25	–	–	Topical gel (negligible)	Decubitus ulcer
Cetrorelix (Cetrotide)	1.43	1.2	5–63, depending on dose	SC (0.85)	GNRH antagonist (delays ovulation in women undergoing controlled ovarian stimulation to increase fertility)
Coagulation factor VIIa (NovoSeven)	50	0.103	2.3	IV injection (1.0)	Hemophilia
Coagulation factor IX (Christmas factor)	55–71	–	17–32	IV injection (1.0)	Hemophilia
Cyclosporin (Sandimmune, Neoral)	1.2	3–5	Variable ~ 10–20 (shorter in children)	Sandimmune: IV infusion (1.0); oral (~ 0.28 [0.1–0.9]) Neoral: oral (~ 34–42 based on comparative AUC data)	Immunosuppressant
Darbepoetin alfa (Aransep)	37.0	3.39–5.98 L	Distribution half life 1.4 h; true elimination half life (IV study) 21 h; apparent elimination half life (SC) 49 h (patients with renal failure) to 74 h (cancer patients)	SC (adult 0.37; children 0.54); IV injection (1.0)	Anemia in chronic renal failure or in cancer patients receiving chemotherapy

Drug					
Desmopressin (DDAVP, Stimate, Minirin)	1.18	–	1.5–2.5	Oral (0.0016); intranasal (0.03)	Synthetic antidiuretic hormone
Digoxin immune fab, ovine (Digibind)	46.2	~0.1	15–20	IV injection (1.0)	Digoxin overdose
DNase; dornase alfa (Pulmozyme)	29.3	–	–	Inhalation (nebulizer) (negligible)	Breathing difficulty in cystic fibrosis
Drotrecogin alfa (Xigris)	55	–	<2	IV infusion (1.0)	Activated protein C (severe sepsis)
Epoetin alpha (Epogen)	30.4	0.12–0.38	4–13	SC (–); IV injection (1.0)	Anemia caused by chemotherapy
Etanercept (Enbrel)	150	–	102 (±30)	SC (0.58–0.76)	Fusion protein that binds and inhibits TNF-α (autoimmune diseases, including rheumatoid arthritis; Alzheimer's disease, investigational)
Follitropin alfa (Gonal-F)	22.67	~0.14	24	SC (~0.70)	Infertility
Follitropin beta (Follistim, Puregon)	22.67	–	27–30	SC (~0.70), IM (~0.70)	Infertility
Galsulfase; N-acetylgalactosamine-4-sulfatase (Naglazyme)	56	0.103; decreasing to 0.069 over time	0.15, increasing to 0.43 over time	IV infusion (1.0)	Mucopolysaccharidosis VI (Maroteaux–Lamy syndrome I)
Glucagon	3.5	0.25	0.13–0.30	IV injection (1.0); SC (–); IM (–)	For severe hypoglycemia
Goserelin (Zoladex)	1.27	20.3 L (females); 44.1 L (males)	2.3 (females); 4.2 (males)	SC (–)	LHRH (GNRH) agonist (inhibits pituitary gonadotropin secretion; treatment of endometriosis; prostate cancer; breast cancer)
Hepatitis B vaccine, recombinant (Engerix-B; Recombivax HB)	(Surface antigen of virus; HBsAg)	–	–	IM (–)	Hepatitis B prevention
Human growth hormone; HGH; somatotropin, recombinant (Genotropin, Humatrope, Serotrostim)	22.1	0.07	True half life 0.33–0.5 (IV study); apparent half lives 3.8 (SC), 4.9 (IM)	SC (0.75); IM (0.63)	Growth hormone deficiency

(Continued)

Table 18.1 (Continued)

Compound	Molecular mass (kDa)	Volume of distribution (L kg^{-1})	Elimination half life (h)	How administered (systemic availability)	Use
Imiglucerase; r-glucocerebrosidase (Cerezyme)	60.4	0.09–0.15	0.06–0.17	IV infusion (1.0)	Gaucher's disease type I and type III
Insulin, human, recombinant; rh-I (Humulin) (values for regular insulin)	5.8	0.26–0.36	True half life 0.08–0.12 (IV studies); apparent half life 1.5 (SC)	SC (0.55–0.77)	Diabetes
Insulin, human (recombinant DNA origin) inhalation powder, Exubera (marketed then withdrawn); other brands in development	5.8	–	Same as SC insulin	Inhalation (dry powder inhaler) (0.06–0.10)	Diabetes
Insulin-like growth factor 1; rh-IGF-1; somatomedin C; mecasermin (Increlex)	7.65	0.26	5.8	SC (~1.0, in healthy subjects)	IGF-1 deficiency, severe
Insulin-like growth factor 1/insulin growth factor-binding protein 3 complex; IGF-1/IGFBP-3; mecasermin rinfabate (IPLEX)	36.4	–	13.4 (IGF-1); 54.1 (IGFBP-3)	SC (–)	IGF-1 deficiency, severe; myotonic muscular dystrophy (phase II)
Interferon alpha; IFNα (Veldona)	19.24	–	5.1 (IV study); 7 (IM)	Oral (lozenge) (–); SC (–); IM (–)	Oral warts; chronic hepatitis C; fibromyalgia (investigational)
Interferon alfa 2a, pegylated (Pegasys)	60	–	80	SC (0.84)	Hepatitis C
Interferon alpha 2b (Intron A)	19.3	–	2–3	SC (–); IM (–)	Hepatitis B; hepatitis C; various cancers
Interferon beta 1a; IFNβ1a (Avonex, Rebif)	22.5	–	10 (Avonex); 70 (Rebif)	Avonex: IM (–); Rebif: SC (–)	Multiple sclerosis
Interferon beta 1b; IFNβ1b (Betaseron)	18.5	0.25–2.88	0.133–4.3	SC (0.5)	Multiple sclerosis
Interferon gamma 1b; IFNγ1b (Actimmune)	32.9 (dimer)	–	2.9 (IM); 5.9 (SC)	SC (>0.89)	Improve leukocyte status for serious infections associated

Drug					Indication
					with granulomatous disease; delay progression of severe malignant osteoporosis
Keratinocyte growth factor (recombinant, human); palifermin (Kepivance)	16.3	–	4.5	IV injection (1.0)	Mucositis
Laronidase; rh-alpha-L-iduronidase precursor; rh-IDU (Aldurazyme)	69.9	0.24–0.60	1.5–3.6	IV infusion (1.0)	Mucopolysaccharidosis I (Hurler and Scheie syndromes)
Octreotide acetate (Sandostatin)	1.02	13.6L	1.7–1.9	SC (1.0); IM (0.60–0.63)	Severe diarrhea caused by carcinoid tumors or tumors secreting vasoactive intestinal peptide; acromegaly
Oxytocin, synthetic (Syntocinon, Pitocin)	1.007	0.17	0.017–0.10	IV infusion (1.0)	Oxytocic (facilitates childbirth)
Oprelvekin; interleukin 11; (Neumega)	19	–	6.9	SC (> 0.8)	Thrombocytopenia caused by myelosuppressive chemotherapy
Pegaspargase (Oncaspar)	31.7	$2.4\,L\,m^{-2}$	140–360	IM (–); IV infusion (1.0)	Acute lymphoblastic leukemia
Pegfilgrastim; pegylated GCSF (Neulasta)	39	–	15–80 (variable)	SC (–)	Chemotherapy-induced neutropenia
Sargramostim; rhu-GMCSF (leukine; Leucomax; Immunex)	14.4	–	1.0 (IV); 2.77 (SC)	IV infusion (1.0); SC (–)	Myeloid stimulation; engraftment (bone marrow transplant)
Tenecteplase; modified tPA (TNKase)	58.95	Plasma volume (4.7 L) (initial)	0.33–0.44 (initial); 1.5–2.17 (terminal)	IV bolus (1.0)	Thrombolytic agent used in acute myocardial infarction
Teriparatide; modified parathyroid hormone (Forteo)	4.12	0.12	True half life (IV) 0.083 h; apparent half life (SC) 1.0	SC (0.95)	Osteoporosis
Tissue plasminogen activator; tPA; alteplase (Activase)	59.04	Plasma volume ($0.05\,L\,kg^{-1}$)	0.083 (initial)	IV bolus injection followed by IV infusion (1.0 in both)	Thrombolytic agent used in acute myocardial infarction, acute ischemic stroke and pulmonary embolism

IV, intravenous; SC, subcutaneous; IM, intramuscular; rh, recombinant, human; GCSF, granulocyte colony-stimulating factor; GMCSF, granulocyte-macrophage colony-stimulating factor; TNF, tumor necrosis factor.

absorption in order to exert its therapeutic effect is the inhalable form of human insulin, Exubera, which was on the market briefly in 2007. After administration to the lungs by dry powder inhaler, its disposition and efficacy were found to be comparable to those of subcutaneously administered insulin, while its absorption was somewhat faster. Other inhaled insulin products are in development.

- One small peptide, desmopressin, has sufficiently bioavailability after intranasal administration to elicit a systemic therapeutic response.
- Sizes of compounds in the table range from 1 to 320 kDa. The smallest substance, oxytocin, is a peptide of nine amino acid residues that is produced by chemical synthesis. The largest compound in the table, antihemophilic factor, is a large glycoprotein produced by recombinant DNA technology. Many of the large peptides and proteins in the table were at one time extracted from blood or urine; however, in order to prevent possible infection, these are now produced recombinantly. There is even an example in the table of a recombinantly produced hepatitis B vaccine, which can claim the advantage of being "free of association with human blood or blood products."
- Apparent volumes of distribution of these proteins and peptides are relatively small (rarely exceeding the volume of extracellular fluid) and roughly inversely correlated with their molecular weights. However, irrespective of the value of the distribution volume, each protein is distributed to the tissue containing receptors for its therapeutic activity in an amount adequate to elicit effect. This specific distribution, though most important for effect, is often of too small in magnitude to affect the value of the overall volume of distribution.
- For proteins, the total volume of distribution at steady state (representative of both central and tissue compartments) is usually not more than twice the initial volume of distribution (representative of the vasculature and the well perfused organs and tissues).
- Pegylation often decreases the volume of distribution of a protein drug.

- Several of these protein and peptide drugs have short elimination half lives, as recorded in intravenous studies. However, when these drugs are administered by subcutaneous or intramuscular injection, delayed absorption causes plasma drug concentrations to remain high for an appreciable period of time. Other drugs with short elimination half lives have been glycosylated or pegylated to increase their molecular weight and extend their half life. Bioengineering of the native proteins (by glycosylation, deglycosylation, pegylation, cyclization, conjugation, or by amino acid substitutions, deletions or additions) often can produce a protein with the therapeutic and pharmacokinetic properties that are desired.

Other information about the pharmacokinetics and pharmacodynamics of peptide and protein drugs follows.

- The site and mechanism of elimination may be determined by charge, oil/water partition coefficient, the presence of sugars or other functional groups associated with the protein and, to a large extent, by molecular weight. For example, proteins that are small enough to be filtered by the glomerulus in the kidney (< 60 kDa) may either be absorbed by endocytosis into proximal tubule cells followed by lysosomal degradation (complex polypeptides and proteins) or (in the case of very small, linear peptides such as bradykinin) may be metabolized by enzymes at the luminal brush border membrane. Other proteins and peptides (including insulin, parathyroid hormone and vasopressin) may be extracted from postglomerular capillaries and then degraded by peritubular receptors. Receptor-mediated endocytosis in the kidney is also an important mechanism of degradation of those proteins that are too large to be filtered by the glomerulus. This is a particularly relevant mechanism for proteins with the appropriate charge on their surface or proteins that are associated with sugar molecules.
- Some proteins are degraded in the liver by intracellular catabolism within hepatocytes. Small polypeptides (< 1 kDa) can be transported to these cells by passive diffusion (if sufficiently lipophilic) or by carrier-mediated

uptake (for more polar molecules). Receptor-mediated endocytosis in the liver is important for moderate-sized proteins (50–200 kDa), depending on surface charge or the presence of sugar molecules. Even though it has a molecular weight of 5.8 kDa, which is below that range, insulin is eliminated to a considerable extent by receptor-mediated endocytosis in the liver.

- The largest proteins (200–400 kDa) are opsonized by association with immunoglobulins and then subject to phagocytosis. Protein complexes or aggregates (> 400 kDa) are also eliminated by phagocytosis.

- For certain proteins, elimination via receptor-mediated endocytosis can occur outside of the liver. This process often occurs at receptors that are very specific for the protein involved. For example, granulocyte colony-stimulating factor (GCSF) binds to receptors in bone marrow, which can eliminate this protein by a saturable process. In contrast, macrophage colony-stimulating factor (MCSF) is eliminated, in part, by binding to macrophages. Since MCSF itself produces macrophages, a negative feedback loop exists in which MCSF induces its own metabolism.

- Elimination of these drugs may be complex processes with dose-dependent, saturable pharmacokinetics.

- Plasma concentrations of these protein drugs may, in fact, correlate poorly with therapeutic effect. The drug may be cleared from blood not because of an elimination process but instead because it is taken up by a receptor, where it may reside for some time, exerting its therapeutic effect. The concentration of drug at this receptor will not be reflected by its blood concentration.

- The curve of therapeutic effect as a function of time may be temporally displaced with respect to the curve of plasma drug concentration over time, requiring the use of indirect pharmacokinetic/pharmacodynamic modeling. Other complicating factors may be at play. For example, over time the formation of antibodies to a protein may neutralize the protein or change its pharmacokinetic profile. At times, the blood concentration–effect relationship is so inaccessible for a particular therapeutic protein that dosing adjustments of the protein is based directly on observed therapeutic or toxic effect rather than by following blood concentrations and employing pharmacokinetic principles.

18.3 Monoclonal antibodies

A monoclonal antibody is an antibody (immunoglobulin molecule) that is produced by recombinant DNA technology; this results in all molecules being identical in structure. These monoclonal antibodies are of high purity and are produced in sufficiently large quantities for use as therapeutic agents.

Table 18.2 summarizes information about the 21 therapeutic monoclonal antibodies approved by the US Food and Drug Administration (FDA) as of 2007.

Several points are worth noting.

- With the exception of two modified products, abciximab and ranibizumab, the molecular weights of these antibodies are around 150 kDa (fairly large proteins).

- Many of these monoclonal antibodies are humanized to prevent the incidence of hypersensitivity reactions that can occur from antibodies from foreign species.

- Volumes of distribution generally do not exceed two times the volume of plasma water.

- Many of the elimination half lives of these compounds are measured in days, ensuring long physiological exposure after a dose.

- Administration is intravenous, subcutaneous or intramuscular. Ranibizumab is an exception in that it is injected intravitreally into the eye.

- Two monoclonal products, Bexxar and Zevalin, belong to the new class of radioimmunotherapy drugs. These drugs, which act by delivering radioactive isotopes directly to cancer cells to kill them, are exhibiting good results in a high percentage of patients who are treated with them.

- Many of these monoclonal antibodies represent revolutionary therapy for diseases for which no small organic molecule has been effective. The mechanisms of action of these compounds rely on the ability of antibodies

Table 18.2 Monoclonal antibodies in current use

Antibody (brand name)	FDA approval date	Type of monoclonal antibody	Size (kDa)	Volume of distribution	Elimination half life	How administered (systemic availability)	Target	Use
Abciximab (ReoPro)	1994	Chimeric	47.6	8.4 L	0.16–0.5 h (but remains on platelets for weeks)	IV injection and infusion (1.0)	Inhibits platelet aggregation by targeting glycoprotein IIb/IIIa receptor	Prevention of thrombosis in percutaneous coronary intervention
Adalimumab (Humira)	2002	Fully human	144	4.7–6 L	10–20 days	SC (0.64)	TNF-α	Rheumatoid arthritis; other autoimmune diseases
Alemtuzumab (Campath)	2001	Humanized	145	$0.18\,L\,kg^{-1}$	Non-linear elimination, 12 days at steady state	IV infusion (1.0)	CD 52 on lymphocytes	Chronic (B cell) lymphocytic leukemia
Basiliximab (Simulect)	1998	Chimeric	144	8.6 L (adults); 5.2 L (children)	7.2 days (adults); 11.5 days (children)	IV injection & infusion (1.0)	IL-2Rα on T lymphocytes	Prevent rejection of kidney transplant
Bevacizumab (Avastin)	2004	Humanized	149	2.66–3.25 L	20 days	IV infusion (1.0)	Vascular endothelial growth factor	Colorectal cancer; advanced non-small cell lung cancer; metastatic breast cancer
Cetuximab (Erbitux)	2004	Chimeric	146	2–$3\,L\,m^{-2}$	4.75 days	IV infusion (1.0)	Epidermal growth factor receptor on cancer cells	Colorectal cancer
Daclizumab (Zenapax)	1997	Humanized	143	$0.074\,L\,kg^{-1}$	20 days	After dilution: by IV infusion (1.0)	CD25 subunit of IL-2Rα on T lymphocytes	Prevent rejection of kidney transplant

Drug	Year	Type	MW	Volume	Half-life	Target	Indication
Eculizumab (Soliris)	2007	Humanized	148	7.7 L	11 days	Complement system protein C5	Paroxysmal nocturnal hemoglobinuria
Efalizumab (Raptiva)	2002	Humanized	150	Central volume $0.058–0.110\,L\,kg^{-1}$	6 days, non-linear	T cell modulator, CD 11a (LFA-1)	Psoriasis
Gemtuzumab ozogamicin (Mylotarg)	2000	Humanized	152	$0.11–0.48\,L\,kg^{-1}$	2.5 days	Antibody targets CD33-positive human leukemia cell line-60; antibody is linked to the cytotoxic agent calicheamicin	Acute myeloid leukemia
Ibritumomab tiuxetan (Zevalin)	2002	Murine	148	Initial volume 3 L	1.25 days	CD20 antigen on (normal and malignant) B cells	Non-Hodgkin lymphoma (used with radionuclides ^{90}Y or ^{111}In)
Infliximab (Remicade)	1998	Chimeric	144	3 L	9.5 days	Inhibition of TNFα signaling	Inflammatory diseases, including Crohn's disease and rheumatoid arthritis
Muromonab-CD3 (Orthoclone OKT3)	1986	Murine	146	–	18 h (harmonic half life)	CD3 receptor on T cells	Transplant rejection
Natalizumab (Tysabri)	2006	Humanized	149	5.7 L	11 days	VLA4 (integrin α4) receptor	Relapsing multiple sclerosis; Crohn's disease
Omalizumab (Xolair)	2004	Humanized	149	$0.078\,L\,kg^{-1}$	26 days	Inhibits binding of IgE to its receptors on the mast cells of basophils	Asthma prophylaxis

(Continued)

Table 18.2 (Continued)

Antibody (brand name)	FDA approval date	Type of monoclonal antibody	Size (kDa)	Volume of distribution	Elimination half life	How administered (systemic availability)	Target	Use
Palivizumab (Synagis)	1998	Humanized	148	–	20 days	IM (–)	Targets fusion protein of respiratory syncytial virus	Prevention of respiratory syncytial virus infection
Panitumumab (Vectibix)	2006	Human	147	$0.054\,L\,kg^{-1}$	7.5 days	IV infusion (1.0)	Epidermal growth factor receptor on cancer cells	Colorectal cancer
Ranibizumab (Lucentis)	2006	Humanized	48	–	3–9 days from vitreous humor	intravitreal injection (low serum concentrations)	Vascular endothelial growth factor	Wet-type macular degeneration
Rituximab (Rituxan, Mabthera)	1997	Chimeric	145	4.3 L	7.25 days at steady state	IV infusion (1.0)	CD20 antigen on B lymphocytes	Non-Hodgkin lymphoma; refractory rheumatoid arthritis; renal transplant (experimental)
Tositumomab (Bexxar)	2003	Murine	144	–	2.79 days (^{131}I)	IV infusion (1.0)	CD20 antigen on B lymphocytes	Non-Hodgkin lymphoma (used with radionuclide ^{131}I)
Trastuzumab (Herceptin)	1998	Humanized	146	$0.044\,L\,kg^{-1}$	1.7–12 days, variable and increasing with dose	IV infusion (1.0)	HER2/neu (ErbB2) receptor	Breast cancer

IV, intravenous; SC, subcutaneous; IM, intramuscular; IL-2Rα, interleukin 2 receptor α; TNF, tumor necrosis factor; LFA, lymphocyte function-associated antigen; HER, human epidermal growth factor receptor.

to target and to inactivate some rather basic biochemical processes. Consequently, these compounds are very potent, and their use represents a trade off between their therapeutic and potentially toxic activities.

- Since the first monoclonal antibody, muromonab-CD3, was approved by the FDA in 1986, the average rate of approval has been exactly one monoclonal antibody per year. There are currently many more therapeutic monoclonal antibodies under development and in phase II and III trials. As science and technology provide us with even more of these unique compounds over the years, great promise exists for the treatment and even cure of diseases that have proven to be refractory so far. One notable recent development in this field is the research being conducted on bapineuzumab, a monoclonal antibody with the potential to treat Alzheimer's disease.

18.4 Oligonucleotides

Therapeutic oligonucleotides are short strands of nucleotides (approximately 20 to 30 nucleotides in length) that interfere with unwanted or pathogenic proteins. As with other new biotechnologies, there are at present only a few oligonucleotides that have been approved as drug products or whose approval is imminent. Other compounds of this type have not been able to translate positive early results into compelling results in large clinical trials. However, intensive research continues apace to overcome the obstacles for the clinical use of these promising drug candidates. Moreover, since these compounds can often be engineered in the laboratory with some degree of facility, they can be quickly produced and screened for activity. Then oligonucleotides showing activity can serve as the basis for the production of monoclonal antibodies or other compounds that may more easily be approved for clinical use.

The first of only two therapeutic oligonucleotides that have been approved for human use as of writing is fomvirsen (Vitravene). It was approved by the FDA in 1998 for the local treatment of cytomegalovirus retinitis. This compound represents the original type of therapeutic oligonucleotide: an antisense compound. It is a single-stranded DNA nucleotide chain, 21 nucleotides long, with the substitution of a phosphorothioate backbone for greater stability. This molecule is complementary to, and therefore interferes with, a messenger RNA (mRNA) sequence in the human cytomegalovirus. This inhibits the production of some viral proteins that are essential for viral replication. The compound is injected intravitreally on a monthly basis.

The second oligonucleotide to be approved is pegaptanib (Macugen). This compound is an antagonist to vascular endothelial growth factor (VEGF). It was approved by the FDA in 2004 for the treatment of neovascular (wet) age-related macular degeneration. This oligonucleotide, 28 bases in length, is classed as an aptamer, or nucleic acid ligand. Aptamers, like their protein counterparts the monoclonal antibodies, bind with high affinity to various molecular targets, thereby inactivating them. Pegaptanib binds with high affinity to the protein VEGF and this inhibits the binding of VEGF to its receptor, thus inactivating it. The objective is to suppress the neovascularization that is characteristic of wet age-related macular degeneration. Pegaptanib is pegylated to extend its elimination half life. This product is also administered by intravitreal injection. Two monoclonal antibodies are also used in this condition: Lucentis and (off-label) Avastin.

Other oligonucleotides are currently in clinical trials. Genasense is an antisense oligonucleotide, comprising a short segment of DNA with a phosphorothioate backbone. This compound inhibits production of the Bcl-2 protein, which is produced by cancer cells and facilitates their survival. Phase III clinical trials for the use Genasense in the treatment of melanoma are currently being evaluated.

Resten-CP, an antisense compound that interferes with the mRNA of a gene involved in the stenosis of vein grafts in coronary artery bypass grafting, is currently undergoing clinical trials.

OGX-011, an antisense compound that inhibits clusterin, a cancer cell survival molecule, is currently in phase II trials for metastatic breast and prostate cancers.

Ampligen is a double-stranded RNA compound undergoing phase III testing for the treatment of severe debilitating chronic fatigue syndrome.

Bevasiranib (C and 5) represents a different class of oligonucleotide. It is a short interfering RNA (siRNA). This compound interferes with the mRNA that produces VEGF protein, responsible for wet age-related macular degeneration. It has completed phase II testing for this indication. It is administered by injection into the eye.

Another siRNA moving into phase II testing for the treatment of wet age-related macular degeneration is the compound Sirna-027.

An oligonucleotide-related therapy on the horizon is the use of toll-like receptor (TLR) agonists to direct the immune system to attack certain cancers, as well as to ameliorate other medical conditions. TLRs are a family of specialized immune receptors that induce protective immune responses when they detect highly conserved pathogen-expressed molecules (unmethylated C_pG dinucleotides) that are not present in vertebral genomes. These TLRs can be stimulated by synthetic oligonucleotides containing unmethylated C_pG dinucleotides. ProMune is an example of this therapy that will be undergoing phase III trials.

An emerging use of aptamers, or nucleic acid ligands, is in the field of targeted drug delivery. For example, progress has been made in the study of nanoparticle–aptamer bioconjugates. Nanoparticles, 50 to 250 nm in diameter, can act to facilitate the entry of encapsulated drug across biological membranes. Aptamers conjugated to these nanoparticles seek out cancer cells and direct the nanoparticles to the cancer cells, which they can then enter and introduce their anticancer drug "payload." Payloads can include cytotoxic small molecules as well as anti-cancer siRNAs.

Considerations regarding the effective production and use of oligonucleotide drugs include stability, delivery and pharmacokinetics.

Along with the usual protection from extremes of temperature, pH and exposure to light, oligonucleotides need to be protected from organic and reactive molecules as well as from nucleases in the body. Most oligonucleotides are stable indefinitely when stored in lyophilized form at

$-20°C$. The drug Vitravene is stable for some time in a buffered, preservative-free solution of fixed osmolality if the usual precautions are observed.

Unlike proteins and peptides, oligonucleotides can be administered by topical/local delivery. Oral delivery is even possible. Because of nucleases in the blood, systemic delivery by intravenous injection or infusion has been challenging. However, newer backbones and other bioengineering innovations have enhanced the *in vivo* stability of oligonucleotides. Early on, several techniques (transfection, electroporation and liposomal encapsulation) were used to place oligonucleotides directly into their target cells. Recent developments in the engineering of the nucleotide backbone render these techniques mostly unnecessary. The newer classes of oligonucleotide can enter cells naturally by receptor-mediated endocytosis.

Systemically administered oligonucleotides distribute particularly to the liver, which is useful for the targeting of liver diseases. There is also good distribution to kidney, spleen and bone marrow. The challenge has been to get distribution to the brain. Most oligonucleotides under development incorporate technologies that assure reasonably long elimination half lives for these compounds. Moreover, systemic bioavailability of most oligonucleotides is adequate. Surprisingly, unlike the complex pharmacokinetics of proteins and peptides, the pharmacokinetics of oligonucleotides are usually quite classic; that is they distribute to one or two compartments and undergoing linear (first-order) elimination.

For oligonucleotides administered directly into the eye, systemic exposure is low. This obviates the concern that oligonucleotides administered in this fashion will display off-target effects, in which unintended silencing of non-target genes may occur.

18.5 Vaccines (immunotherapy)

The use of immunotherapy to treat disorders other than microbiological infections is increasingly being studied. For example, a vaccine called NicVAX, which stimulates the production of anti-nicotine antibodies, is currently in phase IIB testing for the treatment of nicotine addiction. There is also much current interest the use of vaccines for the treatment of various cancers. Several of these anticancer vaccines that are currently in phase III clinical trials or for which phase III trials are imminent will now be discussed.

- MyVax and BiovaxID are two similar vaccines showing activity against follicular non-Hodgkin's lymphoma. These vaccines are both examples of active idiotype, or personalized, anticancer vaccines since they are based on the genetic makeup of an individual patient's tumor. Besides a protein derived from the patient's own tumor, these vaccines contain an antigenic carrier protein, called KLH, and an adjuvant, granulocyte–macrophage colony-stimulating factor (GM-CSF). They are currently in phase III trials.
- In contrast, a vaccine called Gvax, which has shown promise in the treatment of prostate cancer, is not personalized. It employs allogeneic prostate cancer cells expressing the gene for GM-CSF. As of writing, Gvax is preparing for phase III clinical trials.
- Oncophage (vitespen) is a vaccine that contains gp96 heat shock protein/peptide complex from an individual patient's tumor. It has been evaluated in phase III trials for kidney cancer and metastatic melanoma.
- Provenge (sipuleucel T) is a prostate cancer vaccine made from antigen-presenting cells from the patient's own immune system, which are fused to a protein (prostate-secreted acid phosphatase) made from prostate cells. It is currently being evaluated in phase III trials.
- TroVax immunotherapy for renal cell carcinoma consists of the gene for the 5T4 tumor-associated antigen, which is delivered to the body by means of a viral vector. This vaccine is currently undergoing phase III trials.
- Phase III trials of a vaccine therapy for stage II melanoma of the skin are currently being conducted in Europe. In this vaccine, GM2, a common antigen on melanoma cells, is combined with the antigenic carrier KLH (keyhole limpet hemocyanin).
- In the USA, a vaccine for more advanced melanoma of the skin (stages III and IV) is undergoing phase III trials. This vaccine combines MDX-1379 (gp100 melanoma peptides) with MDX-010, a monoclonal antibody that blocks the immunosuppressive molecule CTLA-4 (T-lymphocyte-associated antigen 4).
- Vaccines for ocular melanoma are undergoing phase III testing in both the USA and Europe. These studies are particularly designed to see whether liver metastases of this ocular cancer can be prevented. Both compounds contain melanoma differentiation peptides and adjuvants.
- Two vaccines for the treatment of multiple myeloma developed at the University of Arkansas for Medical Sciences are being prepared for phase III trials. Each vaccine contains peptide fragments from a tumor protein found on myeloma cells.

Finally, mention should be made of a promising new class of cancer immunotherapy undergoing early-stage testing. In this therapy, called adoptive cell transfer (ACT), tumor-reactive lymphocytes are harvested from a patient with melanoma, activated and expanded *ex vivo*, and then infused back into the patient. The result, in many patients, is the production of lymphocytes with increased tumor-fighting capacity. Research is ongoing to optimize clinical results from this type of treatment.

18.6 Gene therapies

As each year passes, science uncovers the genetic basis of more and more diseases. Oligonucleotides and monoclonal antibodies, discussed above, can play a role in inactivating the protein products of defective genes. When a disease has been shown to be caused by missing genes, research can be started to determine a way to supply these genes to the patient in the most effective way. Gene therapy consists of the introduction of genetic material into a patient in order to treat a disease. This process is usually accomplished by the use of a suitable vector, such as a virus. Since the first use of gene therapy in 1990, for the treatment of adenosine deaminase (ADA) deficiency, many different gene therapy trials have been performed,

Table 18.3   Gene therapy products under development

Name	Gene	Disease	Administration	Status
Advexin	p53 tumor suppressor gene delivered via adenoviral vector	Head and neck cancer; Li-Fraumeni syndrome	Intratumoral	Phase III data under analysis by FDA
Biostrophin	Miniaturized gene for dystrophin delivered via biological nanoparticles derived from adeno-associated virus	Duchenne muscular dystrophy	Injected into bicep	First clinical trial underway (2006)
Cerepro	Herpes simplex virus gene for thymidine kinase delivered via adenoviral vector	Malignant glioma	Into healthy brain tissue surrounding resected tissue	In Phase III trials
Gendicine	Containing the p53 tumor-suppressor gene delivered via adenoviral vector	Head and neck squamous cell carcinoma	Intratumoral	Approved by SFDA (China) 2004
(gp91 phox gene)	Gene that produces gp91 phox enzyme delivered via retroviral vector	X-linked chronic granulomatous disease	Transfer into hematopoietic stem cells	Phase I

INGN 241	Melanoma differentiation-associated gene 7 (*mda-7*) delivered via adenoviral vector	Melanoma	Intratumoral	Phase II
Rexin-G	Gene that interferes with the gene for cyclin G_1 in the cancer cell, delivered via proprietary tumor-targeted vector system	Pancreatic cancer; osteosarcoma; solid tumors	Intravenous infusion	Pancreatic cancer: phase I/II (US); Osteosarcoma: phase II (US); Solid tumors: approved (Philippines)
TNFerade	Gene for TNFα under control of radio- and chemo-inducible Egr-1 promoter	Esophageal cancer; head and neck cancer	Intratumoral	Phase II

TNF, tumor necrosis factor.

with some notable successes. There were also some early setbacks, such as the production of leukemia (which ultimately responded to treatment) in two patients cured of severe combined immunodeficiency disease (SCID) by gene therapy, as well as a death in a trial of gene therapy for ornithine transcarboxylase (OTC) disease. As the field has matured, the ability to avoid these types of outcome has greatly increased.

At the time of writing, there is yet to be a gene therapy treatment approved by the FDA for use as a prescription drug. However, at present, some candidate therapies are approaching this status. Difficulties in creating approvable gene therapy products have included:

- difficulty in selecting an effective and safe vector
- rejection of the genetic material by the immune system

- untoward side effects
- transient nature of effect and need for multiple dosing.

Currently, vectors are being used that experience has shown to be safer and that better distribute the genetic material to its target tissue. A recent development may help to decrease rejection of gene therapy products by the immune system. MicroRNAs (miRNAs) are endogenous non-coding RNAs 21 to 23 nucleotides in length. Their function is to repress translation of target cellular transcripts. Recently it was shown that miRNAs can be used to de-target transgene expression from hematopoietic lineages and thus prevent immune-mediated vector clearance. This will be a very useful way to enable stable gene transfer.

Table 18.3 provides a summary of the status of some gene therapy products under development.

Appendix

Statistical moment theory in pharmacokinetics

Objectives

Upon completion of the Appendix, you will have the ability to:

- understand the basis of non-compartmental (model-independent) pharmacokinetic analysis
- describe the most common applications of statistical moment theory.

A.1 Introduction

In recent years, non-compartmental or model-independent approaches to pharmacokinetic data analysis have been increasingly utilized since this approach permits the analysis of data without the use of a specific compartment model. Consequently, sophisticated, and often complex, computational methods are not required. The statistical or non-compartmental concept was first reported by Yamaoka in a general manner and by Cutler with specific application to mean absorption time. Riegelman and Collier reviewed and clarified these concepts and applied statistical moment theory to the evaluation of *in vivo* absorption time. This concept has many additional significant applications in pharmacokinetic calculations.

The theory and application of statistical moment rest on the tenet that the movement of individual drug molecules through a body compartment is governed by probability. The residence time of a molecule of drug in the body, therefore, can be regarded as a random statistical variable. The mean and the variance of the retention times of a mass of drug molecules reflect the overall behavior of these drug molecules in the body. The mean residence time (MRT) is interpreted as the mean (average) time for a mass of intact drug molecules to transit through the body. MRT involves a composite of all disposition processes and, when applicable, drug release from the dosage form and absorption. Therefore, at any given time after a dose of a drug has been administered to a subject, some of the drug molecules will have been excreted, while other drug molecules will still reside in the body. We can, however, observe only the overall properties of a large mass of drug molecules, not individual molecules. Furthermore, the application of statistical moment theory is more commonly applied in linear elimination pharmacokinetics, although this is not an absolute prerequisite. Additionally, the time course of plasma concentration data can usually be regarded as a frequency distribution curve proportional to the probability of a drug molecule residing in the body for a given time.

This Appendix presents the general treatment and derivation of equations for the plasma concentration versus time data following the administration of a drug by intravascular (both intravenous bolus and infusion) and extravascular routes of administration. Derivation of equations is limited to one- and two-compartment pharmacokinetic models. The equations use terms frequently used in the main text and so these are not redefined for every equation. Particular attention is given to the interpretation of MRT in these cases. In this way we hope to provide the reader with an intuitive grasp of the physical reality of the processes that are occurring and that give rise to the equations. We conclude with a discussion of several useful applications of statistical moment theory.

A.2 Statistical moment theory

In many cases pharmacokinetic data (i.e. plasma drug concentration versus time data) cannot be fitted to an explicit equation equivalent to a system containing a discrete number of compartments into which drug distributes. This data analysis requires some form of non-compartmental analysis (also referred to as model-independent analysis.) This is achieved by the use of statistical moment theory.

A function of time, $f(t)$, has a series of statistical moments equal to:

$$\int_0^\infty t^m f(t)dt \tag{A.1}$$

where the exponent m refers numerically to the moment that is being considered. For example, if m equals 1, the first statistical moment is involved. Pharmacokinetics generally deals with only two statistical moments, the 0th moment ($m=0$) and the first moment ($m=1$).

For the case when $m=0$, we have the formula:

$$\int_0^\infty t^0 f(t)dt = \int_0^\infty f(t)dt = (\text{AUC})_0^\infty = \tag{A.2}$$
the area under the curve for $f(t)$
from time 0 to time ∞

Specifically, the pharmacokinetic curve involved in this case is the curve representing the plasma drug concentration versus time function; and, even when this function is not explicitly known, the area under the curve (AUC) can be estimated by a technique called the trapezoidal approximation. Briefly stated, this divides the

area into a series of segments between each observed data point. These have the general shape of trapezoids, whose area can be calculated by geometric formula. In order to estimate $(\text{AUC})_0^\infty$, these areas are summed and added to the area of the final segment from the last observed point to time infinity. This final segment can be shown to equal the ratio of the final plasma drug concentration divided by the rate constant for the final exponentially declining portion of the curve. $(\text{AUC})_0^\infty$ is a very important parameter in pharmacokinetics, even when an explicit compartmental analysis is applicable.

Another statistical moment is employed in pharmacokinetics, namely the first statistical moment. Setting $m=1$ in the general formula (Eq. A.1), yields:

$$\int_0^\infty t^1 f(t)dt = \int_0^\infty tf(t)dt \tag{A.3}$$

This first moment (or, more strictly speaking, according to Yamaoka *et al.*, the unnormalized first moment) is called the AUMC (area under the [first] moment curve). It is estimated by the trapezoidal approximation of the area under the curve having the product of plasma drug concentration multiplied by time on the ordinate and time on the abscissa. AUMC is rarely used per se in pharmacokinetics. However, the ratio of AUMC/AUC is widely used in non-compartmental pharmacokinetic analysis. This ratio, the MRT, is described in considerable detail below.

After a dose of drug has been administered, its mean residence time (MRT) is defined as the mean (average) time a typical drug molecule spends in the body before it is eliminated. In reality, a distribution of residence times occurs, with large numbers of drug molecules staying in the body for either longer or shorter times than this average time.

In order to obtain an equation for determination of MRT, consider the situation where a particular group of molecules of a drug resides in the body, after dosing, for a specific length of time (t_i). If these drug molecules are measured by their mass, this individual group of drug molecules can be represented by the mass (ΔX_i). And, when this mass of the drug exits the body, after having resided in the body for exactly t_i time units, the letter e can be appended to the term ΔX_i in order to accentuate this fact. Thus, the term $(\Delta X_i)_e t_i$ defines the product of the mass of a group of molecules having a given residence time multiplied by this residence time.

Since there exist many groups of molecules with differing residence times, a list of these mass × time) products could be compiled (ordered from shortest to longest residence times, as follows:

$$\ldots \{(\Delta X_i)_{e1} t_1, (\Delta X_i)_{e2} t_2, \ldots (\Delta X_i)_{en} t_n\} \quad (A.4)$$

This list is n items long, indicating that there are n groups of molecules with different residence times. Once this list is envisioned, it can be used to find the MRT of a typical group of molecules of the drug in question.

An analogy may make this concept a little more intuitive. If we surveyed 1000 workers to record the number of hours each worked during a single week, we could then obtain a grand total by adding the number of worker-hours for all the workers. If, for example, we found this sum to equal 40 000 worker-hours, we could then divide this value by the total number of workers and find the average number of hours worked during the week (40 h).

Determination of mean residence time

The average residence time can then be calculated by summing all these (mass × time) products on the list and then dividing by the sum of all the masses of drug (i.e. by the absorbed dose, FX_0). Thus:

$$\text{MRT} = \frac{\sum_{i=1}^{n} \Delta X_{e_i} t_i}{\sum_{i=1}^{n} \Delta X_{e_i}} = \frac{\sum_{i=1}^{n} \Delta X_{e_i} t_i}{FX_0} \quad (A.5)$$

In reality, however, there is not a finite number of groups of drug molecules with differing residence times; there is a continuum of drug molecules, each having, or being capable of having, at least a slightly different residence time from any other molecule. Recognizing this, the expression for MRT becomes:

$$\text{MRT} = \frac{\int_0^{X_e^\infty} (dX_e)(t)}{FX_0} = \frac{\int_0^{X_e^\infty} t \, dX_e}{FX_0} \quad (A.6)$$

The numerator of this expression (Eq. A.6) represents the sum of the masses of an infinite

number of infinitesimally small groups of drug molecules ready to exit the body multiplied by their individual residence times. The MRT is the ratio of this value to the dose of drug. Note that the unit corresponding to the numerical value of MRT will be some unit of time.

Intravenous bolus administration, one-compartment model

In order to simplify Eq. A.6 for the determination of MRT of a drug that exhibits the characteristics of the first-order process, one-compartment model, and administered as an intravenous bolus dose, the rate of drug elimination must be calculated first:

$$\frac{dX_e}{dt} = -\frac{dX}{dt} = KX = KX_0 e^{-Kt} \quad (A.7)$$

Therefore, $dX_e = KX_0 e^{-Kt} dt \quad (A.8)$

Substitution of the expression on the right side of Eq. A.8 for the term dX_e in Eq. A.6, yields:

$$\text{MRT} = \frac{\int_0^\infty t \, KX_0 e^{-Kt} dt}{X_0} \quad (A.9)$$

Compared with Eq. A.6, Eq. A.9 is integrated over time: therefore, the upper limit of the integral has changed from X_e^∞ to ∞. Next, the two constants are pulled out of the integral, which allows D_0 to be canceled in the numerator and denominator:

$$\text{MRT} = \frac{KX_0 \int_0^\infty t \, e^{-Kt} dt}{X_0}$$

$$= K \int_0^\infty t \, e^{-Kt} dt \quad (A.10)$$

Integration by parts, with $u = t$, $v = e^{-Kt}$, $du = d$, and $-dv/dt = e^{-Kt} dt$, yields:

$$\text{MRT} = \left[(K)\left(-\frac{te^{-Kt}}{K} - \frac{e^{-Kt}}{K^2} \right) \right]_0^\infty$$

$$= \left[-\frac{Ke^{-Kt}}{K^2} \right]_0^\infty = \left[-\frac{e^{-Kt}}{K} \right]_0^\infty$$

$$= \frac{1}{K} \quad (A.11)$$

Therefore, the MRT for an intravenous bolus that exhibits single-compartment distribution

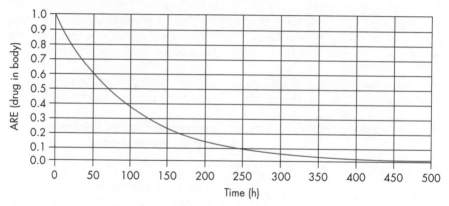

Figure A.1   Amount of drug remaining to be eliminated (ARE) versus time: one-compartment drug, intravenous bolus dose.

and first-order elimination is simply the reciprocal of the first-order elimination rate constant.

The MRT can also be thought of as the ratio:

$$\frac{\text{Area under the amount of drug}}{\text{remaining to be eliminated } vs \text{ time curve}}{\text{Total amount of drug eliminated}}$$

(A.12)

For intravenous administration of a drug that follows the first-order process and one-compartment model, this definition yields the same result as in the previous derivation for Eq. A.11: $1/K$. Symbolically, Eq. A.12 then becomes:

$$\text{MRT} = \frac{\int_0^\infty (FX_0 - X_e)dt}{FX_0}$$

(A.13)

In Eq. A.13, X_e is the cumulative mass of drug eliminated by time t. For any intravenous bolus, the amount of drug remaining to be eliminated, that is $(X_0 - X_e)$, is simply the amount of drug remaining in the body, X. For an intravenous bolus of a drug that exhibits the characteristics of a one-compartment model, this equals $(X_0)e^{-Kt}$ (Fig. A.1).

Substituting this expression into Eq. A.13, and recognizing that $F = 1$ for an intravenous bolus, yields:

$$\begin{aligned}
\text{MRT} &= \frac{\int_0^\infty (X_0)(e^{-Kt})dt}{X_0} \\
&= \int_0^\infty (e^{-Kt})dt = \left[\frac{-1}{K}(e^{-Kt})\right]_0^\infty \\
&= \frac{1}{K}
\end{aligned}$$

(A.14)

There is a third way to determine MRT. This method generally yields the simplest expression to evaluate and is based on the equality:

$$\text{MRT} = \frac{\text{AUMC}}{\text{AUC}} = \frac{\sum \frac{\Lambda}{\lambda^2}}{FX_0/\text{Cl}}$$

(A.15)

The term AUMC in the numerator of Eq. A.15 represents the area under the first moment curve. Each term in the polyexponential equation defining plasma drug concentration for a given compartmental pharmacokinetic model consists of a coefficient Λ multiplied by a monoexponential expression containing a rate constant λ. AUMC can be expressed as the sum of the ratios of each coefficient Λ to the square of its corresponding rate constant λ, as seen in the numerator of Eq. A.15. The AUC in the denominator of this equation is evaluated as the ratio of absorbed dose to systemic drug clearance (Cl). Figure A.2 shows the AUMC and AUC for a one-compartment drug administered as an intravenous bolus.

Application of Eq. A.15 for a drug that exhibits one-compartment model, first-order process, and administered intravenously produces a single term in the expression for plasma drug concentration as a function of time, namely:

$$C_p = (C_p)_0 e^{-Kt} = \frac{X_0}{V}e^{-Kt}$$

(A.16)

$$\text{Therefore,} \sum \frac{\Lambda}{\lambda^2} = \frac{\Lambda}{\lambda^2} = \frac{(C_p)_0}{K^2}$$

$$= \frac{X_0/V}{K^2}$$

(A.17)

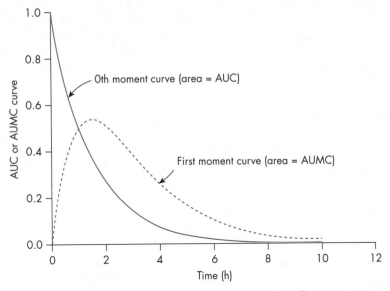

Figure A.2 Area under the curve (AUC) or area under the first moment curve (AUMC) versus time: one-compartment drug, intravenous bolus dose.

and, since $F = 1$ for an intravenous bolus and $Cl = KV$, Eq. A.15 becomes:

$$\text{MRT} = \frac{X_0/V/K^2}{X_0/KV} = \frac{1}{K} \qquad (A.18)$$

where K is the elimination rate constant and V is the apparent volume of distribution. It is demonstrated here that the three methods yield identical results in the case of an intravenous bolus of a drug exhibiting the characteristics of a one-compartment model.

Figure A.3 shows the frequency distribution of residence times for a typical one-compartment

intravenous bolus model. The MRT is also indicated in the figure.

Intravenous bolus administration, two-compartment model

The equation for mass of drug in the body as a function of time for an intravenous bolus administration and two compartment model is:

$$X = Je^{-\alpha t} + We^{-\beta t} \qquad (A.19)$$

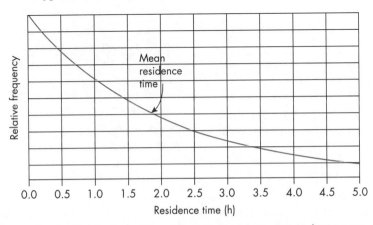

Figure A.3 Distribution of residence times and mean residence time: one-compartment drug, intravenous bolus dose.

where

$$\text{where } J = \frac{(X_0)(k_{10} - \beta)}{\alpha - \beta} \quad \text{and}$$

$$W = \frac{(X_0)(\alpha - k_{10})}{\alpha - \beta} \tag{A.20}$$

The elimination rate equals:

$$\frac{dX_e}{dt} = -\frac{dX}{dt} = \alpha J e^{-\alpha t} + \beta W e^{-\beta t} \tag{A.21}$$

and

$$dX_e = \alpha J e^{-\alpha t} dt + \beta W e^{-\beta t} dt \tag{A.22}$$

Substitution of the expression on the right side of Eq. A.22 for dX_e in Eq. A.6 yields:

$$\text{MRT} = \frac{\int_0^\infty t\alpha J e^{-\alpha t} dt + \int_0^\infty t\beta W e^{-\beta t} dt}{X_0}$$

$$= \frac{\alpha J \int_0^\infty t e^{-\alpha t} dt + \beta W \int_0^\infty t e^{-\beta t} dt}{X_0}$$

$$\tag{A.23}$$

Employing integration by parts on each integral in a manner similar to that used in Eq. A.11 yields:

$$\text{MRT} = \frac{J/\alpha + W/\beta}{X_0} \tag{A.24}$$

Substitution of the equalities for J and W from Eq. A.20 into Eq. A.24 and cancellation of X_0 in the numerator and denominator yields:

$$\text{MRT} = \frac{(k_{10} - \beta)}{(\alpha - \beta)(\alpha)} + \frac{(\alpha - k_{10})}{(\alpha - \beta)(\beta)} \tag{A.25}$$

A little algebraic legerdemain will transform Eq. A.25 to:

$$\text{MRT} = \frac{1}{\alpha} + \frac{1}{\beta} - \frac{k_{10}}{\alpha\beta} \tag{A.26}$$

However, since $\alpha\beta = k_{10}k_{21}$, Eq. A.26, following substitution and cancellation of terms, becomes:

$$\text{MRT}_{2\text{-C IVB}} = \frac{1}{\alpha} + \frac{1}{\beta} - \frac{1}{k_{21}} \tag{A.27}$$

where $\text{MRT}_{2\text{-C IVB}}$ is the MRT for a two-compartment drug administered by intravenous bolus. For any intravenous bolus, ARE (the amount of

drug remaining to be eliminated; i.e. $X_0 - X_e$), is simply the mass of drug in the body, X. For an intravenous bolus of a two-compartment drug, this is:

$$X = Je^{-\alpha t} + We^{-\beta t} \tag{A.28}$$

Employing Eq. A.13, the following expression can be produced for MRT:

$$\text{MRT} = \frac{\int_0^\infty (Je^{-\alpha t} + We^{-\beta t})dt}{X_0}$$

$$= \frac{(J/\alpha) + (W/\beta)}{X_0} \tag{A.29}$$

The right hand side of Eq. A.29 is the same as that in Eq. A.24, which simplifies to yield the same result as in Eq. A.27.

The third method, in the case of a two-compartment-model drug administered as an intravenous bolus, requires the use of the plasma concentration equations,

$$Cp = Ae^{-\alpha t} dt + Be^{-\beta t}$$

and Eq. A.15 becomes:

$$\text{MRT} = \frac{\dfrac{A}{\alpha^2} + \dfrac{B}{\beta^2}}{FX_0/\text{Cl}} \tag{A.30}$$

where $A = \dfrac{X_0(\alpha - k_{21})}{V_c(\alpha - \beta)}$ and

$$B = \frac{X_0(k_{21} - \beta)}{V_c(\alpha - \beta)} \tag{A.31}$$

Since $F = 1$ for an intravenous bolus, and since $\text{Cl} = k_{21}V_c$ for a two-compartment model, Eq. A.30 becomes:

$$\text{MRT} = \frac{k_{10}}{\alpha - \beta}\left(\frac{\alpha - k_{21}}{\alpha^2} + \frac{k_{21} - \beta}{\beta^2}\right) \tag{A.32}$$

Following some algebraic manipulation, Eq. A.32 yields the familiar result Eq. A.27:

$$\text{MRT}_{2\text{-C IVB}} = \frac{1}{\alpha} + \frac{1}{\beta} - \frac{1}{k_{21}}$$

Equation A.27 represents the *total* MRT for an intravenous bolus injection of a two-

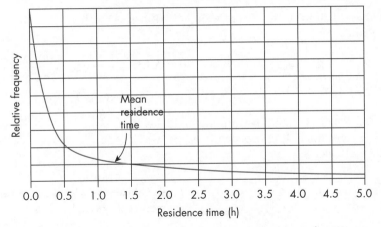

Figure A.4 Distribution of residence times and mean residence time: two-compartment drug, intravenous bolus dose.

compartment drug. It is the sum of the time the drug is present in the central compartment (indicated in terms by a subscript C) plus the time it is present in the peripheral (tissue) compartment (indicated in terms by a subscript peri).

Figure A.4 shows the frequency distribution of residence times for a typical two-compartment intravenous bolus model, with total MRT indicated.

The next task is, therefore, to determine how much of the total MRT is spent in each of these two compartments: the MRT in the central compartment ($\mathrm{MRT_C}$) and the MRT in the peripheral compartment ($\mathrm{MRT_{peri}}$).

Mean residence time in the central compartment ($\mathrm{MRT_C}$)

For the central compartment, Eq. A.6 becomes:

$$\mathrm{MRT_C} = \frac{\int_0^{D_e^\infty} t\, d(X_e)_C}{X_0} \quad (A.33)$$

where $d(X_e)_C$ is the net loss of drug from the central compartment over an infinitesimal time period; this net loss equals eliminated drug plus drug distributed to the peripheral compartment minus drug re-entering the central compartment from the peripheral compartment.

Therefore:

$$d(X_e)_C = -dX_C \quad (A.34)$$

where $-d(X)_C$ is an infinitesimal mass of drug lost from the central compartment. Therefore:

$$\mathrm{MRT_C} = \frac{-\int_0^{D_e^\infty} t\, dX_C}{X_0} \quad (A.35)$$

The rate of change of mass of drug in the central compartment after an intravenous bolus of a two-compartment drug has been determined (Gibaldi and Perrier, 1975) to be equal to:

$$\frac{dX_C}{dt} = k_{21}X_{\mathrm{peri}} - k_{12}X_C - k_{10}X_C \quad (A.36)$$

where X_{peri} is the mass of drug in the peripheral (tissue) compartment. X_{peri} is known to be equal to $\left(\frac{k_{12}X_0}{\alpha-\beta}\right)(e^{-\beta t} - e^{-\alpha t})$ and X_C is known to equal $\left(\frac{X_0(\alpha-k_{21})}{\alpha-\beta}\right)(e^{-\alpha t}) + \left(\frac{X_0(k_{21}-\beta)}{\alpha-\beta}\right)(e^{-\beta t})$.

Substituting these expressions into Eq. A.36, canceling terms and simplifying the result yields the following expression:

$$dX_C = \left(\frac{X_0}{\alpha-\beta}\right)(Pe^{-\alpha t} + Qe^{-\beta t})(dt) \quad (A.37)$$

where $P = (-k_{12}\alpha - k_{10}\alpha + k_{10}k_{21})$ and $Q = (-k_{12}\beta - k_{10}k_{21} + k_{10}\beta)$.

Substitution of the term dX_C from Eq. A.37 into Eq. A.35 yields:

$$\mathrm{MRT_C} = -\left(\frac{1}{\alpha-\beta}\right)\left(\int_0^\infty tPe^{-\alpha t}dt + \int_0^\infty tQe^{-\beta t}dt\right) \quad (A.38)$$

Solutions to these definite integrals are well known, resulting in:

$$\text{MRT}_C = -\left(\frac{1}{\alpha-\beta}\right)\left(\frac{P}{\alpha^2}+\frac{Q}{\beta^2}\right)$$

Substituting for P and Q, and performing several simplifying steps (including the identity $\beta^2 - \alpha^2 = [\beta+\alpha][\beta-\alpha]$), yields:

$$\text{MRT}_C = \frac{k_{12}+k_{10}-\alpha-\beta}{-\alpha\beta} = \frac{-k_{21}}{-\alpha\beta}$$
$$= \frac{1}{k_{10}} \tag{A.39}$$

It has been reported (Shargel *et al.* 2005) that $\text{MRT}_C = \frac{(\text{AUC})_0^\infty}{(C_p)_0}$; however, this is exactly equal to $1/k_{10}$.

The result obtained in Eq. A.39 can be confirmed by using the "amount remaining to be eliminated" method. In the case, the numerator of the expression for MRT_C represents the area under the curve for the amount of drug in the central compartment (rather than drug in the whole body) remaining to be eliminated. This equals $V_C C_p$, which equals $V_C(Ae^{-\alpha t}+Be^{-\beta t})$, where A and B are as defined in Eq. A.31. Therefore:

$$\text{MRT}_C = \frac{\int_0^\infty (V_c\,Ae^{-\alpha t}+V_c\,Be^{-\beta t})dt}{X_0} \tag{A.40}$$

Substitution of the equalities for A and B from Eq. A.31 into Eq. A.40 and integrating the resulting expression between $t=0$ and $t=\infty$, yields:

$$\text{MRT}_C = \left(\frac{1}{\alpha-\beta}\right)\left(\frac{-(\alpha-k_{21})}{-\alpha}-\frac{-(k_{21}-\beta)}{-\beta}\right)$$
$$= \frac{k_{21}}{\alpha\beta} = \frac{1}{k_{10}}$$
$$\tag{A.41}$$

Finally, the same result is obtained by applying Eq. A.15 to this case. In this instance, the coefficients Λ_i are A and B; and λ equals the rate constant for elimination from the central compartment, namely k_{10}.

More specifically:

$$\text{MRT}_C = \frac{\frac{A}{k_{10}^2}+\frac{B}{k_{10}^2}}{X_0/\text{Cl}} = \frac{(C_p)_0/k_{10}^2}{X_0/k_{10}V_c}$$
$$= \frac{(C_p)_0/k_{10}}{X_0/V_c} = \frac{X_0/V_c/k_{10}}{X_0/V_c}$$
$$= \frac{1}{k_{10}} \tag{A.42}$$

Mean residence time in the peripheral compartment (MRT$_{\text{peri}}$)

Now that we have proved that $\text{MRT}_C = 1/k_{10}$ we can solve for MRT_{peri}, the MRT for drug in the peripheral (tissue) compartment. This equals the difference between total MRT and MRT in central compartment. Therefore:

$$\text{MRT}_{\text{peri}} = \text{MRT} - \text{MRT}_C = \frac{1}{\alpha}+\frac{1}{\beta}-\frac{1}{k_{21}}-\frac{1}{k_{10}}$$
$$= \frac{\beta k_{21}k_{10}+\alpha k_{21}k_{10}-\alpha\beta k_{10}-\alpha\beta k_{21}}{\alpha\beta k_{21}k_{10}}$$

Since $\alpha\beta$ is equal to $k_{21}k_{10}$, substitution of $k_{21}k_{10}$ for $\alpha\beta$ in the above expression, followed by cancellation of common factors in the numerator and denominator, yields:

$$\text{MRT}_{\text{peri}} = \frac{\beta+\alpha-k_{10}-k_{21}}{k_{21}k_{10}} = \frac{k_{12}}{k_{21}k_{10}}$$
$$= \frac{k_{12}}{\alpha\beta} \tag{A.43}$$

Extravascular administration, one-compartment model

Let us now explore the applications of these methods to calculate the MRT for another important pharmacokinetic model, namely the one-compartment model with extravascular route of administration. In the following discussion, though the oral route is specified in the derivations, the results apply to any other extravascular route of drug administration. For a one-compartment drug administered orally, the equation for mass of drug in the body (excluding the gastrointestinal tract, which is treated by pharmacokinetic convention as an extracorporeal compartment) as a function of time is:

$$X = I'e^{-Kt} - I'e^{-K_a t} \tag{A.44}$$

where $\quad I' = (V)(I) = (FX_0)\left(\dfrac{K_a}{K_a - K}\right) \tag{A.45}$

The rate of decrease of mass of drug present in the body (exclusive of the gastrointestinal tract) for this model is:

$$\frac{-dX}{dt} = K I'e^{-Kt} - K_a I'e^{-K_a t} \tag{A.46}$$

and, therefore:

$$-dX = (K I'e^{-Kt} - K_a I'e^{-K_a t})dt \tag{A.47}$$

Substitution of the expression on the right side of Eq. A.47 for dX_e in Eq. A.6 provides the following expression for MRT_b, the MRT in the body, exclusive of time spent in the gastrointestinal tract:

$$MRT_b = \frac{K I' \int_0^\infty t\, e^{-Kt}dt - K_a I' \int_0^\infty t\, e^{-K_a t}dt}{FX_0} \tag{A.48}$$

Using Eq. A.45 and substituting for the term I' in Eq. A.48, and cancellation of the term FX_0 in numerator and denominator yields:

$$MRT_b = \left(\frac{KK_a}{K_a - K}\right)\int_0^\infty te^{-Kt}dt - \left(\frac{K_a^2}{K_a - K}\right)\int_0^\infty te^{-K_a t}dt \tag{A.49}$$

Using integration by parts gives:

$$MRT_b = \left(\frac{K_a}{K_a - K}\right)\left(\frac{K}{K^2} - \frac{K_a}{K_a^2}\right) = \frac{1}{K} \tag{A.50}$$

Interestingly, MRT_b for an oral dose (Eq. A.50) yields the same result as the MRT after an intravenous bolus (Eqs A.11, A.14 and A.18), namely $1/K$. A little reflection, however, shows the logic of this situation, as follows.

For an oral dose of drug, MRT_b represents the time spent in the body once drug has been absorbed. Therefore, the time spent in the body corresponding to MRT_b after an oral dose and to MRT after an intravenous bolus of the same drug should be identical since these residence times both have the same starting point.

However, MRT_b, as reported in Eq. A.50, is not the total MRT for a one-compartment model for the oral route. The total MRT in this case is the sum of the MRT in the gastrointestinal tract (GIT) or the site of drug administration, MRT_{GIT}, plus the MRT in the body, MRT_b. Therefore, it is first necessary to calculate MRT_{GIT}. Then, total MRT may be calculated by adding MRT_{GIT} to MRT_b. Accordingly, total MRT will then also equal MRT_{GIT} plus $1/K$.

For first-order absorption, the equation for mass of drug in the gastrointestinal tract as a function of time is:

$$X_{GIT} = FX_0 e^{-K_a t} \tag{A.51}$$

The rate of transfer out of the gastrointestinal tract is:

$$\frac{d(X_e)_{GIT}}{dt} = \frac{-dX_{GIT}}{dt} = K_a FX_0 e^{-K_a t} \tag{A.52}$$

Therefore:

$$d(X_e)_{GIT} = K_a FX_0 e^{-K_a t}\, dt \tag{A.53}$$

Substitution of the right side of Eq. A.53 for dX_e in Eq. A.6, followed by cancellation of FX_0 in numerator and denominator, yields the following expression for MRT in the gastrointestinal tract (more commonly expressed as mean absorption time [MAT]):

$$MAT = MRT_{GIT} = K_a \int_0^\infty t\, e^{-K_a t}dt \tag{A.54}$$

Again, employing integration by parts yields:

$$MAT = (K_a)\left(\frac{1}{K_a^2}\right) = \frac{1}{K_a} \tag{A.55}$$

Recalling that MRT for a one-compartment oral model is the sum of MAT and MRT$_b$, the following is obtained:

$$\text{MRT} = \text{MAT} + \text{MRT}_b = \frac{1}{K_a} + \frac{1}{K} \qquad (A.56)$$

This MRT represents the average time a drug molecule spends in the gastrointestinal tract or the site of administration and in the rest of the body after an oral dose.

Earlier, for this one-compartment oral model, dX_e was equated with $-dX$ from Eq. A.47. This resulted in the formula for MRT$_b$, that is the MRT in the body (except for the gastrointestinal tract). Now let us instead focus on elimination of drug from the body as a whole, for which:

$$\frac{dX_e}{dt} = +KX \qquad (A.57)$$

and

$$dX_e = KX dt \qquad (A.58)$$

Substitution of the expression on the right side of Eq. A.58 for dX_e in Eq. A.6 provides the following expression for MRT:

$$\text{MRT} = \frac{K \int_0^\infty tX dt}{FX_0} \qquad (A.59)$$

Further substitution of the expression on the right side of Eq. A.44 for X in Eq. A.59 produces:

$$\text{MRT} = \frac{K \int_0^\infty (tI'e^{-Kt} - tI'e^{-K_a t})dt}{FX_0}$$

$$= \frac{KI' \int_0^\infty (te^{-Kt})dt - \int_0^\infty (te^{-K_a t})dt}{FX_0} \qquad (A.60)$$

Substitution of I' from Eq. A.45 and cancellation of the term FX_0 in the numerator and denominator yields:

$$\text{MRT} = \frac{(KK_a)}{(K_a - K)} \left(\int_0^\infty te^{-Kt}dt - \int_0^\infty te^{-K_a t}dt \right) \qquad (A.61)$$

Integration by parts, with $-\frac{dV}{K} = e^{-Kt}dt$ for the first term and $-\frac{dV}{K_a} = e^{-K_a t}dt$ for the second term, yields:

$$\text{MRT} = \left(\frac{KK_a}{K_a - K} \right) \left(\frac{1}{K} \int_0^\infty e^{-Kt}dt - \frac{1}{K_a} \int_0^\infty e^{-K_a t}dt \right) \qquad (A.62)$$

Further simplification produces:

$$\text{MRT} = \left(\frac{KK_a}{K_a - K} \right) \left(\left[\frac{-1}{K^2}e^{-Kt} \right]_0^\infty - \left[\frac{-1}{K_a^2}e^{-K_a t} \right]_0^\infty \right)$$

$$= \left(\frac{KK_a}{K_a - K} \right) \left(\frac{1}{K^2} - \frac{1}{K_a^2} \right)$$

$$= \frac{K_a}{(K_a - K)K} - \frac{K}{(K_a - K)K_a}$$

$$= \frac{K_a^2 - K^2}{(K_a - K)KK_a} = \frac{K_a + K}{KK_a} = \frac{1}{K} + \frac{1}{K_a} \qquad (A.63)$$

Therefore, a derivation regarding dX_e in terms of elimination from the body as a whole yields total MRT for a one-compartment extravascular system.

Confirmation of this result may be obtained by employing an ARE (amount remaining to be eliminated) derivation. Using Eq. A.13, for an oral dosage form, the amount of drug remaining to be eliminated at any time (i.e. $F(X_0) - X_e$) is the mass of drug in the body (X) plus the mass of drug in the gastrointestinal tract, X_{GIT}. For an oral dose of a one-compartment drug, this equals:

$$I'e^{-Kt} - I'e^{-K_a t} + FX_0 e^{-K_a t} \qquad (A.64)$$

Figure A.5 is a plot of ARE for a one-compartment drug administered orally.

Substitution of I' from Eq. 45, followed by algebraic rearrangement, produces:

$$\frac{FX_0}{K_a - K}(K_a e^{-Kt} - Ke^{-K_a t}) \qquad (A.65)$$

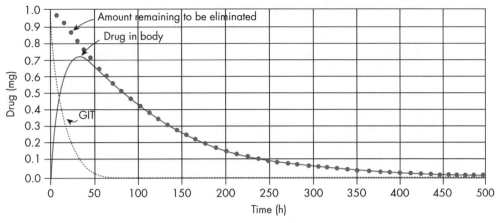

Figure A.5 Amount remaining to be eliminated (ARE): one-compartment drug, oral dose.

Substitution of Eq. A.65 for $[F(X_0) - X_e]$ in Eq. A.13, and cancellation of FX_0 in numerator and denominator, yields:

$$\text{MRT} = \frac{1}{K_a - K}\left(K_a \int_0^\infty e^{-Kt}\,dt - K\int_0^\infty e^{-K_a t}\,dt\right)$$

(A.66)

Integration of Eq. A.66 and algebraic manipulation produces the familiar result:

$$\text{MRT} = \frac{1}{K_a} + \frac{1}{K}$$

(A.67)

Finally, a proof can be pursued using Eq. A.15.
For a one-compartment oral model:

$$C_p = Ie^{-Kt} - Ie^{-K_a t}$$

(A.68)

where,

$$I = \left(\frac{FX_0}{V}\right)\left(\frac{K_a}{K_a - K}\right)$$

(A.69)

I represents the y-axis intercept of a plasma drug concentration versus time plot. By Eq. A.15,

$$\text{MRT} = \frac{\frac{I}{K^2} - \frac{I}{K_a^2}}{FX_0/\text{Cl}}$$

(A.70)

The numerator of Eq. A.70 equals AUMC; while the denominator equals AUC (Fig. A.6).

Substitution of the expression for I from Eq. A.69 into Eq. A.70, followed by substitution of

KV for clearance (Cl) and cancellation of FX_0/V in numerator and denominator, yields:

$$\text{MRT} = \left(\frac{KK_a}{K_a - K}\right)\left(\frac{1}{K^2} - \frac{1}{K_a^2}\right)$$

$$= \frac{1}{K} + \frac{1}{K_a}$$

(A.71)

which concurs with our previous results (Eqs A.56 and A.67).

Figure A.7 shows the frequency distribution of residence times for a typical one-compartment extravascular model, with total MRT indicated.

Extravascular administration, two-compartment model

As in the one-compartment extravascular situation, total MRT for a two-compartment drug administered extravascularly is the sum of MRT in the gastrointestinal tract (MRT_{GIT}; also called MAT) plus MRT for the rest of the body (MRT_b). Because of this principle of additivity, an equation can be constructed for total MRT for a two-compartment drug administered extravascularly, e.g. orally, by adding MAT (Eq. A.55) to $\text{MRT}_{2\text{-C IVB}}$ (Eq. A.27).

Thus:

$$\text{MRT}_{2-\text{C PO}} = \text{MAT} + \text{MRT}_{2-\text{C IVB}}$$

$$= \frac{1}{K_a} + \frac{1}{\alpha} + \frac{1}{\beta} - \frac{1}{K_{21}}$$

(A.72)

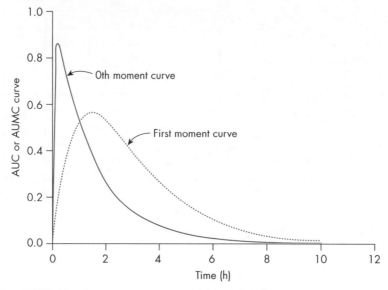

Figure A.6   AUC or AUMC versus time: one-compartment drug, oral dose.

where $MRT_{2\text{-}C\ IVB}$ is the MRT for the two-compartment drug in the intravenous bag and $MRT_{2\text{-}C\ PO}$ is the MRT for the two-compartment drug for the oral dose.

Figure A.8 shows the frequency distribution of residence times for a typical two-compartment extravascular model, with total MRT indicated.

Intravenous infusion, one-compartment model

For an intravenous infusion, where a drug in solution is infused intravenously into a patient at a constant (zero-order) rate, the discussion here is limited to a drug that both distributes to a single compartment and is eliminated by a first-order process.

The MRT of drug in this situation will be the sum of the MRT in the intravenous bag $(MRT)_{bag}$ plus the MRT in the patient. For a one-compartment drug with first-order elimination, it has been shown previously that MRT in the patient equals $1/K$. Therefore, the task is to calculate MRT_{bag} and then add this result to $1/K$ to yield the total MRT.

The MRT for zero-order transfer between the intravenous bag and the patient reflects the situation where the total amount of drug in the

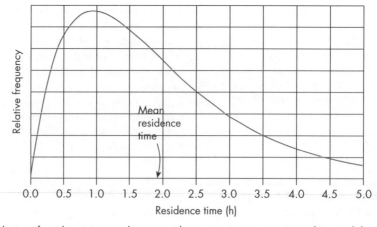

Figure A.7   Distribution of residence times and mean residence time: one-compartment drug, oral dose.

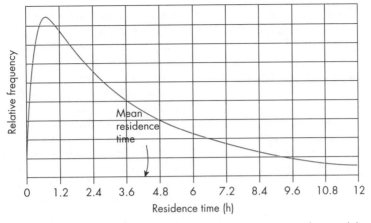

Figure A.8   Distribution of residence times and mean residence time: two-compartment drug, oral dose.

intravenous bag at time zero $(X_{bag})_0$ will be infused into the patient over the finite infusion time (t_{inf}). Moreover, the constant rate of transfer means that the amount of drug in the bag will decline linearly over time. Thus, a plot of X_{bag} versus time will be a straight line with negative slope. There will be zero mass of drug remaining in the intravenous bag at $t = t_{inf}$ (Fig. A.9).

The slope in Fig. A.9 represents the constant rate of change of mass of drug in the intravenous bag over time. This slope (rate) equals $(X_{bag})_0/t_{inf}$. If

the minus sign is dropped, this gives the rate of infusion of drug into the patient, which also equals the rate of loss of drug from the intravenous bag:

$$\frac{dX_e}{dt} = \frac{(X_{bag})_0}{t_{inf}} \qquad (A.73)$$

Rearranging Eq. A.73,

$$dX_e = \frac{(X_{bag})_0}{t_{inf}} dt \qquad (A.74)$$

Applying the definition of MRT from Eq. A.6 and substituting the right-hand side of Eq. A.74 for dX_e:

$$MRT_{bag} = \frac{\int_0^{t_{inf}} \left(\frac{(X_{bag})_0}{t_{inf}} t \right) dt}{X_0}$$

$$= \frac{\frac{(X_{bag})_0}{t_{inf}} \int_0^{t_{inf}} t\,dt}{(X_{bag})_0} = \left[\frac{1}{t_{inf}} \frac{t^2}{2} \right]_0^{t_{inf}}$$

$$= \frac{t_{inf}}{2} \qquad (A.75)$$

MRT_{bag} can also be calculated by using the amount remaining to be removed approach, as follows. The amount of drug remaining to be removed from the intravenous bag at any time equals:

$$(X_{bag})_0 - (\text{rate of loss})(\text{time})$$
$$= (X_{bag})_0 - \frac{(X_{bag})_0}{t_{inf}} t$$

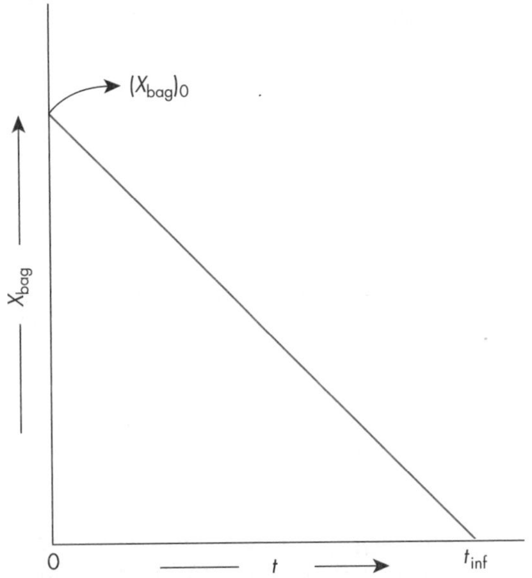

Figure A.9   Mass of drug remaining in the intravenous infusion bag (D_{bag}) versus time: one-compartment drug.

Substitution for this latter expression for $(FX_0 - X_e)$ in Eq. A.13 then yields the following:

$$\text{MRT}_{\text{bag}} = \int_0^{t_{\text{inf}}} \left((X_{\text{bag}})_0 - \frac{(X_{\text{bag}})_0}{t_{\text{inf}}} t \right) dt$$

The upper limit, t_{inf}, suggests that this process does not go on until time infinity; rather, drug has been completely removed from the intravenous bag at $t = t_{\text{inf}}$. Simplifying the above equation gives:

$$\text{MRT}_{\text{bag}} = \frac{(X_{\text{bag}})_0}{(X_{\text{bag}})_0} \int_0^{t_{\text{inf}}} \left(1 - \frac{t}{t_{\text{inf}}} \right) dt$$

$$= \left[t - \frac{t^2}{2t_{\text{inf}}} \right]_0^{t_{\text{inf}}}$$

$$= \left(t_{\text{inf}} - \frac{t_{\text{inf}}^2}{2t_{\text{inf}}} \right) = \frac{t_{\text{inf}}}{2} \tag{A.76}$$

Both of the above solutions agree that $\text{MRT}_{\text{bag}} = t_{\text{inf}}/2$. This means that the total MRT for the intravenous infusion of a one-compartment drug will equal:

$$\text{MRT} = \text{MRT}_{\text{bag}} + \text{MRT}_{\text{patient}}$$

$$= \frac{t_{\text{inf}}}{2} + \frac{1}{K} \tag{A.77}$$

A.3 Applications

The $(\text{AUC})_0^\infty$ has been shown above to be the 0th statistical moment. It can be calculated for plasma drug concentration data that are not describable by an explicit pharmacokinetic equation, even in cases when the curve has an irregular shape. If the assumption is made that all the underlying processes of absorption, distribution, and elimination follow linear kinetics (are mono-exponential functions), $(\text{AUC})_0^\infty$ can provide us with the most important parameter in all pharmacokinetics, the systemic clearance of drug (Cl_s). Here is the relationship:

$$\text{Cl}_\text{S} = \frac{FX_0}{(\text{AUC})_0^\infty} \tag{A.78}$$

where F is the bioavailability fraction and X_0 is the dose of the drug.

Clearance is defined as the volume of plasma from which drug, at concentration $(C_\text{p})_t$ is removed per unit time. For first-order kinetics, and for a patient receiving a particular drug, clearance has a constant value, making it a very useful parameter for calculating an effective drug dosing regimen for an individual patient. Knowledge of a patient's drug clearance allows the dosing rate to be calculated (FX_0/τ), which will produce a given average steady-state plasma drug concentration, by the following equation:

$$(\bar{C}_\text{p})_\infty = \frac{FX_0}{\text{Cl}_\text{S}\tau} \tag{A.79}$$

where $(\bar{C}_\text{p})_\infty$ is average-steady state plasma drug level, τ is the dosing interval, and other symbols are as previously defined.

The $(\text{AUC})_0^\infty$ is an important parameter in bioequivalency studies, where it is used for the calculation of the relative extent of absorption of two oral dosage forms of the same drug. Rearrangement of Eq. A.78 yields:

$$(\text{AUC})_0^\infty = \frac{FX_0}{\text{Cl}_\text{S}} \tag{A.80}$$

If the same individual, on two separate occasions, receives the same dose of a reference standard (trade name) and a generic formulation of the same drug, a ratio of the AUC values can be calculated:

$$\frac{(\text{AUC}_\text{G})_0^\infty}{(\text{AUC}_\text{S})_0^\infty} = \frac{\frac{F_\text{G}X_0}{\text{Cl}_\text{S}}}{\frac{F_\text{S}X_0}{\text{Cl}_\text{S}}} = \frac{F_\text{G}}{F_\text{S}} \tag{A.81}$$

where subscript G refers to generic drug and subscript S refers to standard

This ratio of AUC values equals the relative bioavailability F_G/F_S. The term Cl_s in Eq. A.81 could be canceled since the test subject's clearance will not change for two formulations of the same drug.

Another application of AUC is in the area of metabolite pharmacokinetics. In the case of an intravenously administered drug undergoing biotransformation to a metabolite that, in turn, does not undergo sequential metabolism, measurement of the AUC and measurement of cumulative metabolite excreted into the urine $(m_1)_u$ allows the calculation of the formation clearance of the metabolite, $(Cl_F)_{m1}$:

$$(Cl_F)_{m_1} = \frac{(m_1)_u}{AUC} \qquad (A.82)$$

If the area under the plasma metabolite concentration versus time curve $(AUC)_m$ is also measured, the (elimination) clearance of metabolite can also be calculated:

$$(Cl)_{m_1} = \frac{(m_1)_u}{AUC_{m_1}} \qquad (A.83)$$

The MRT is the other model-independent parameter with several applications in pharmacokinetics. Once calculated, MRT can be used for the calculation of a very important parameter, V_{ss} (the apparent volume of distribution at steady state):

$$V_{ss} = MRT \times Cl_s \qquad (A.84)$$

The value of Cl_s in the above equation may be calculated from Eq. A.78.

The apparent volume of distribution at steady state is a true measure of the extent of a drug's distribution at steady-state equilibrium, since this parameter is independent of any changes in elimination. At any time after steady-state equilibrium has been achieved, it can be viewed as a proportionality constant between mass of drug in the body and plasma drug concentration.

Since the calculated value of MRT is the average time a typical drug molecule is present in the body, from the time it is administered up to the time it is eliminated, MRT will have a different physical significance depending on how the drug was administered and whether or not there is an absorption step.

As seen above, MRT for an intravenous infusion includes the average time spent in the infusion bag. For multicompartmental distribution, MRT includes time spent in the central compartment as well as in any tissue compartments. For an orally administered drug, MRT includes average time spent in the gastrointestinal tract.

All these individual contributions to total MRT are additive. This property permits us to separately calculate each component of total MRT. For example, in the case of a drug administered by intravenous infusion, Eq. A.77 shows that MRT inside the patient equals the total calculated MRT minus $t_{inf}/2$. This is an important parameter for drugs that cannot be modeled compartmentally. Computer programs, such as WinNonlin, can calculate AUC and AUMC without assuming a given number of compartments. The ratio of these parameters, MRT, once adjusted for time drug spends in the infusion bag, can then give an idea of the time required for disposition (distribution and elimination processes) for a given drug in a patient.

Similarly, in the case of a two-compartment drug given by intravenous bolus, total MRT is the sum of MRT in the central compartment (MRT$_C$; Eqs A.39, A.41 and A.42) plus MRT in the tissue compartment (MRC$_{peri}$; Eq. A.43). The reciprocal of MRT$_C$ is k_{10}, a pure rate constant for elimination of drug. Even when compartmental analysis cannot be used, MRT$_{peri}$ can provide important information about a drug's distribution into tissue. For example, the ratio MRT$_{peri}$/MRT indicates the percentage of time a drug spends in tissue; while MRT$_C$/MRT shows the percentage of time the drug spends in that part of the body which is in fast equilibrium with blood.

For a drug administered orally, MRT is the sum of time spent in the gastrointestinal tract (mean absorption time) as well as time spent in the rest of the body. In the case of a one-compartment model drug, the mean absorption time is actually equal to the reciprocal of the absorption rate constant (Eq. A.55) and is, therefore, proportional to the absorption half life. For non-compartmental analysis, the mean absorption time is still a good indicator of the rate of drug absorption. In order to get an estimate of mean absorption time in the non-compartmental situation, the drug is administered both orally and intravenously to a subject. Then:

$$MAT = MRT_{oral} - MRT_{IV} \qquad (A.85)$$

Since all distribution and elimination processes are the same for the same drug administered to the same subject, the only difference between the oral and intravenous doses will be the absorption occurring with the oral dosage form. Since an

MRT is the sum of the MRT values for each individual process, MRT_{IV} represents the distribution and elimination processes occurring for both the oral and intravenous doses. Therefore, subtracting MRT_{IV} from MRT_{oral} will yield the MRT for the absorption process, namely the mean absorption time (MAT).

Further advantage can be taken of the additive property of MRT values to determine another important non-compartmental parameter. Mean dissolution time (MDT) is a useful parameter reflecting the time for dissolution of a solid oral dosage form (tablet or capsule) in the human subject, rather than *in vitro*. At different times, the solid dosage form and a solution of the same drug are administered to the same human subject. MRT values are recorded in each case. Then:

$$MDT = MRT_{solid} - MRT_{solution} \qquad (A.86)$$

Glossary

Notation

A   coefficient in the equation for plasma drug concentration over time for a two-compartment intravenous bolus model

AUC   area under the plasma drug concentration versus time curve

$(\mathbf{AUC})_0^\infty$ the area under the plasma concentration-time versus curve from $t = 0$ to time $t = \infty$

ARE   amount of drug remaining to be eliminated at time t

AUMC (area under the [first] moment curve)   a synonym for the first statistical moment: $\int_0^\infty tf(t)dt$. It is estimated by the trapezoidal approximation of the area under the curve having the product of plasma drug concentration multiplied by time on the ordinate and time on the abscissa. The ratio AUC/AUMC is equal to MRT.

B   coefficient in the equation for plasma drug concentration over time for a two-compartment intravenous bolus model; it is the y-axis intercept of the terminal log linear segment of the plasma drug concentration versus time curve

Cl or **Cl$_s$**   systemic clearance of a drug

Cl$_H$ hepatic clearance of a drug

Cl$_{int}$ intrinsic clearance of a drug

Cl$'_{int}$ intrinsic free (unbound) clearance of a drug

Cl$_{NR}$ non-renal clearance of a drug

Cl$_R$ renal clearance of a drug

C_p   plasma drug concentration at time t following drug administration

$(C_p)_0$ plasma drug concentration at $t = 0$ (immediately) following drug administration)

$(C_p)_{max}$ peak plasma concentration after a single oral dose of drug

$(C_p)_\infty$ [also **$(C_p)_{ss}$**]   concentration of drug in the plasma at steady state

$(\overline{C}_p)_{ss}$ average steady-state plasma drug concentration

$(C_{p\infty})_{max}$ [also **$(C_{pss})_{max}$**]   peak steady-state plasma drug concentration

$(C_{p\infty})_{min}$ [also **$(C_{pss})_{min}$**]   minimum or trough, steady-state plasma drug concentration

$(C_{pn})_t$ plasma drug concentration at a time t after the administration of the nth dose of a multiple dosing regimen

$(C_p)_{t'}$ plasma drug concentration at a time t' after the cessation of an intravenous infusion

$(C_p)_{HI}$ for multiple intravenous infusion, a "peak" concentration that is collected late and that requires mathematical adjustment to estimate the "peak" concentration that would have been recorded if the blood sample had been collected on time

$(C_p)_{LO}$ for multiple intravenous infusion, a trough concentration that is collected early and that requires mathematical adjustment to estimate the trough concentration that would have been recorded if the blood sample had been collected on time

$(C_p)_{\text{"PK"}}$ the *useable* peak concentration for a two-compartment drug administered by multiple intravenous infusion; this occurs when a semilogarithmic plot of plasma drug concentration versus time becomes linear (for vancomycin: approximately 1–2 h after the infusion is stopped)

dX/dt   instantaneous rate of change in the mass of drug present in the body (exclusive of the gastrointestinal tract) at time t (if dX/dt is positive, mass is increasing over time; if it is negative, mass is decreasing over time)

dX$_e$/dt   the rate of drug elimination; the rate of loss of drug from the body as a whole; it is equal to $(+)KX$ for one-compartment drugs (both intravenous bolus and oral) and is equal to $(+)k_{10}X_{C}$ for two-compartment drugs (both intravenous bolus and oral); moreover, it is equal to $-(dX/dt)$ for intravenous bolus, but not for oral, dosing

dX_{u}/dt the rate of change of drug eliminated by the body by urinary excretion

des   subscript indicating a desired, or target, plasma drug concentration

D_{L} loading dose of drug

$(D_{L})_{inf}$ administered dose of a loading intravenous infusion

$(D_{L})_{IV}$ loading dose administered as an intravenous bolus injection

E the hepatic extraction ratio for a drug; it is the fraction drug metabolized (and eliminated) by the liver during a single pass through the liver

f fraction of an oral dose absorbed from the gastrointestinal tract into the portal (not the systemic) circulation; affected predominately by dissolution of drug in the gastrointestinal tract

f [in context] fraction drug remaining in the body at time t after an intravenous bolus dose of drug

F the fraction of an extravascularly administered dose of drug that is absorbed into the systemic circulation; it is the extent of a drug's bioavailability

f_{C} fraction of total drug in the body that is present in the central compartment at time t

f_{C}^{*} fraction of total drug in the body that is present in the central compartment in the post-distribution phase

F_{G} extent of systemic absorption for a generic formulation of drug

F_{IV} fraction of an intravenous dose reaching the general circulation; by definition, this equals 1.0

F_{PO} [or F_{oral}]   fraction of an oral dose reaching the general circulation; it is the product: $f \times F^{*}$

F_{S} extent of systemic absorption for a standard (trade name) formulation of drug

f_{ss} for multiple dosing, the ratio of plasma drug concentration at time t to plasma drug concentration that would be achieved at steady-state; fraction of steady state achieved at time t

f_{up} fraction drug unbound in the plasma

f_{ut} fraction drug unbound in the tissue

F^{*} fraction of drug in the portal circulation that goes on to survive the first-pass effect and enter the systemic circulation; it equals $1 - E$, where E is the hepatic extraction ratio for the drug

I coefficient in the equation for plasma drug concentration over time for a one-compartment extravascular model; it is the intercept on the y-axis of the extrapolated terminal linear segment of a semilogarithmic plot of plasma drug concentration (C_{p}) versus time after an oral dose of drug

K (or K_{el})   the first-order elimination rate constant for a one-compartment drug

K_{a} the first-order absorption rate constant

K_{e} the first-order rate constant for renal excretion of drug

K_{m} the first-order rate constant for metabolism of drug; or [in context] the Michaelis constant in non-linear pharmacokinetics

K_{0} the zero-order elimination rate constant

K_{other} the first-order rate constant for elimination of drug by a process other than metabolism or renal excretion

K_{10} for a two-compartment drug, the first-order rate constant for elimination of drug from the central compartment

K_{12} for a two-compartment drug, the first-order rate constant for transfer from the central to the peripheral compartment

K_{21} for a two-compartment drug, the first-order rate constant for transfer from the peripheral to the central compartment

MAT   mean absorption time; mean residence time in the gastrointestinal tract; synonymous with MRT_{GIT}

MDT   mean dissolution time *in vivo* of a solid oral dosage form administered to a human subject

MRT   mean residence time; the mean (average) time for a mass of intact drug molecules to transit through the body; it is a composite of all disposition processes and, when applicable, drug release from the dosage form and absorption

n the dose number (e.g. the fifth dose for $n = 5$)

NaPH   abbreviation used for sodium phenytoin

PH abbreviation used for phenytoin (free acid)

Q intravenous infusion rate rate (mass/time units)

Q_H hepatic plasma flow

Q_L the infusion rate of a loading intravenous infusion

r the Dost ratio

R accumulation factor; [in context] the rate of administration of drug

S the salt form correction factor

t time; [in context] time since the latest dose in a series of multiple doses was administered

t' time following the cessation of an infusion

T time at which the infusion is stopped

t_{inf} the duration of an intravenous infusion (time during which the intravenous infusion is being infused into the patient)

t_0 lagtime (time elapsed after oral dosing until C_p begins to rise above zero

t_p time of peak plasma drug concentration after a single oral dose

t'_p time of peak plasma drug concentration after multiple oral doses to steady state

$t_{1/2}$ first-order elimination half life

V apparent volume of distribution

V_β ($V_{d\beta}$) for a two-compartment model drug, the apparent total volume of distribution in the post-distribution phase after a single dose of drug

V_C apparent volume of distribution of the central compartment for a two-compartment drug

V_{circ} actual circulatory volume

V_{max} maximal velocity (rate) of elimination in non-linear (Michaelis–Menten) kinetics

V_{ss} (V_{dss}) for a two-compartment model drug, the apparent total volume of distribution at steady state

V_{TBW} volume of total body water

X the mass, or amount, of drug present in the body at time t; this does not include any drug that may be present in the gastrointestinal tract

X_a the mass, or amount, of drug capable of being absorbed present in the absorption site (e.g. the gastrointestinal tract) at time t

$(X_a)_{t=0}$ the mass, or amount, of absorbable drug present in the absorption site (e.g. the gastrointestinal tract) at time $t=0$; this is equal to FX_0

X_{bag} for statistical moment analysis, the mass of drug remaining in the intravenous infusion bag at time t

X_C for a two-compartment model drug, the mass of drug present in the central compartment at time t

$(X_C)_0$ for a two-compartment model drug, the mass of drug present in the central compartment at time $t=0$

X_{GIT} mass of drug in the gastrointestinal tract at time t

$(X_{GIT})_0$ mass of drug in the gastrointestinal tract at $t=0$

X_0 the dose of drug administered

$(X_{inf})_0$ administered dose of a multiple intermittent intravenous infusion

$(X_m)_t$ mass of metabolite present in the blood at time t

$(X_{mu})_t$ mass of metabolite present in the urine at time t

X_{peri} for a two-compartment drug, the mass of drug present in the peripheral compartment at time t

$X_{t=0}$ mass of drug present in the body at $t=0$ (immediately) following drug administration

$(X_u)_{cum}$ cumulative mass of drug excreted in the urine at time t

$(X_u)_{cum}^\infty$ cumulative mass of drug excreted in the urine at time $=\infty$

X* for a two-compartment model drug, the mass of drug present in the body in the post-distribution phase

α the fast disposition rate constant for a two-compartment drug (usually representing the rate of drug distribution)

β the slow disposition rate constant for a two-compartment drug; it is derived from the slope of the terminal linear segment of C_p versus time and, in this phase, is usually indicative of elimination of drug from the body as a whole

λ general term for a rate constant, e.g. K, K_a, β, etc.

τ fixed dosing interval for a multiple intermittent dose regimen

Φ fluctuation factor at steady state

Definitions

active transport a type of specialized transport where energy is used to move a drug molecule against a concentration gradient

ADME acronym for the pharmacokinetic processes absorption, distribution, metabolism, and excretion

absorption the process by which an extravascularly administered drug gets into the systemic circulation

adsorption binding on to a surface

AUC (area under the [plasma drug concentration versus time] curve) an indicator of extent of absorption of an orally administered drug formulation

binding, plasma protein drug binding to albumin and other proteins in the blood; since bound drug is inactive, displacement of drugs from binding sites by other drugs may be important, especially for drugs with a high degree (>90%) of binding

bioavailability, extent the fraction (F) of orally administered drug that reaches (is absorbed into) the systemic circulation; it is also called absolute bioavailability

bioavailability, rate the rate of absorption of an orally administered drug

bioavailability, relative the extent of orally administered drug reaching the systemic circulation compared with that of another extravascular formulation

bioequivalence study a study that compares the relative rate and extent of bioavailability (systemic absorption) of a generic drug with the rate and extent of bioavailability of the standard formulation of the same drug; it is the basis of approval of a generic formulation by the US Food and Drug Administration (FDA)

bioequivalent a formulation deemed by the FDA to have essentially the same rate and extent of absorption as the standard (*see also* therapeutic equivalent)

circulation, portal blood vessels draining the gastrointestinal tract; orally administered drug traversing the gastrointestinal tract membrane goes into the portal circulation, which conveys it to the liver, where it may then undergo elimination via the first-pass effect

circulation, systemic blood vessels that distribute absorbed drug throughout the body; intravenously administered drug goes directly into the systemic circulation

clearance a pharmacokinetic parameter that indicates the volume of plasma from which all drug is removed (cleared) per unit time

compartment a virtual space into which absorbed drug can be considered to be distributed; some drugs remain in a central compartment comprising the vasculature and the well-perfused organs and tissues, while other drugs undergo a further transfer into a more peripheral space termed the tissue compartment

conjugate acid the substance produced when a weak base gains a proton

deaggregation a process by which granules from the disintegration of tablets or capsules are further decreased in size to fine particles

diffusion movement of drug molecules that is powered by a concentration gradient; (*see* passive diffusion and facilitated diffusion]

disintegration a process by which a tablet or capsule is broken down into particles called granules

dissociation in solution, the physical separation of anions and cations of an acid, a base or a salt; dissociation approaches 100% for most salts and for strong acids and bases, while the degree of dissociation of weak acids and bases is governed by their dissociation constants

dissolution the process by which a drug goes into solution in which individual drug molecules are separated by molecules of solvent (water)

distribution the process in which a drug molecule is carried by the circulation to well-perfused organs and tissues and, depending on the drug, even more extensively to distant tissues

effect response of the body to a pharmacological agent; this response may be either therapeutic or toxic; it is characterized by an onset, intensity, and duration

elimination   removal of active drug from the body by metabolism and/or excretion processes

elimination half life   for a drug with linear elimination pharmacokinetics, the time it takes for 50% of drug present to be eliminated; it is constant for a given patient receiving a particular drug

elimination pharmacokinetics, *linear*   elimination following a first-order process; in this situation, AUC is a linear function of dose

elimination pharmacokinetics, non-*linear*   elimination following a process other than a first-order process; in this situation, AUC is not a linear function of dose; large changes in steady-state plasma drug concentrations can occur for relatively small changes in dose

excretion   physical removal of a drug molecule or a metabolite from the body; excretion is predominantly by the kidney (renal excretion) and in the bile (biliary excretion)

excipient   ingredients in a pharmaceutical formulation, other than the active ingredient, which confer useful properties to the formulation (e.g. disintegrants, lubricants, stabilizing agents)

extraction ratio   the fraction of drug eliminated from the body during a single pass through an organ of elimination (e.g. the liver)

facilitated diffusion   diffusion of a drug molecule across a membrane aided by a carrier molecule

Fick's first law   law that governs the rate of diffusion across a membrane

first-order process   a process whose rate is directly proportional to the current amount of the compound being transferred by the process; linear elimination pharmacokinetic is an example of a first-order process

first pass effect   the situation whereby the fraction of a dose of orally administered drug that reaches the systemic circulation is equal to 1 minus its hepatic extraction ratio

formulation   a dosage form of a particular drug

generic   a formulation of drug prepared by a company that did not innovate the drug; the company will present bioequivalency data to the FDA for its approval, with a view to marketing the generic formulation when the innovator drug formulation comes off patent

hydrophilic   "water-loving," possessing a low octanol/water partition coefficient

ionization   charge separation in a molecules, producing electron-depleted cations and electron-rich anions; salts can be fully ionized in the dry state

kinetics   rate

lipid bilayer   biological membrane

lipophilic   "fat-loving;" possessing a high octanol/water partition coefficient

metabolism   effective removal of a parent drug molecule by converting it to a chemically different species; usually this results in an inactive molecule that is more readily excreted than the parent; phase I and phase II metabolism pathways exist

micronization   reduction of a drug's particle size to the μm range; necessary for rapid dissolution of some drugs

minimum effective concentration (MEC)   the plasma drug concentration below which, on the average, no therapeutic effect occurs

minimum toxic concentration (MTC)   the plasma drug concentration above which, on the average, toxicity occurs

nephron   the functional unit of the kidney, comprising glomerulus, tubules and surrounding vasculature

Noyes–Whitney equation   equation that governs the rate of dissolution of particles of drug

octanol/water partition coefficient   the amount of drug that goes into the octanol phase compared with the amount of drug that goes into the aqueous phase in a two-phase system; having a larger value for more lipophilic drugs

parameter   a pharmacokinetic constant for a given patient receiving a particular drug

parenteral   by injection

passive diffusion   movement of drug molecules that is powered by a concentration gradient; diffusion occurs across the lipid bilayer (membrane) for lipophilic drugs and via aqueous channels (pores) for small hydrophilic drugs

peak concentration after an oral dose of drug, $(C_p)_{max}$ affected by rate of absorption and/or extent of absorption

pH   the negative log of the hydronium ion (H_3O^+) concentration; a lower number indicates greater acidity of a solution

pK_a of a weak acid   the negative log of the dissociation constant of the weak acid; value decreases with strength (degree of dissociation) of the acid

pK_a of the conjugate acid of weak base   14 minus the pK_b of the weak base; value increases with strength (degree of dissociation) of the base

pK_b of a weak base   the negative log of the dissociation constant of a weak base; value decreases with strength (degree of dissociation) of the base

pore   aqueous channel through which small polar drug molecules are able to traverse a membrane

potency   a measure of a drug molecule's ability to exert therapeutic effect; the more potent a drug molecule, the lower the plasma drug concentration necessary to elicit therapeutic effect

regimen, drug   how much drug in a dose and how often it is given

salt   a molecule containing at least one positively charged cation and at least one negatively charged anion

site of action   the area of the body where the drug exerts its therapeutic activity; it is often inferred rather than defined as a well-demarcated physiological space

solubility (thermodynamic, or equilibrium)   the amount of drug that goes into solution after steady state has been reached; it is a state function, unaffected by agitation etc.

solubility, rate   how quickly a compound reaches its equilibrium solubility concentration; may be affected by agitation, etc. (*see* dissolution)

solution   a single-phase system containing a solute dispersed at the molecular level in a solvent; in pharmaceutics, a system containing individual drug molecules separated by water molecules

specialized transport   carrier-mediated transfer across a membrane (*see* facilitated diffusion and active transport)

statistical moment $\int_0^\infty t^m f(t)dt$, where $f(t)$ is some function of time and the exponent m refers numerically to the moment with which you are dealing

steady state   an equilibrium state in which rate of drug input equals rate of drug elimination; for all practical purposes, can be considered to occur after a constant-input-rate multiple dose has been given for more than five half lives

suspension   a two-phase system that contains particles of solute dispersed in solvent

therapeutic equivalent   a bioequivalent formulation of drug that produces essentially the same therapeutic and toxic activity profile as the standard formulation (*see also* bioequivalent)

therapeutic range (therapeutic window)   difference between the minimum effective concentration and the minimum toxic concentration

volume of distribution, apparent   the volume of plasma that would be required to dilute a given dose of drug, resulting in its observed plasma drug concentration

References

Aguir AJ *et al*. (1967). Effect of polymorphism on the absorption of chloramphenicol palmitate. *J Pharm Sci* 56: 847.

American Pharmaceutical Association (1972). *Guideline for Biopharmaceutical Studies in Man* Washington, DC American Pharmaceutical Association.

Anonymous (1973). Pharmacokinetics and biopharmaceutics: a definition of terms. *J Pharmacokin Biopharm* 1: 3–4.

Brodie RR *et al*. (1986). Pharmacokinetics and bioavailability of the anti-emetic agent Bromopride. *Biopharm Drug Disp* 7: 215–222.

Burkhardt RT *et al*. (2004). Lower phenytoin serum levels in persons switched from brand to generic phenytoin. *Neurology* 63: 1494–1496.

Crawford P, Hall WH, Chappell B, Collings J, Stewart A (1996). Generic prescribing for epilepsy. Is it safe?. *Seizure* 5: 1–5.

Ereshefsky L, Glazer W (2001). Comparison of the bioequivalence of generic versus branded clozapine. *J Clin Psychol* 62 (Suppl 5): 25–28.

Foord RD (1976). Cefuroxime: human pharmacokinetics. *Antimicrob Agents Chemother* 9: 741–747.

Gibian H *et al*. (1968). Effect of particle size on biological activity of norethisterone acetate. *Acta Physiol Lat Am* 18: 323–326.

Griffith RS, Black HR (1969). Comparison of blood levels following pediatric suspensions of erythromycin estolate and erythromycin ethyl succinate. *Clin Med* 76: 16–18.

Higuchi T, Ikeda M (1974). Rapidly dissolving forms of digoxin:hydroquinone complex. *J Pharm Sci* 63: 809.

Hollister LE (1972). Measuring measurin: problems of oral prolonged-action medications. *Clin Pharmacol Ther* 13: 1.

Israel KS *et al*. (1975). Cinoxacin: pharmacokinetics and the effect of probenecid. *J Clin Pharmacol* 18: 491–499.

Jounela AJ *et al*. (1975). Effect of particle size on the bioavailability of digoxin. *Eur J Clin Pharmacol* 8: 365–370.

Katchen B, Symchowicz S (1967). Correlation of dissolution rate and griseofulvin absorption in man. *J Pharmaceut Sci* 56: 1108–1110.

Khalil SA *et al*. (1972). GI absorption of two crystal forms of sulfameter in man. *J Pharm Sci* 61: 1615–1617.

Kluznik JC *et al*. (2001). Clinical effects of a randomized switch of patients from Clozaril to generic clozapine. *J Clin Psychiatry* 62 (Suppl 5): 14–17.

Langlois Y *et al*. (1972). A bioavailability study on three oral preparations of the combination trimethoprim–sulfamethoxazole. *J Clin Pharmacol New Drugs* 12: 196–200.

Lesko LJ *et al*. (1979). Pharmacokinetics and relative bioavailability of oral theophylline capsules. *J Pharm Sci* 68: 1392–1394.

Levy G (1961). Comparison of dissolution and absorption rates of different commercial aspirin tablets. *J Pharm Sci* 50: 388–392.

Levy G, Gumtow RH (1963). Effect of certain tablet formulation factors on dissolution rate of the active ingredient III. *J Pharm Sci* 52: 1139.

Lott RS, Hayton WL (1978). Estimation of creatinine clearance from serum creatinine concentration. *Drug Intel Clin Pharm* 12: 140–150.

MacDonald JT (1987). Breakthrough seizure following substitution of Depakene capsules (Abbott) with a generic product. *Neurology* 37: 1885.

McAllister RG (1976). Intravenous propranolol administration: a method for rapidly achieving and sustaining desired plasma levels. *Clin Pharmacol Ther* 20: 517–523.

Mellinger TJ (1965). Serum concentrations of thioridazine after different oral medication forms. *Am J Psychiatry* 121: 1119–1122.

Mellinger TJ, Bohorfoush JG (1966). Blood levels of dipyridamole (Persantin) in humans. *Arch Int Pharmacodyn Ther* 163: 471.

Meyer MC *et al.* (1992). The bioinequivalence of carbamazepine tablets with a history of clinical failures. *Pharm Res* 9: 1612–1616.

Mullins JD, Macek TJ (1960). Some pharmaceutical properties of novobiocin. *J Am Pharm Assoc* 49: 245.

Nash JF *et al.* (1979). Linear pharmacokinetics of orally administered fenoprofen calcium. *J Pharm Sci* 68: 1087–1090.

Neuvonen PJ *et al.* (1977). Factors affecting the bioavailability of phenytoin. *Int J Clin Pharmacol Biopharm* 15: 84.

Olling M *et al.* (1999). Bioavailability of carbamazepine from four different products and the occurrence of side effects. *Biopharm Drug Dispos* 20: 19–28.

Oser BL *et al.* (1945). Physiological availability of vitamins. study of methods for determining availability in pharmaceutical products. *Ind Eng Chem Anal Ed* 17: 401–411.

Pedersen *et al.* (1985). *Ugeskr Laeger* 147: 2676–2677.

Poole J (1968). Physicochemical factors influencing the absorption of the anhydrous and the trihydrate forms of ampicillin. *Curr Ther Res* 10: 292–303.

Prescott LF *et al.* (1970). The effects of particle size on the absorption of phenacetin in man. A correlation between plasma concentration of phenacetin and effects on the central nervous system. *Clin Pharmacol Ther* 11: 496–504.

Reinhold JG *et al.* (1945). A comparison of the behavior of microcrystalline sulfadiazine with that of regular sulfadiazine in man. *Am J Med Sci* 210: 141.

Ritschel WA, Kearns GL (2004). *Handbook of Basic Pharmacokinetics*. 6th edn. Washington, DC: American Pharmaceutical Association.

Rosenbaum DH *et al.* (1994). Comparative bioavailability of a generic phenytoin and Dilantin. *Epilepsia* 35: 656–660.

Shull BC *et al.* (1978). A useful method for predicting creatinine. clearance in children. *Clin Chem* 24: 1167–1169.

Simons KJ, Briggs CJ (1983). The pharmacokinetics of HI-6 in beagle dogs. *Biopharm Drug Dispos* 4: 375–388.

Singh P *et al.* (1966). Effect of inert tablet ingredients on drug absorption I: Effect of PEG 4000 on intestinal absorption of four barbiturates. *J Pharm Sci* 55: 63.

Sjogren J *et al.* (1965). Studies on the absorption rate of barbiturates in man. *Acta Med Scand* 178: 553.

Tawashi R, Piccolo J (1972). Inhibited dissolution of drug crystals by certified water soluble dyes: in vivo effect. *J Pharm Sci* 61: 1857.

Tembo AV *et al.* (1977). Bioavailability of prednisolone tablets. *J Pharmacokinet Biopharm* 5: 257–270.

Teorell T (1937). Kinetics of distribution of substances administered to the body. *Arch Intern Pharmacodyn* 57: 205–240.

Thomson W (Lord Kelvin) (1889). *Popular Lectures and Addresses*, Vol 1. London: Macmillan 1889, 254 (lecture delivered 1883).

Tse FLS, Szeto DW (1982). Theophylline bioavailability in the dog. *J Pharm Sci* 71: 1301–1303.

US Food and Drug Administration (1977). *Bioavailability/Bioequivalence Regulations*. Rockville, MD: US Food and Drug Administration.

US Food and Drug Administration http:www.fda.gov/cder/drug/infopage/clozapine.htm(3/8/01) [NB this webpage no longer exists]..

Wagner J (1961). Biopharmaceutics; absorption aspects. *J Pharm Sci* 50: 359.

Wagner JG (1964). Biopharmaceutics; gastrointestinal absorption aspects. *Antibiot Chemother Adv* 12: 53–84.

Welling PG, Craig WA (1976). Pharmacokinetics in disease state modifying renal function. In Benet LZ ed., *The Effect of Disease States on Drug Pharmacokinetics*. Washington, DC: Academy of Pharmaceutical Sciences and American Pharmaceutical Association 173.

Welty TE *et al.* (1992). Loss of seizure control associated with generic substitution of carbamazepine. *Ann Pharmacother* 26: 775–777.

Wolters Kluwer. *Facts and Comparison*. http://www.factsandcomparisons.com/.

Yacobi A (1981). The assessment of intersubject variability in digoxin absorption in man from two oral dosage forms. *J Clin Pharmacol* 21: 301–310.

Zamen R *et al.* (1986). Bioequivalency and dose proportionality of three tableted promethazine products. *Biopharm Drug Dispos* 7: 281–291.

Selected reading

Introduction and overview

Gibaldi M (1984). *Biopharmaceutics and Clinical Pharmacokinetics*. 3rd edn. Philadelphia, PA: Lea and Febiger.

Koch-Weser J (1972). Serum drug concentrations as therapeutic guides. *New Engl J Med* 287: 227–231.

Rescigno A (2003). *The Foundations of Pharmacokinetics*. New York: Springer.

Rescigno A, Segre G (1966). *Drugs and Tracer Kinetics*. Waltham: Blaisdell.

Ritschel W, Kearns G (2004). *Handbook of Basic Pharmacokinetics*. 6th edn. Washington, DC: American Pharmaceutical Association.

Shargel L *et al.* (2005). *Applied Biopharmaceutics and Pharmacokinetics*. 5th edn. New York: McGraw-Hill.

Troy D (2005). *Remington: The Science and Practice of Pharmacy*. 21st edn. Baltimore, MD: Lippincott, Williams & Wilkins.

von Dost H (1953). *Der Blutspiegel* Leipzig: Thieme.

Mathematical review

Ansel H, Stocklosa M (2005). *Pharmaceutical Calculations*. 12th edn. Baltimore, MD: Lippincott, Williams, and Wilkins.

Polya G (1957). *How to Solve It*. 2nd edn. Princeton, CT: Princeton University Press.

Segel I (1976). *Biochemical Calculations*. 2nd edn. Hoboken: Wiley.

Smith S, Rawlins M (1973). *Variability in Human Drug Response*. London: Butterworths.

Zwillinger D (2003). *CRC Standard Mathematical Tables and Formulae*. 31st edn. New York: Chapman & Hall.

Intravenous bolus administration (one-compartment model)

Benet L (1972). General treatment of linear mammillary models with elimination from any compartment as used in pharmacokinetics. *J Pharm Sci* 61: 536–541.

Benet L *et al.* (2006). Appendix II In: Brunton L Lazo J Parker K ed. *Goodman & Gilman's The Pharmacological Basis of Therapeutics*. 11th edn. New York: McGraw-Hill.

Teorell T (1937). Kinetics of distribution of substances administered to the body II. The intravascular modes of administration. *Arch Int Pharmacodyn Ther* 57: 226–240.

Wagner J (1975). *Fundamentals of Clinical Pharmacokinetics*. Hamilton, IL Drug Intelligence Publications.

Clearance concepts

Bauer L (2001). *Applied Clinical Pharmacokinetics*. New York: McGraw-Hill.

Jeliffe RW, Jeliffe SM (1972). A computer program for estimation of creatinine clearance from unstable creatinine levels, age, sex, and weight. *Math Biosci* 14: 17–24.

Pang KS, Rowland M (1977). Hepatic clearance of drugs, 1. Theoretical considerations of a 'well-stirred' model and a 'parallel tube' model. Influence of hepatic blood flow, plasma, and blood cell binding, and the hepatocellular enzymatic activity on hepatic drug clearance. *J Pharmacokinet Biopharmacol* 5: 625.

Rowland M *et al.* (1973). Clearance concepts in pharmacokinetics. *J Pharmacokinet Biopharmacol* 1: 123–136.

Salazar DE, Corcoran GB (1988). Predicting creatinine clearance and renal drug clearance in obese patients from estimated fat-free body mass. *Am J Med* 84: 1053–1060.

Wilkinson G, Shand D (1975). A physiological approach to hepatic drug clearance. *Clin Pharmacol Ther* 18: 377–390.

Drug absorption from the gastrointestinal tract

Albert K (1983). *Drug Absorption and Disposition: Statistical Considerations*. Washington, DC: American Pharmaceutical Association and Academy of Pharmaceutical Sciences.

Dressman J, Lennernas H (2000). *Oral Drug Absorption: Prediction and Assessment*. New York: Marcel Dekker.

Martinez M, Amidon G (2002). A mechanistic approach to understanding the factors affecting drug absorption: a review of fundamentals. *J Clin Pharmacol* 42: 620–643.

Saunders L (1974). *The Absorption and Distribution of Drugs*. Baltimore, MD: Williams & Wilkins.

Extravascular routes of drug administration

Teorell T (1937). Kinetics of distribution of substances administered to the body I. The extravascular modes of administration. *Arch Int Pharmacodyn Ther* 57: 205–225.

Wagner J (1975). *Fundamentals of Clinical Pharmacokinetics* Hamilton, IL: Drug Intelligence Publications.

Wagner J, Nelson E (1963). Percent unabsorbed time plots derived from blood level and/or urinary excretion data. *J Pharm Sci* 52: 610–611.

Bioavailability/bioequivalence

Chen M *et al.* (2001). Bioavailability and bioequivalence: An FDA Regulatory Overview. *Pharm Res* 18: 1645–1650.

Schuirmann D (1987). A comparison of the two one-sided tests procedure and the power approach for assessing the equivalence of average bioavailability. *J Pharmacokinet Biopharm* 15: 657–680.

Ueda C (1988). *Concepts in Clinical Pharmacology Series: Essentials of Bioavailability and Bioequivalence*. Kalamazoo, MI: Upjohn.

US Food and Drug Administration. *CFR Part 320.26, Bioavailability and Bioequivalency Requirements* (revised 4/1/06). Rockville, MD: US Food and Drug Administration, http://www.accessdata.fda.gov/scripts/cdrh/cfdocs/cfcfr/CFRSearch.cfm.

van de Waterbeemd H *et al.* (2003). *Methods and Principles in Medicinal Chemistry, Vol. 18: Drug Bioavailability: Estimation of Solubility, Permeability, Absorption and Bioavailability* Weinheim Wiley-VCH.

Welling P, *et al.* (1991). *Pharmaceutical Bioequivalence*. New York: Marcel Dekker.

Factors affecting drug absorption: physicochemical factors

Ballard BE (1968). Teaching biopharmaceutics at the University of California. *Am J Pharm Ed* 32: 938.

Curry S, Whelpton R (1983). *Manual of Laboratory Pharmacokinetics*. New York: Wiley.

Florence A, Atwood D (2006). *Physicochemical Principles of Pharmacy,* 4th edn. London: Pharmaceutical Press.

Martini L, Crowley (2007). Physicochemical approaches to enhancing oral absorption. *Pharmaceut Technol Europe*. Nov, online version, http://www.ptemag.com).

Yalkowsky S *et al.* (1980). *Physical Chemical Properties of Drugs*. New York: Marcel Dekker.

Gastrointestinal absorption: role of the dosage form

Allen L *et al.* (2004). *Ansel's Pharmaceutical Dosage Forms and Drug Delivery Systems,* 8th edn. Baltimore, MD: Lippincott, Williams & Wilkins.

Banker G (2007). *Modern Pharmaceutics*. 4th edn. London: Taylor and Francis.

Carstensen J (1998). *Pharmaceutical Preformulation*. Cleveland, OH: CRC Press.

Kim C (1999). *Controlled Release Dosage Form Design*. New York: Informa Health Care.

Kim C (2004). *Advanced Pharmaceutics: Physicochemical Principles*. Boca Raton, FL: CRC Press.

Lambkin I, Pinilla C (2002). Targeting approaches to oral drug delivery. *Expert Opin Biol Ther* 2: 67–73.

Continuous intravenous infusion (one-compartment model)

DiPiro J *et al.* (2005). Theophylline *Concepts in Clinical Pharmacokinetics*. 4th edn. Bethesda American Society of Health System Pharmacists, 187–192.

Wagner J (1974). A safe method of rapidly achieving plasma concentration plateaus. *Clin Pharmacol Ther* 16: 691–700.

Multiple dosing: intravenous bolus administration

Gibaldi M, Perrier D (1982). *Pharmacokinetics,* 2nd edn. New York: Marcel Dekker.

Krueger-Thiemer E, Bunger P (1965–66). The role of the therapeutic regimen in dosage form design I. *Chemotherapeutics* 10: 61.

Levy G (1966). Kinetics of pharmacologic effect. *Clin Pharmacol Ther* 7: 362.

van Rossum J, Tomey A (1968). Rate of accumulation and plateau plasma concentration of drugs after chronic medication. *J Pharm Pharmacol* 20: 390.

Multiple dosing: extravascular routes of drug administration

Alexanderson B (1972). Pharmacokinetics of nortriptyline in man after single and multiple oral doses: the predictability of steady-state plasma concentrations from single dose plasma-level data. *Eur J Clin Pharmacol* 4: 82.

Gibaldi M, Perrier D (1982). *Pharmacokinetics*. 2nd edn. New York: Marcel Dekker.

Two-compartment model

Gibaldi M, Perrier D (1975). *Pharmacokinetics*. New York: Marcel Dekker.
Levy G *et al.* (1968). Multicompartment pharmacokinetic models and pharmacologic effects. *J Pharm Sci* 58: 422–424.
Notari R (1980). *Biopharmaceutics and Clinical Pharmacokinetics,* 3rd edn. New York: Marcel Dekker.
Welling P (1986). *ACS Monograph 185: Pharmacokinetics: Processes and Mathematics* Washington, DC: American Chemical Society.

Multiple intermittent infusions

Moise-Broder P (2006). In: Burton ME *et al.* ed. *Applied Pharmacokinetics and Pharmacodynamics.*4th edn. Baltimore, MD: Lippincott, Williams & Wilkins.
Rowland R, Tozer T (1995). *Clinical Pharmacokinetics: Concepts and Applications,* 3rd edn. Baltimore, MD: Williams & Wilkins, 313–339.

Non-linear pharmacokinetics

Gerber N, Wagner J (1972). Explanation of dose-dependent decline of diphenylhydantoin plasma levels by fitting to the integrated form of the Michaelis–Menten equation. *Res Commun Chem Pathol Pharmacol* 3: 455.
Mehvar R (2001). Principles of nonlinear pharmacokinetics. *Am J Pharm Ed* 65: 178–184.
Michaelis L, Menten M (1913). Die kinetic der invertinwirkung. *Biochem Z* 49: 333–369.
Wagner J (1971). A new generalized nonlinear pharmacokinetic model and its implications. *Biopharmaceutics and Relevant Pharmacokinetics*, Ch. 40. Hamilton, IL, Drug Intelligence Publications.
Wagner J (1975). *Fundamentals of Clinical Pharmacokinetics.* Hamilton, IL Drug Intelligence Publications.
Winter M (2003). Phenytoin In: *Basic Clinical Pharmacokinetics,* 4th edn. Baltimore, MD: Lippincott, Williams & Wilkins, 321–363.

Drug interactions

Aithal G *et al.* (1999). Association of polymorphisms in the cytochrome P450 CYP2C9 with warfarin dose requirement and risk of bleeding complications. *Lancet* 353: 714–719.
Ayrton A, Morgan P (2001). Role of transport proteins in drug absorption, distribution, and excretion. *Xenobiotica* 31: 469–497.
Bukaveckas B (2004). Adding pharmacogenetics to the clinical laboratory. *Arch Pathol Lab Med* 128: 1330–1333.
Dresser G, Bailey D (2002). A basic conceptual and practical overview of interactions with highly prescribed drugs. *Can J Clin Pharmacol* 9: 191–198.
Dresser M (2001). The MDR1 C3434T polymorphism: effects on P-glycoprotein expression/function and clinical significance. *AAPS Pharm Sci3 Commentary* 3: 1–3, http://www.aapspharmsci.org.
Giacomini KM *et al.* (2007). The Pharmacogenetics Research Network: from SNP discovery to clinical drug response. *Clin Pharmacol Ther* 81: 328–345.
Hansten P, Horn J (2007).Top 100 Drug Interactions. Freeland, WA: H and H Publications.
Hansten P, Horn J (2007). *Drug Interactions Analysis and Management (DIAM) 2007*. St Louis, MO: Drug Intelligence Publications.
Ho R, Kim R (2005). Transporters and drug therapy: implications for drug disposition and disease. *Clin Pharmacol Ther* 78: 260–277.

Indiana University School of Medicine (2006). *Cytochrome P450 Table* (Dr. David Flockhart). Indianapolis, IA: Indiana University School of Medicine http://medicine/iupui.edu/flockhart/ table.htm (accessed 15 June 2007).

Kartner N, Ling V (1989). Multidrug resistance in cancer. *Medicine* March: 110–117.

Lacy C *et al.* (2005). *Drug Information Handbook: A Comprehensive Resource for All Clinicians and Healthcare Professionals,*13th edn. Hudson, OH Lexicomp.

Ma J *et al.* (2004). Genetic polymorphisms of cytochrome P450 enzymes and the effect on inter-individual, pharmacokinetic variability in extensive metabolizers. *J Clin Pharmacol* 44: 447–456.

MacKichan J (1984). Pharmacokinetic consequences of drug displacement from blood and tissue proteins. *Clin Pharmacokinet* 9 (Suppl 1): 32–41.

Mayersohn M (1992). Special pharmacokinetic considerations in the elderly. In: Evans W, Schentag J, Jusko W, eds. *Applied Pharmacokinetics: Principles of Therapeutic Drug Monitoring.* Baltimore: Lippincott,Williams & Wilkins, Ch. 9, 1–43.

McKinnon R, Evans A (2000). Cytochrome P450: 2. Pharmacogenetics. *Aust J Hosp Pharm* 30: 102–105.

Meyer U (2000). Pharmacogenetics and adverse drug reactions. *Lancet* 356: 1667–1671.

Rogers J *et al.* (2002). Pharmacogenetics affects dosing, efficacy, and toxicity of cytochrome P450-metabolized drugs. *Am J Med* 113: 746–750.

Schaeffeler E *et al.* (2001). Frequency of C3435T polymorphism of MDR1 gene in African people. *Lancet* 358: 383–384.

Shapiro L, Shear N (2002). Drug interactions: proteins, pumps, and P-450s. *J Am Acad Dermatol* 47: 467–484.

Zanger U *et al.* (2004). Cytochrome P450 2D6: overview and update on pharmacology, genetics, biochemistry. *Naunyn Schmiedebergs Arch Pharmacol* 369: 23–37.

Zucchero F *et al.* (2004). *Pocket Guide to Evaluation of Drug Interactions.* 5th edn. Washington, DC: American Pharmacists' Association.

Pharmacokinetics and pharmacodynamics

Bourne D (1995). *Mathematical Modeling of Pharmacokinetic Data.* Lancaster, PA: Technomic Publishing.

Derendorf H, Hochhaus G (1995). *Handbook of Pharmacokinetic/Pharmacodynamic Correlation.* Boca Raton, FL: CRC Press.

Gabrielsson J, Weiner D (1994). *Pharmacokinetic/Pharmacodynamic Data Analysis: Concepts and Applications.* Uppsala: Swedish Pharmaceutical Press.

Smith R *et al.* (1986). *Pharmacokinetics and Pharmacodynamics: Research Design and Analysis* Cincinnati, OH: Harvey Whitney.

Tozer T, Rowland R (2006). *Introduction to Pharmacokinetics and Pharmacodynamics.* Baltimore, MD: Lippincott Williams & Wilkins.

Pharmacokinetics and pharmacodynamics of biotechnology drugs

Allen T, Cullis P (2004). Drug delivery systems: entering the mainstream. *Science* 303: 1818–1822.

Amgen (2007). Amgen science pipeline. Thousand Oaks, CA: Amgen. http://www.amgen.com/ science/pipe.jsp (accessed 11 May 2007).

Ansel H *et al.* (1999). Products of bioechnology. *Pharmaceutical Dosage Forms and Drug Delivery Systems.* Media, PA: Williams & Wilkins 503–534.

Booy E *et al.* (2006). Monoclonal and biospecific antibodies as novel therapeutics. *Arch Immunol Ther Exp* 54: 85–101.

Braekman R (1997). Pharmacokinetics and pharmacodynamics of peptide and protein drugs, In: Crommelin D Sindelar R, eds. *Pharmaceutical Biotechnology.* Newark, NJ: Harwood Academic 101–121.

Brown B *et al.* (2006). Endogenous microRNA regulation suppresses transgene expression in hemato-poietic lineages and enables stable gene transfer. *Nat Med* 12: 585–591.

Cochlovius B *et al.* (2003). Therapeutic antibodies. *Modern Drug Discovery* October: 33–38.

Couzin J (2004). RNAi shows cracks in its armor. *Science* 306: 1124–1125.

Cross D, Burmester J (2006). Gene therapy for cancer treatment: past, present, and future. *Clin Med Res* 4: 218–227.

Eurekalert (2005). *Targeted Drug Delivery Achieved with Nanoparticle–Aptamer Bioconjugates.* Washington, DC: American Association for the Advancement of Science, http://eurekalert.org/pub_releases/2005–11/foec-tdd110105.php (accessed 4 June 2007).

Glick B, Pasternak J (1994). *Molecular Biotechnology: Principles and Applications of Recombinant DNA.* Washington, DC: American Society of Medicine Press.

Harris J (2003). Peptide and protein pegylation II: clinical evaluation. *Adv Drug Delivery Rev* 55: 1259–1260.

Howstuffworks (2007). How cancer vaccines will work. http://health.howstuffworks.com/cancer-vaccine2.htm (accessed 6 March 2007).

Kim C *et al.* (2002). Immunotherapy for melanoma. *Cancer Control* 9: 22–30.

Krieg A (2007). Development of TLR9 agonists for cancer therapy. *J Clin Invest* 117: 1184–1194.

Krimsky S (2005). China's gene therapy drug. *GeneWatch* 18: 10–13.

Lobo E *et al.* (2004). Antibody pharmacokinetics and pharmacodynamics. *J Pharm Sci* 93: 2645–2668.

Lockman P *et al.* (2002). Nanoparticle technology for drug delivery across the blood–brain barrier. *Drug Dev Ind Pharm* 28: 1–13.

Mascelli M *et al.* (2007). Molecular, biologic, and pharmacokinetic properties of monoclonal antibodies: impact of these parameters on early clinical development. *J Clin Pathol* http://jcp.sagepub.om/cgi/content/full/47/5/553 (accessed 25 April 2007).

Medarex (2007). Antibodies as therapeutics. Princeton, NJ: Medarex, http://www.medarex.com/Development/Therapeutics.htm (accessed 26 May 2007).

Meibohm B (2007). *Pharmacokinetics and Pharmacodynamics of Biotech Drugs: Principles and Case Studies in Drug Development.* Wiley-VCH: New York.

National Cancer Institute (2003). Cancer vaccine fact sheet. London: National Cancer Institute, http://www.cancer.gov/cancertopics/factsheet/cancervaccine/ (accessed 25 May 2007).

Ott M *et al.* (2006). Correction of X-linked chronic granulomatous disease by gene therapy, augmented by insertional activation of MDS1-EVI1, PRDM16, or SETBP1. *Nat Med* 12: 401–409.

Ross J *et al.* (2003). Anticancer antibodies. *Am J Clin Pathol* 119: 472–485.

Senzer N *et al.* (2006). Bi-modality induction of TNFα: neoadjuvant chemoradiotherapy and TNFerade in patients with locally advanced, resectable esophageal carcinoma. *Mol Ther* 13 (Suppl 1): S110.

Tabrizi M, Roskos L (2007). Preclinical and clinical safety of monoclonal antibodies. *Drug Discovery Today* 12: 540–547.

Tang L *et al.* (2004). Pharmacokinetic aspects of biotechnology products. *J Pharm Sci* 93: 2184–2204.

VIB-RUG Department of Molecular Biomedical Research (2004). Therapeutic monoclonal antibodies used in clinical practice 2004. Ghent: VIB-RUG Department of Molecular Biomedical Research, http://users.pandora.be/nmertens/U11/IM_abs_table.htm (accessed 24 May 2006).

Wills R, Ferraiolo B (1992). The role of pharmacokinetics in the development of biotechnologically derived agents. *Clin Pharmacokinet* 23: 406–414.

Zito S (1997). *Pharmaceutical Biotechnology: A Programmed Text* Lancaster, PA: Technomic Publishing.

Statistical moment theory in pharmacokinetics

Nakashima E, Benet L (1988). General treatment of mean residence time, clearance, and volume parameters in linear mammillary models with elimination from any compartment. *J Pharmacokinet Biopharm* 16: 475–492.

Yamaoka K *et al.* (1978). Statistical moments in pharmacokinetics. *J Pharmacokinet Biopharm* 6: 547–558.

Index